INSTANT

IN

RETINA AND VITREOUS

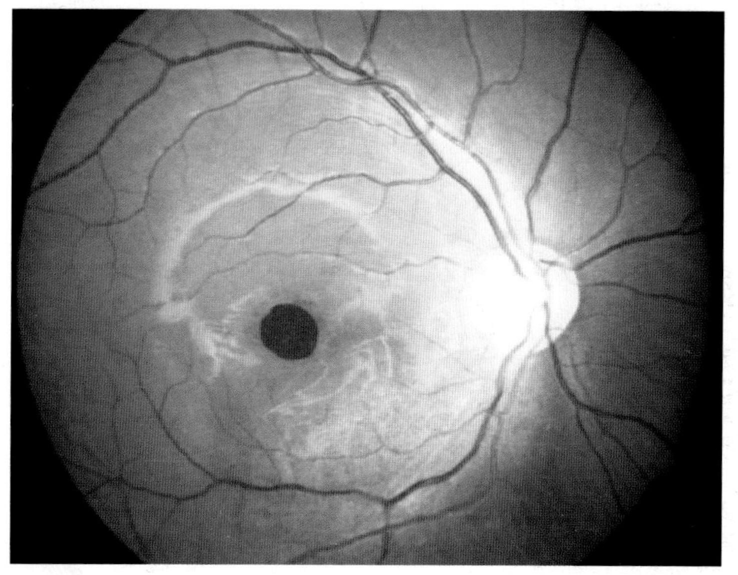

Instant Clinical Diagnosis in Ophthalmology
Retina and Vitreous

Series Editors

Ashok Garg
MS PhD FIAO(Bel) FRSM FAIMS ADM FICA
International and National Gold Medalist
Chairman and Medical Director
Garg Eye Institute and Research Centre
235-Model Town, Dabra Chowk
Hisar-125005 (India)

Emanuel Rosen
MD
Medical Director
Rosen Eye Associates
Harbour City, Salford Quays
M50 3 BH
UK

Editors

Jose Maria Ruiz Moreno
MD PhD
Professor of Ophthalmology
Albacete Medical School
University of Castilla La Mancha
Avendia de Almansa, 14
02006, ALBACETE
Spain

T Mark Johnson
MD FRCS
Consultant
Vitreoretinal Surgeon
National Retina Institute,
Suite 101,
5530 Wisconsin Ave
Chevy Chase 20815, USA

Foreword

Marta S De Figueroa

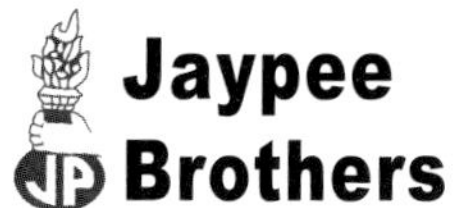

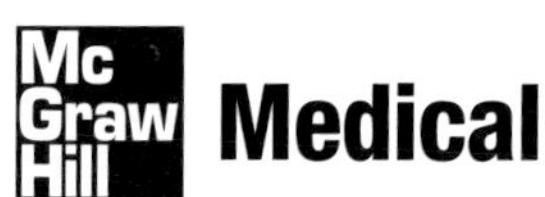

First published in India in 2009 by

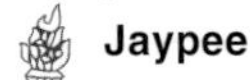

Jaypee Brothers Medical Publishers (P) Ltd.

Corporate Office

4838/24 Ansari Road, Daryaganj, **New Delhi** - 110002, India, +91-11-43574357

Registered Office

B-3 EMCA House, 23/23B Ansari Road, Daryaganj, **New Delhi** 110 002, India
Phones: +91-11-23272143, +91-11-23272703, +91-11-23282021,
+91-11-23245672, Rel: +91-11-32558559 Fax: +91-11-23276490, +91-11-23245683
e-mail: jaypee@jaypeebrothers.com, Visit our website: www.jaypeebrothers.com

First published in USA by The McGraw-Hill Companies, 2 Penn Plaza, New York, NY 10121. Exclusively worldwide distributor except South Asia (India, Nepal, Sri Lanka, Bhutan, Pakistan, Bangladesh, Malaysia).

ISBN-13: 978-0-07-163233-1
ISBN-10: 0-07-163233-6

Dedicated to

- My Respected Param Pujya Guru Sant Gurmeet Ram Rahim Singh Ji for his Blessings and Motivation
- My Respected Parents, Teachers, My Wife Dr. Aruna Garg, Son Abhishek and Daughter Anshul for their Constant Support and Patience during all these Days of Hard Work
- My Dear Friend Dr. Amar Agarwal, A Renowned International Ophthalmologist for his Constant Support, Guidance and Expertise

—Ashok Garg

The Memory of My Step Daughter Nicola Ross who Enjoyed Benefits from Refractive Surgery were Cut Short by A Tragic Fatal Illness

—Emanuel Rosen

My Family (Magali, My Wife and Jorge, Guillermo and Magali My Children) for the Time, Comprehension and Patience that they have had with me during all these Years of Hard Work

—Jose M Ruiz Moreno

My Wife Joanne and My Son Connor for Providing me with their Love, Wisdom and Support throughout the Years

—T Mark Johnson

Contributors

Ajay Aurora MS
Sr. Vitreoretina Consultant and Director, Delhi Retina Centre
Chaudhary Eye Centre and Laser Vision, 4802, Bharat Ram Road
24, Darya Ganj, New Delhi, India

Alay Banker MS
Banker Retina Clinic and Laser Centre
5 - Subhash Society
Behind Ishvar Bhuvan
Navrangpura
Ahmedabad - 380009, India

Anjli Hussain MS
Medical Retina and ROP Specialist
LV Prasad Eye Institute
LV Prasad Marg
Banjara Hills
Hyderabad - 500034
India

Ashok Garg MS PhD FRSM
Chairman and Medical Director
Garg Eye Institute and Research Centre
235-Model Town, Dabra Chowk
Hisar - 125005, India

Avnindra Gupta MD
Consultant
Retina Management Group
Centre for Sight
B-5/24, Safdarjung Enclave
New Delhi - 110029, India

Debraj Shome MD FRCS
Head Deptt. of Ophthalmic and Facial Plastic Surgery
Aditya Jyot Eye Hospital Pvt. Ltd.
Plot No. 153
Road No. 9
Major Parmeshwaran Road
Opp. SIWS College
Gate No. 3
Wadala, Mumbai - 400031
India

Dinesh Talwar MD
Sr. Consultant Ophthalmologist
Apollo Hospitals
Director Vitreoretina Services
Centre for Sight
B-5/24, Safdarjung Enclave
(Opp. Deer Park)
New Delhi - 110029
India

Emanuel Rosen MD FRCS
Rosen Eye Associates
Harbour City
Salford Quays
M50 3 BH
UK

Francisco L Lugo MD
Consultant
Vitreoretinal Department
Alicante Institute of Ophthalmology
Alicante
Spain

HK Tewari MD
Ex-Chief
Dr RP Centre for Ophthalmic Sciences
AIIMS, Retina Management Group
Centre for Sight
B-5/24, Safdarjung Enclave
New Delhi - 110029
India

Hsi Kung Kuo MD
Department of Ophthalmology
Chang Gung Memorial Hospital
Kaohsiung Medical Centre
123, Tapei Road, Niaosung
Hsein, Kaohsiung, Hsein
883, Taiwan ROC

Javier A Montero MD PhD
Vitreoretina Department
Alicante Institute of Ophthalmology
Alicante
Spain

Jose M Ruiz Moreno MD
Professor
Department of Ophthalmology
Albacete Medical School
Castilla La Macha University
Avendia de Almansa, 14
02006, Albacete
Spain

Lalit Verma MD
Senior Vitreoretina Consultant
Apollo Hospitals and Center for Sight
B-5/24, Safdarjung Enclave
(Opp. Deer Park)
New Delhi-29
India

Madhu Karna MD
Associate Consultant
Retina Management Group
Centre for Sight
B-5/24, Safdarjung Enclave
New Delhi - 110029
India

Nazimul Hussain MS, DNB
Consultant Vitreoretina Specialist
Al Zahra Pvt. Hospital
Sharjah/Dubai, UAE

Neeraj Sanduja MD
Consultant Vitreoretinal Surgeon
Dr. Chaudhary Eye Centre and Laser Vision
4802, Bharat Ram Road
24 Daryaganj, New Delhi
India

Nikoloz Labauri MD
Aditya Jyot Eye Hospital Pvt. Ltd.
Plot No. 153, Road No. 9
Major Parmeshwaran Road
Opp. SIWS College, Gate No. 3
Wadala, Mumbai - 400031
India

Pedro Amat Peral MD
Vitreoretinal Department
Alicante Institute of Ophthalmology
Alicante, Spain

Priyanka Doctor MS
Aditya Jyot Eye Hospital Pvt. Ltd.
Plot No. 153, Road No. 9
Major Parmeshwaran Road
Opp. SIWS College, Gate No. 3
Wadala, Mumbai - 400031
India

Rajpal Vohra MD
Professor of Ophthalmology
Dr RP Centre for Ophthalmic Sciences
AIIMS, Ansari Nagar
New Delhi - 110029
India

Rupesh Aggarwal MS
Consultant
LV Prasad Eye Institute
LV Prasad Marg
Banjara Hills
Hyderabad - 500034
India

S Natarajan MS
Chairman and Medical Director
Aditya Jyot Eye Hospital Pvt. Ltd.
Plot No. 153, Road No. 9
Major Parmeshwaran Road
Opp. SIWS College, Gate No. 3
Wadala, Mumbai - 400031
India

Shaifali Singla MD
Retina Management Group
Centre for Sight
B-5/24, Safdarjung Enclave
New Delhi - 110029
India

Soumen Mondal MS
Aditya Jyot Eye Hospital Pvt. Ltd.
Plot No. 153, Road No. 9
Major Parmeshwaran Road
Opp. SIWS College, Gate No. 3
Wadala, Mumbai - 400031
India

Supriya Dabir MS
Aditya Jyot Eye Hospital Pvt. Ltd.
Plot No. 153, Road No. 9
Major Parmeshwaran Road
Opp. SIWS College, Gate No. 3
Wadala, Mumbai - 400031
India

T Mark Johnson MD, FRCSC
Consultant Vitreoretinal Surgeon
National Retina Institute
Ste 101-5530 Wisconsin
Ave Chevy Chase
MD 20815
USA.

Vikrant Sharma MS
Consultant Ophthalmologist
Grewal Eye Institute
Sector 9-C, Madhya Marg
Chandigarh - 160009
India

Foreword

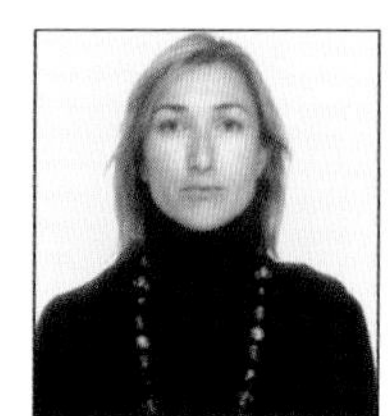

When Dr. Ashok Garg honored me with the opportunity to write the foreword to this book, he sent me the table of contents and the list of contributors. I knew immediately that the textbook he and his team of co-editors had planned to write, edit and publish would be an outstanding and, indeed, invaluable resource for both general ophthalmologists and vitreoretinal specialists.

My initial reaction proved to be right, for the book provides an admirably broad yet detailed overview of retinal diseases. In addition, the contributors have assembled a wonderful collection of illustrative fundus photographs and angiograms; thus, constituting a remarkable educational resource on diseased human fundi. **Dr Garg and co-editors' efforts will be rewarded with the gratitude of clinicians and their patients**.

Marta S De Figueroa
Chairman and Medical Director of Vissum Mirasierra
Santa Hortensia 58
28002 Madrid, Spain
Director of Vitreoretinal Department
Ramony Cajal University Hospital
Carretera de Colmenar Km 9
28034 Madrid, Spain
Professor University Alcalá de Henares
Madrid, Spain
E-mail: figueroa@servicom2000.com

Preface

In modern day busy and fast life ophthalmologists are glued to their clinical and surgical practice and have little time to read large volume books. The need of hour is to have pocket size ready recokner enriched with complete and uptodate information of the diseases in a most comprehensive manner. At present very few quality ready-reference books are available at an International level.

After detail research for the need of ophthalmologists we have developed a series of 10-volume ready-reference books titled as *Instant Clinical Diagnosis in Ophthalmology*. This series covers Oculoplastic and Reconstructive Surgery, Retina and Vitreous, Lens, Glaucoma, Refractive Surgery, Pediatric Ophthalmology, Strabismus, Anterior Segment diseases, Cornea and Neurophthalmology. The present series has been designed to provide uptodate information of concerned disease in a comprehensive and a lucid manner along with high quality clinical photographs in a easy to read format. International masters of concerned subject have contributed chapters in this series covering pathophysiology, clinical signs and symptoms, investigations, differential diagnosis, treatment and prognosis in a simplified manner.

This volume deals with important topic of retina which is the most sensitive, photoreceptive and innermost nervous tunic of the globe. Every ophthalmologists be an anterior or posterior segment surgeon must have complete knowledge of retina. This book covers all the clinical conditions of retina alongwith clinical photographs to serve as visual aid to ophthalmologists. Illustrations are clear and precise and include all the relevant information.

We are highly thankful to our publisher M/s Jaypee Brothers Medical Publishers (P) Ltd. specially Shri Jitendar P Vij (CEO), Mr Tarun Duneja, General Manager (Publishing) and all staff members for their dedication and hard efforts put in for the preparation of high quality series of instant clinical books.

We hope this 10-volume set of ready-reference small size books will provide complete and useful clinical information to ophthalmologists all around the world and will help them accurately and precisely diagnose, treat and manage their clinical cases confidently to the satisfaction and expectations of their valued patients. We also hope this ready reckoner will serve as useful companion on every clinician desk.

Editors

Contents

CHAPTER
ONE

AGE RELATED MACULAR DEGENERATION

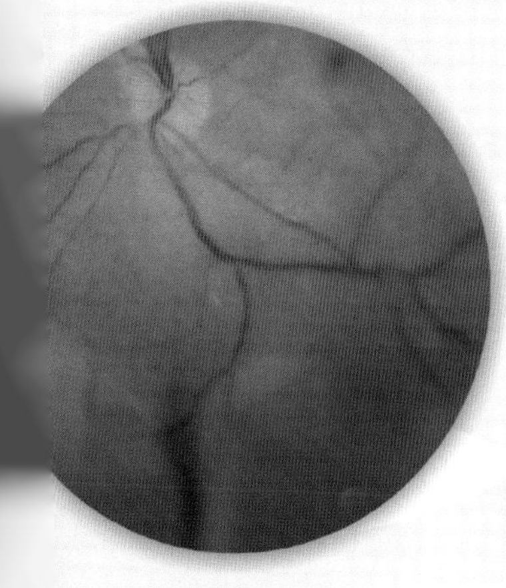

Age Related Macular Degeneration – I

Jose M Ruiz Moreno, Javier A Montero, Francisco L Lugo (Spain)

INTRODUCTION

Age related macular degeneration (AMD) is a degenerative process involving the choriocapillaris, Bruch´s membrane, retinal pigment epithelium (RPE) and photoreceptors in the macula. AMD causes legal blindness in 1.7% of people aged 50 or older and is the leading cause of irreversible vision loss in developed countries in this group of age. AMD is classified as dry or atrophic and exudative or wet.

The prevalence of AMD increases with age from 40 years onwards. The prevalence of both forms among Caucasians is higher than among blacks.

CLINICAL SIGNS AND SYMPTOMS

Atrophic AMD is defined by the appearance of geographic areas of RPE atrophy greater than 175 microns in diameter which permits visualization of the choroidal vessels. Neovascular AMD is defined by RPE detachment associated to other signs of age related maculopathy, subretinal or sub RPE neovascularization, scars, glial tissue, fibrin, subretinal hemorrhages or hard exudates.

Hard drusen are white-yellowish deposits 50 microns in diameter with well defined contour that may appear in the posterior pole. Soft drusen are larger with poorly defined borders, tend to be confluent and appear in the perifoveal area and may cause drusenoid detachments. Pigment changes are hyper or hypo pigmented areas in the outer retina.

Atrophic AMD is a bilateral, slowly progressive condition, characterized by rapidly progressive loss of visual acuity and the appearance of a central or para central scotoma and metamorphopsia. Funduscopy reveals well defined atrophic areas larger than 175 microns with irregular borders. Choroidal vessels may be seen through the atrophic area. FA shows early, well defined hyperfluorescent areas without leakage.

Exudative AMD is characterized by rapidly progressive visual acuity loss with metamorphopsia and central scotoma caused by CNV in the posterior pole, frequently with a severe loss of visual acuity.

INVESTIGATIONS

Biomicroscopy and ophthalmoscopy reveal a grayish-yellowish, rounded or oval subretinal lesion which may be surrounded by a ring of pigment or blood.

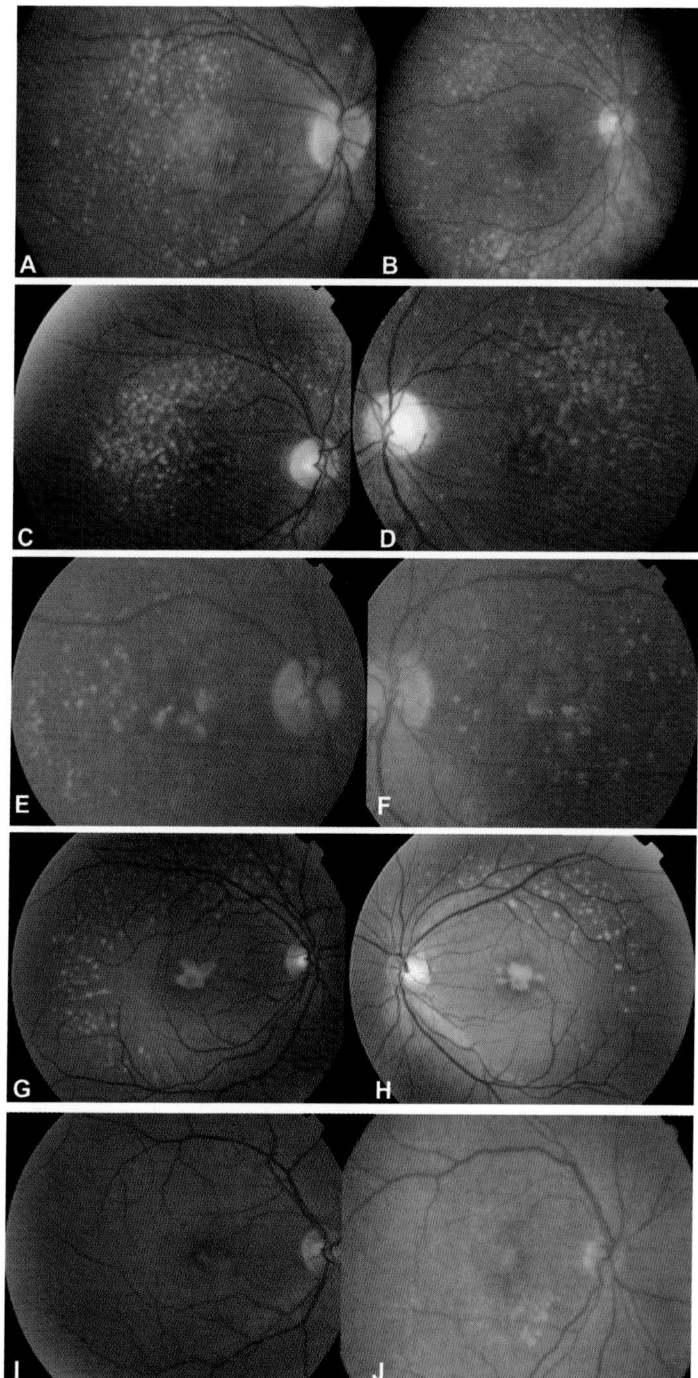

Figs 1A to J: (A and B) Hard drusen with atrophic phenomena. (C and D) soft drusen. (E and F) calcified drusen. (G and H) Drusenoid detachment. (I and J) Pigmentary changes (hyper and hypopigmentation)

Old lesions may show hard exudates or cystoid macular edema. New vessels frequently bleed causing subretinal hemorrhages. RPE detachments are frequent.

FA permits classification of CNV according to the distance to the fovea, the pattern or type of neovascularization and the components of the lesion. According to the distance to the fovea, CNV can be classified as extrafoveal 200 microns or more from the geometric center of the FAZ), juxtafoveal (1 to 199 microns) and subfoveal (affecting the geometric centre of the FAZ). According to the angiographic pattern, two types of CNV are differentiated: classic and occult. Classic CNV is characterized by a well delimited area of intense hyperfluorescence in the early frames with leakage in the intermediate frames which may hide the borders of the CNV. Pathologically they are between the RPE and the neurosensory retina. Early frames show irregular hyperfluorescence, mottled or with irregular elevations of the RPE. Late frames show fluorescein leakage which accumulates in the RPE detachment. RPE may be well or ill defined, and fluorescence is less intense than in classic forms or can be mottled and non homogeneous. These findings originate two FA patterns characteristic of occult CNV: fibrovascular pigment epithelium detachment (FVPED) and late leakage of Undetermined Source (LLUS).

FVPED are characterized by an irregular elevation of the RPE with mottled hyperfluorescence 1 to 2 minutes after fluorescein injection, well or ill defined and with leakage in the late frames. LLUS are characterized by fluorescein leakage in the late frames; the origin can not be determined and is different from classic and FVDEP.

Other components should be considered, such as blood, blocked fluorescence and serous PED.

According to the proportion of lesion occupied by the different components, three main types of lesions can be considered: Predominantly Classic CNV (classic CNV > 50% of entire lesion), Minimally classic CNV(classic CNV < 50%, > 0% area of entire lesion) and Occult with no classic CNV.

OCT reveals soft drusen as elevated RPE with no posterior shadowing towards the choroid whereas PED appears as RPE elevation with shadowing. CNV appears as a hyperreflective band anterior to RPE inducing posterior shadowing. The presence of fluid may be a sign of activity of CNV. Fibrosis appears as a hyperreflective band with no fluid accumulation. Occult lesions present diffuse or cystic intraretinal fluid and PED. OCT provides important information about the persistence of active CNV and the healing process, revealing the presence of RPE rips or changes and elevation of RPE. Presently, the follow up of CNV associated with AMD is performed basically by OCT.

Research is focused on the complement gene which might be responsible for 43% of the cases. Many other genetic studies will be required to confirm the causality of AMD related to this gene.

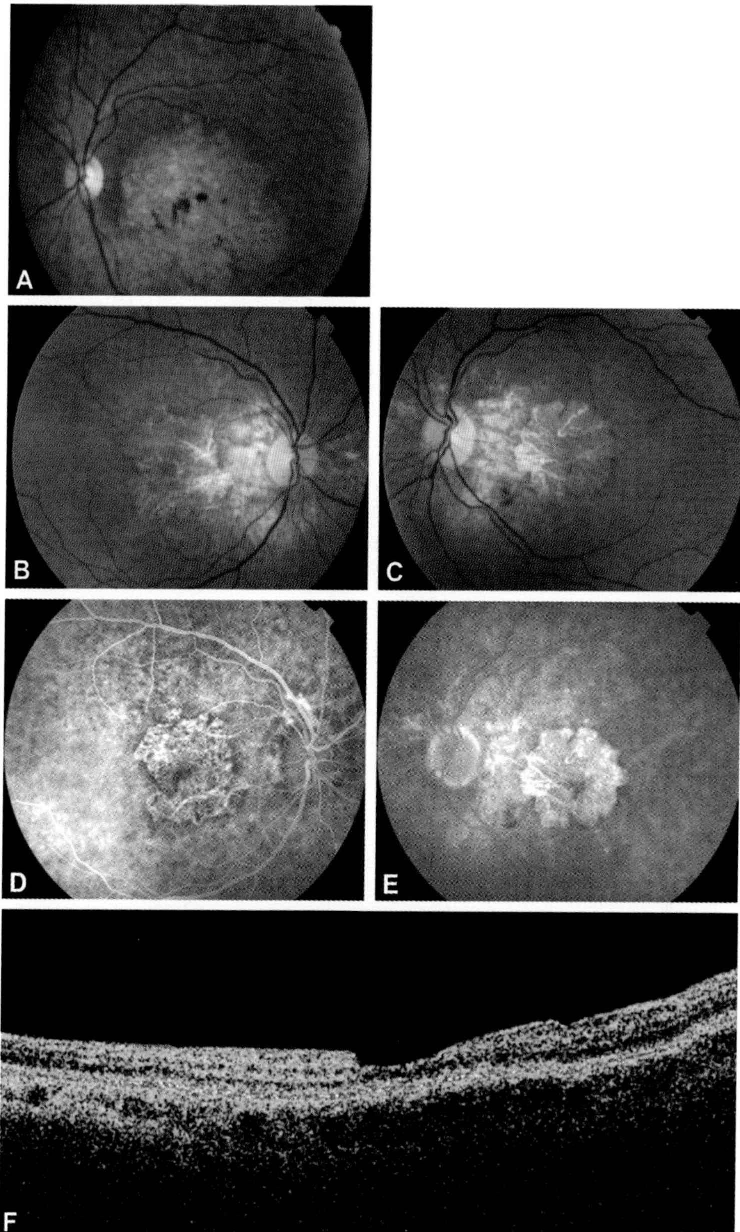

Figs 2A to F: (A) Fundus eye of a patient with atrophic ARMD. (B to E) Fundus eye (right and left) and fluorescein angiography (FA) of a patient with atrophic ARMD in both eyes. (F) OCT of the right eye with thin retina

Oxidative stress causes damage to the RPE and the choriocapillaris. RPE lesions trigger an inflammatory response in Bruch´s membrane and choroid stimulating the production of an abnormal extracellular matrix which further modifies the behavior of RPE increasing the damage to the retina and the choroid.

Pharmacological inhibition of angiogenesis is the new therapeutic modality to treat CNV in AMD. New possibilities of blocking angiogenesis are under research, such as blocking the expression of the genes after DNA transcription (RNA interference).

RNA interference is a cellular mechanism that silences the expression of one protein in a specific a powerful way using short RNA molecules addressed against a specific RNAm. Other therapeutic approach under research is the blockade of cellular receptors for VEGF tirosinkinase 2 and VEGF trap. VEGF trap-eye is a recombinant protein consisting of human VEGF receptor extracellular domains fused to the Fc portion of human immunoglobulin IgG1. VEGF trap is a specific blocker that binds and inactivates circulating VEGF in the blood stream and in the extracellular extravascular space.

DIFFERENTIAL DIAGNOSIS

Differential diagnosis should be established with Polypoidal Choroidal Vasculopathy (PCV) and Retinal Angiomatous Proliferation (RAP).

TREATMENT

Thermal laser has been much restricted presently. The results of the MPS group at 5 years revealed recurrences at 5 years in 41% of the cases, with a marked visual acuity loss in 52% of the treated eyes. Only in cases with well defined extrafoveal CNV distant enough from the fovea to permit treating the whole lesion without damaging the FAZ. Transpupillary thermotherapy has been abandoned.

Verteporfin PDT is known to reduce the patient's perception of scotoma. The appearance of recurrences and the need to retreat is still high. Combined treatment with intravitreal triamcinolone acetonide (TA) and PDT unite the short-term effect of PDT inducing CNV closure with the anti-inflammatory effects of intravitreal TA. Combined treatment PDT and intravitreal antiangiogenic drugs is being tested.

Antiangiogenic drugs: Positive results have been reported with intravitreal injections of an anti VEGF aptamer (Macugen®) to treat wet AMD. A fragment of a humanized monoclonal antibody anti VEGF (ranibizumab, Lucentis®) has been reported to be effective as well as the off label use of the complete antibody (bevacizumab, Avastin®).

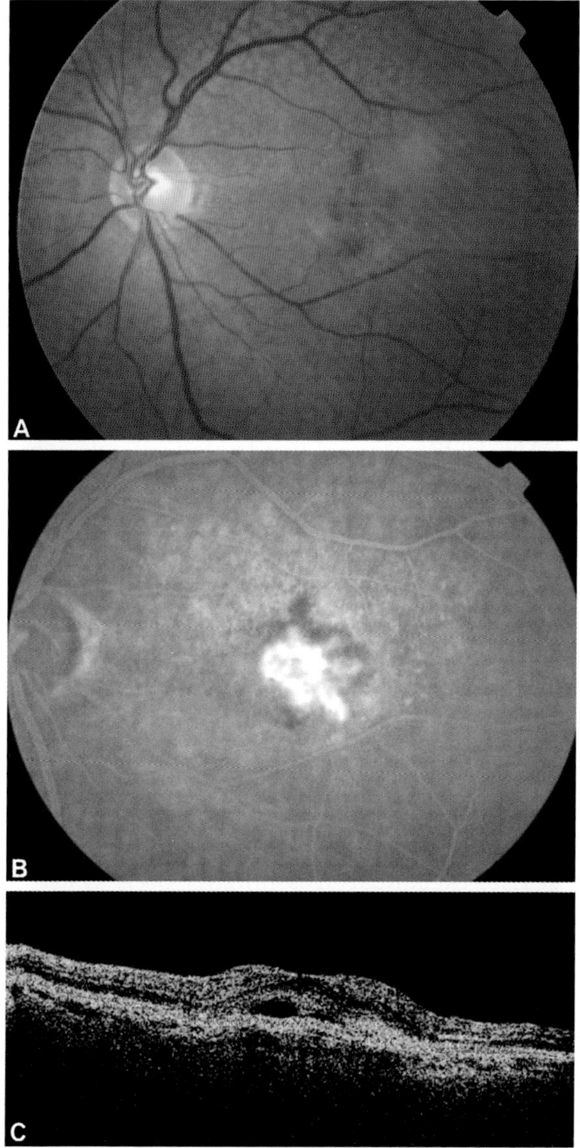

Figs 3A to C: Fundus eye, FA (late phase) and OCT of a patient with predominantly classic subfoveal CNV associated to ARMD

Macugen® (sodium pegaptanib) is a pegylated aptamer with anti VEGF properties and a molecular weight of 50 KD which acts specifically and with high affinity on the isoform 165 of VEGF, which is the most frequent in retinal CNV. The drug is injected intravitreally every six weeks. 0,3 mg Macugen® was useful vs sham injections to avoid 3 lines loss (70% versus 55%; $P < 0,001$). Regarding safety, and after analyzing adverse events related to the drug and the injecting procedure revealed that Macugen® was well tolerated at all concentrations.

Lucentis® inhibits VEGF mediated neovascularization. A molecular weight of 48 kD (smaller than the complete monoclonal antibody, 149 kD) facilitates its penetration into the subretinal space.

The pivotal masked randomized controlled phase III trials with Lucentis® (MARINA and ANCHOR) revealed that treated patients gained an average 6.6 and 5.4 letters with 0.5 and 0.3 mg respectively, vs an average loss of 14.9 letters in the control group after 2 years; ANCHOR presented 11.3 and 8.5 letters gain respectively vs an average loss of 9.5 letters in the PDT group. More than 90% of the treated patients maintained BCVA after 2 years vs 60% in the controls. A new trial was designed (PIER) to reduce the number of injections treating the eyes with 3 injections during the first 3 months, and once every 3 months thereafter. However visual outcome was worse than in MARINA and ANCHOR.

Avastin® is a humanized monoclonal antibody antiVEGF that links to all the biologically active forms of VEGF as occurs with Lucentis®. Bevacizumab was approved by the FDA for the intravenous treatment of metastatic colorectal cancer. Bevacizumab was initially used systemically to treat exudative AMD and was later injected intravitreally. BCVA improves one week after the injection and is maintained for 3 months. Mean retinal thickness is significantly decreased at 3 months follow-up.

It is not clinically feasible to perform intravitreal injections every four weeks for 2 years. The most accepted injecting schedule presently derives from the PRONTO trial: 3 monthly injections with a re injection criteria including increased central retinal thickness > 100 microns, BCVA loss > 5 letters with retinal fluid in OCT, new classic CNV or hemorrhage and persistence of fluid 1 month after the injection. Its results were similar to those of MARINA and ANCHOR with a lower number of injections (average 5.5/year, mean time after the first re-injection 4.3 months).

We have to inform about the advantages, drawbacks, risks and legal situation of each drug. The cardiovascular risk of these patients should be individually considered.

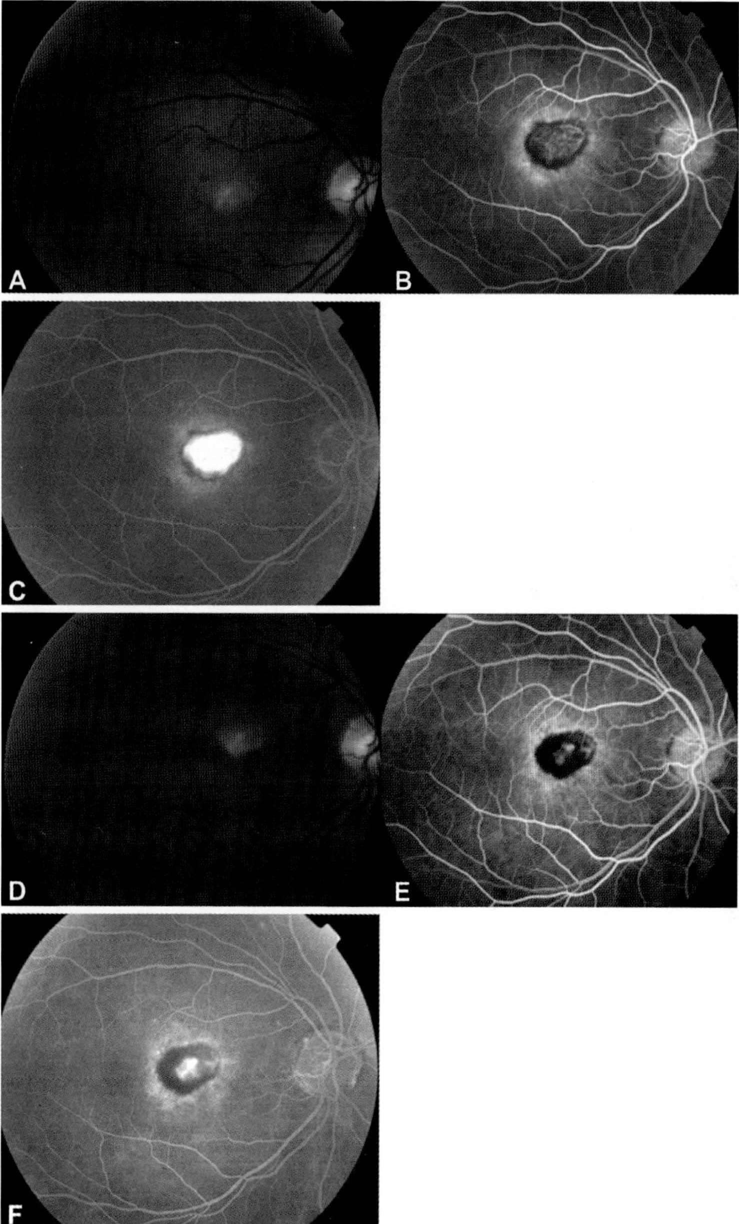

Figs 4A to F: (A to C) Fundus eye and FA (early and late phase) of a patient with predominantly classic subfoveal CNV associated to ARMD. (D to F) fundus eye and FA (early and late phase) of a same patient after three PDT treatments

PROGNOSIS

The natural history of CNV is a fibrous disc shaped scar known as disciform. The presently available therapies may modulate new vessels growth and hyperpermeability, reducing the formation of disciform scars and improving visual outcome. However, we are still not able to modify the atrophic and degenerative changes in RPE and choriocapillaris.

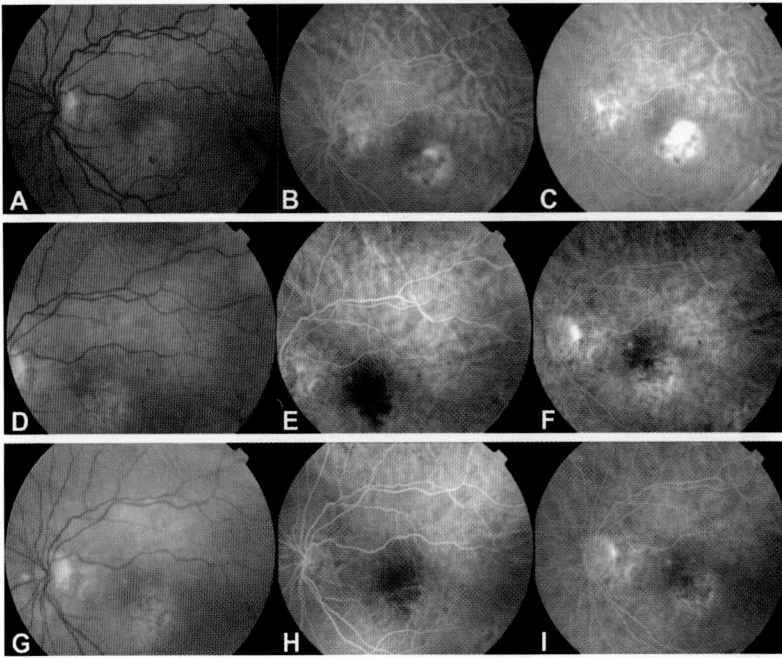

Figs 5A to I: (A to C) Fundus eye and FA (early and late phase) of a patient with minimally classic subfoveal CNV associated to ARMD. (D to F) fundus eye and FA (early and late phase) of a same patient three months after one PDT treatment combined with high dose intravitreal triamcinolone. (G to I) fundus eye and FA (early and late phase) of a same patient six months after one PDT treatment combined with high dose intravitreal triamcinolone

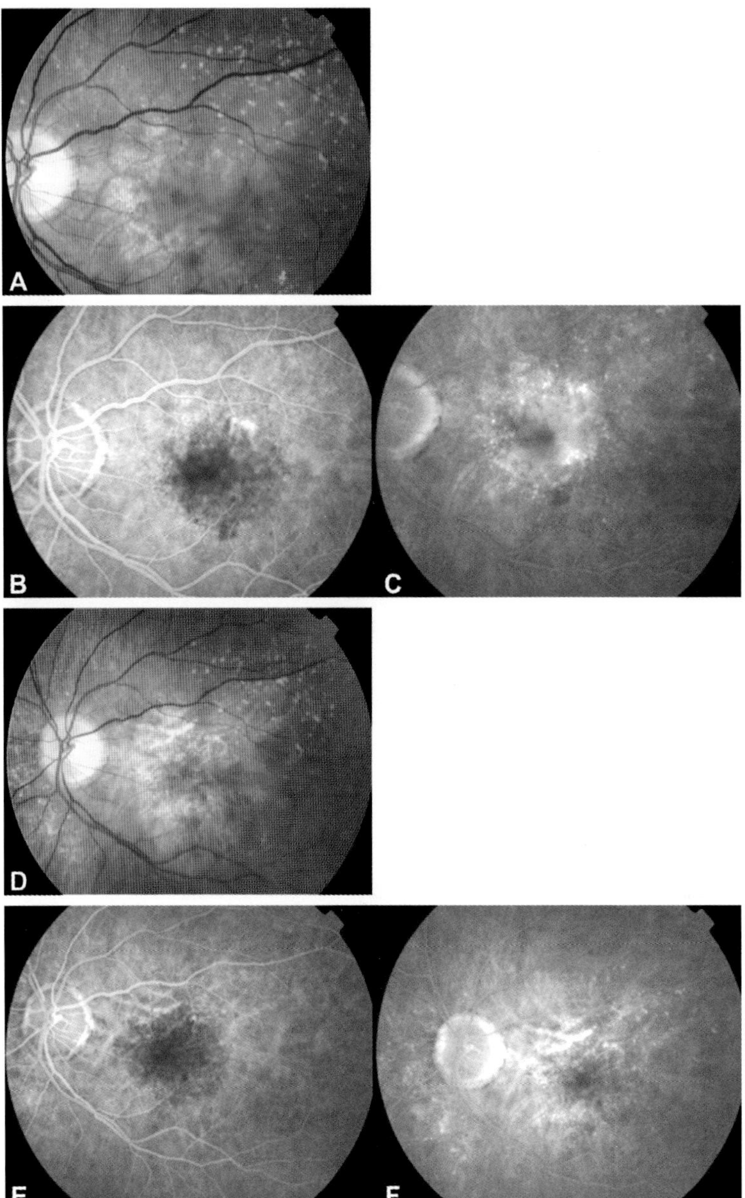

Figs 6A to F: (A to C) Fundus eye and FA (early and late phase) of a patient with occult subfoveal CNV associated to ARMD (late leakage of undetermined source). (D to F) fundus eye and FA (early and late phase) of a same patient after one PDT treatment combined with high dose intravitreal triamcinolone

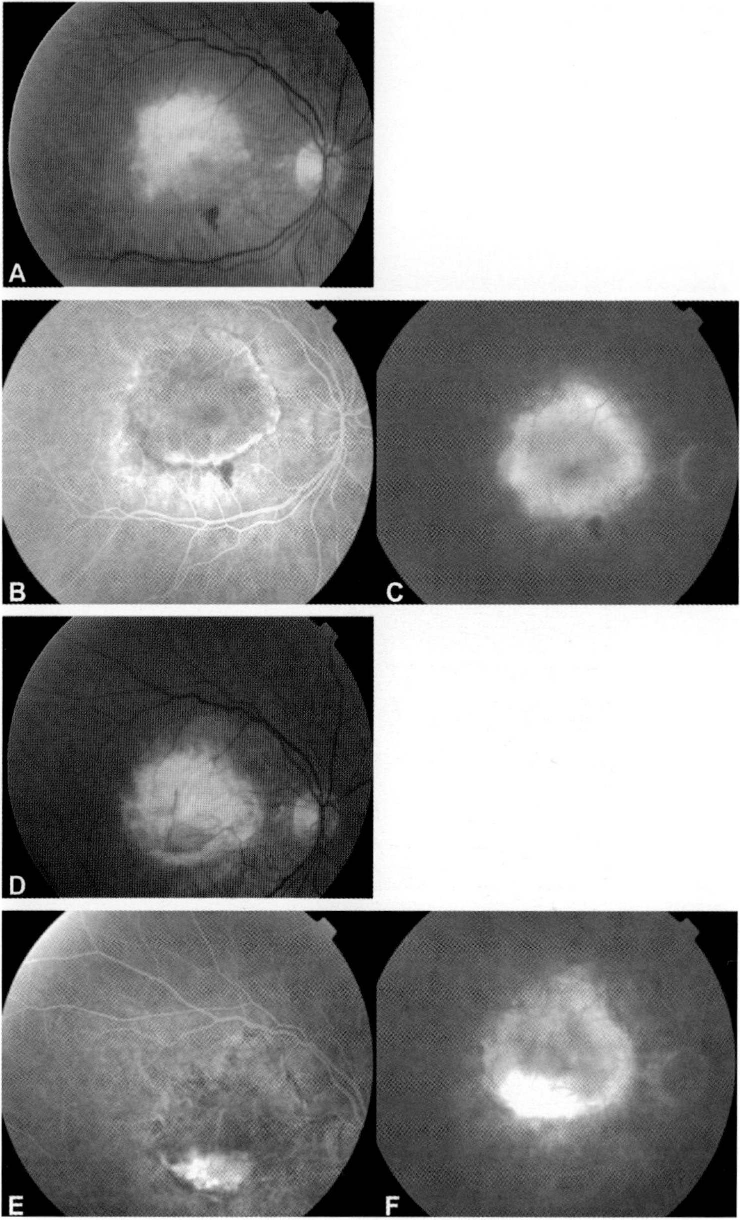

Figs 7A to F: (A to C) Fundus eye and FA (early and late phase) of a patient with occult subfoveal CNV associated to ARMD (fibrovascular PED). (D to F) fundus eye and FA (early and late phase) of a same patient after four PDT treatments with persistent activity of the CNV

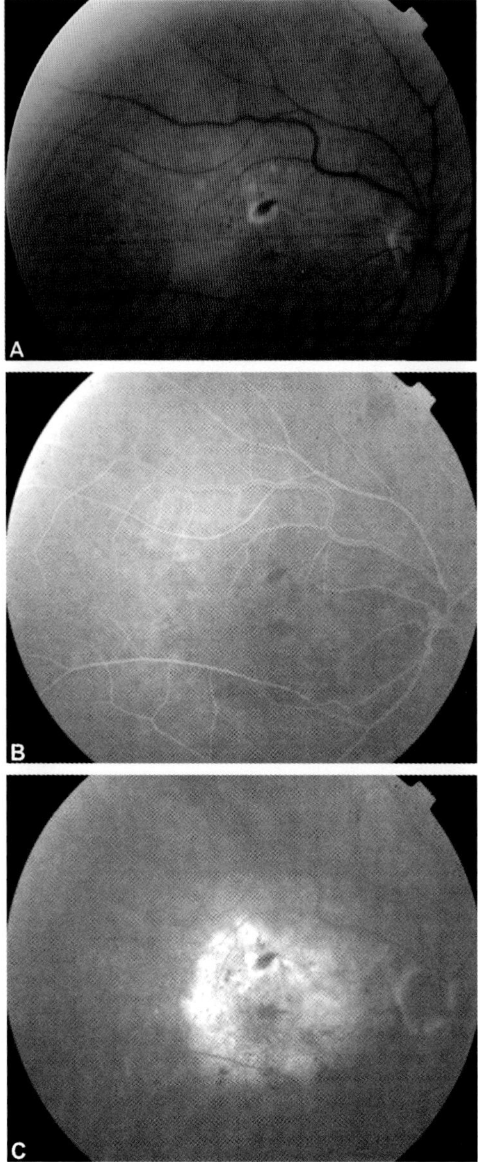

Figs 8A to C: Fundus eye and FA (early and late phase) of a patient with occult subfoveal CNV associated to ARMD (late leakage of undetermined source)

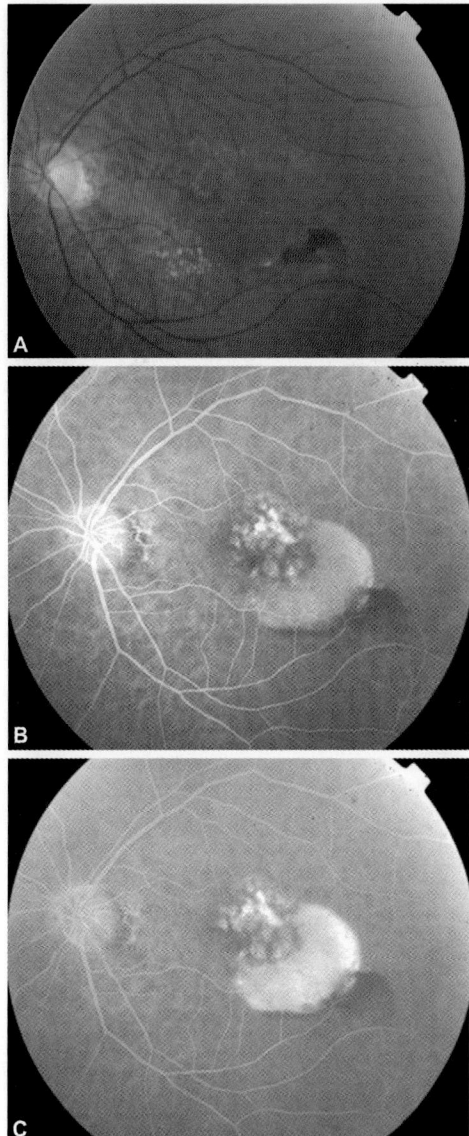

Figs 9A to C: Fundus eye and FA (early and late phase) of a patient with occult subfoveal CNV associated to ARMD (fibrovascular and serous PED)

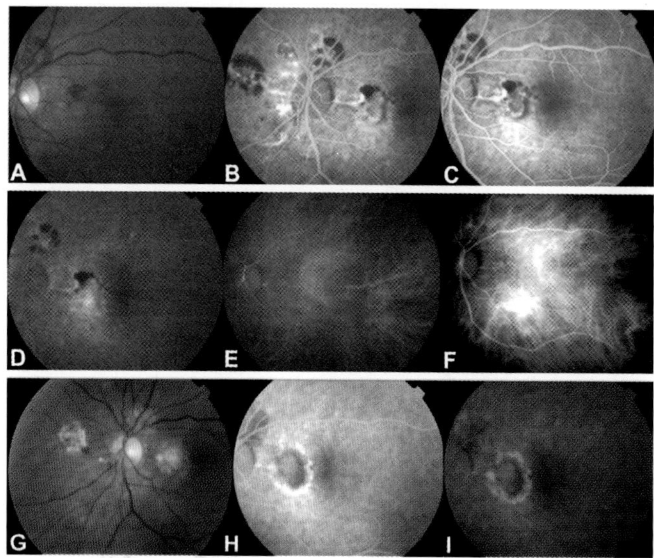

Figs 10A to I: (A to D) Red free fundus eye and FA (early, middle and late phase) of a patient with polypoidal vasculopathy. (E and F) ICG (early and middle phase) showing small hyperfluorescent polyps. (G to I) Fundus eye and FA (early and late phase) of a same patient after treatment by argon green laser photocoagulation

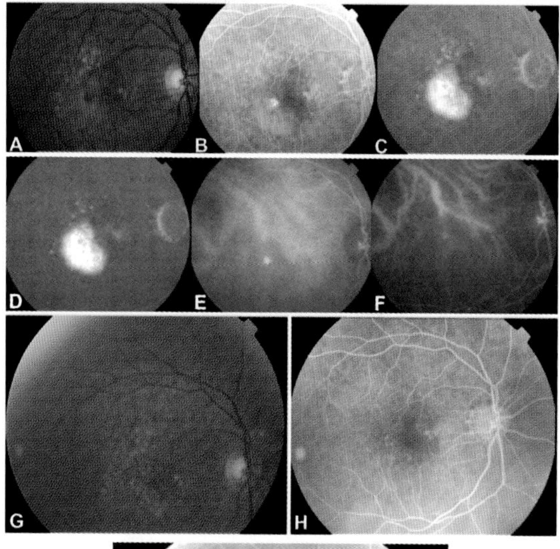

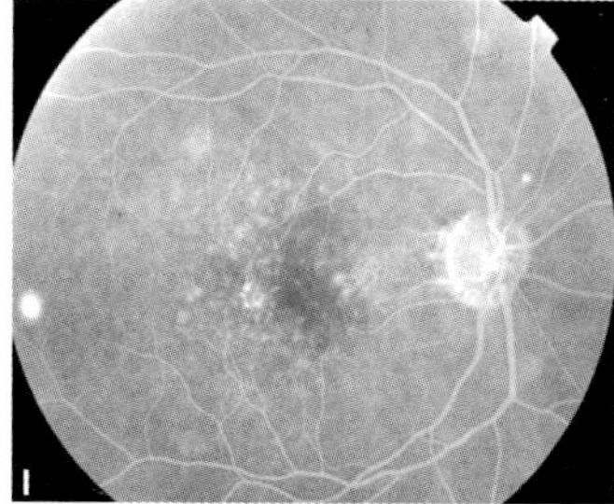

Figs 11A to I: (A to D) Fundus eye and FA (early, middle and late phase) of a patient with Retinal Angiomatous Proliferation stage II (RAP). (E and F) ICG (early and middle phase) showing intraretinal angiomatous proliferation. (G to I) fundus eye and FA (early and late phase) of a same patient after treatment by of a same patient six months after one PDT treatment combined with high dose intravitreal triamcinolone

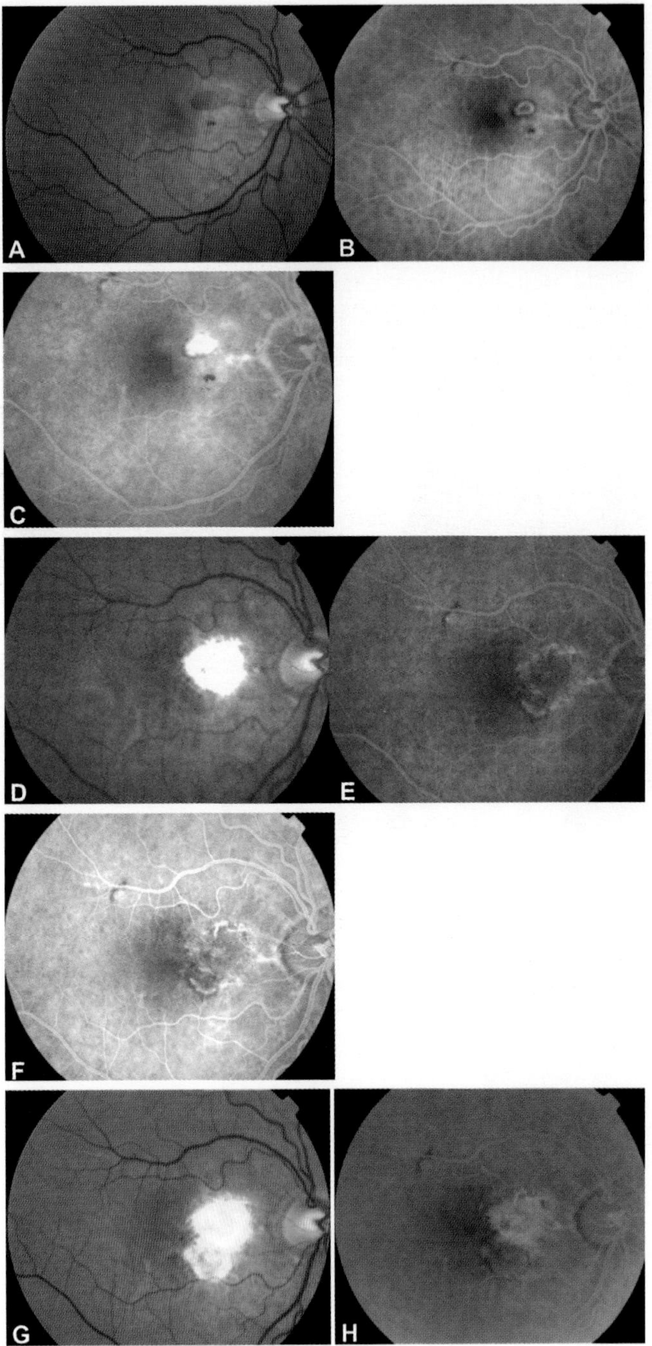

Figs 12A to H: (A to C) Fundus eye and FA (early and late phase) of a patient with predominantly classic subfoveal CNV associated to ARMD. (D to F) red free fundus eye and FA (early and late phase) of a same patient after argon green laser photocoagulation with new CNV re-growth in the edge of a previous scar. (G and H) fundus eye and FA (early and late phase) of the same patient after second argon laser treatment with no activity of the CNV

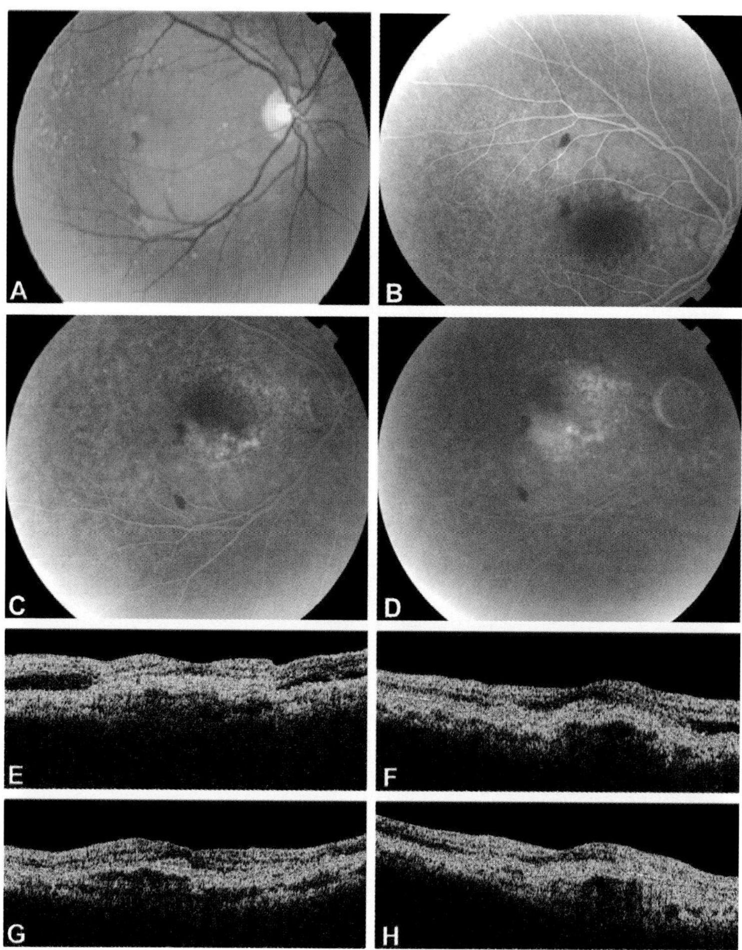

Figs 13A to H: (A to D) Fundus eye and FA (early, middle and late phase) of a patient with occult subfoveal CNV associated to ARMD. (E and F) horizontal and vertical OCT previous treatment. (G and H) OCT of a same patient after one Lucentis® intravitreal injection

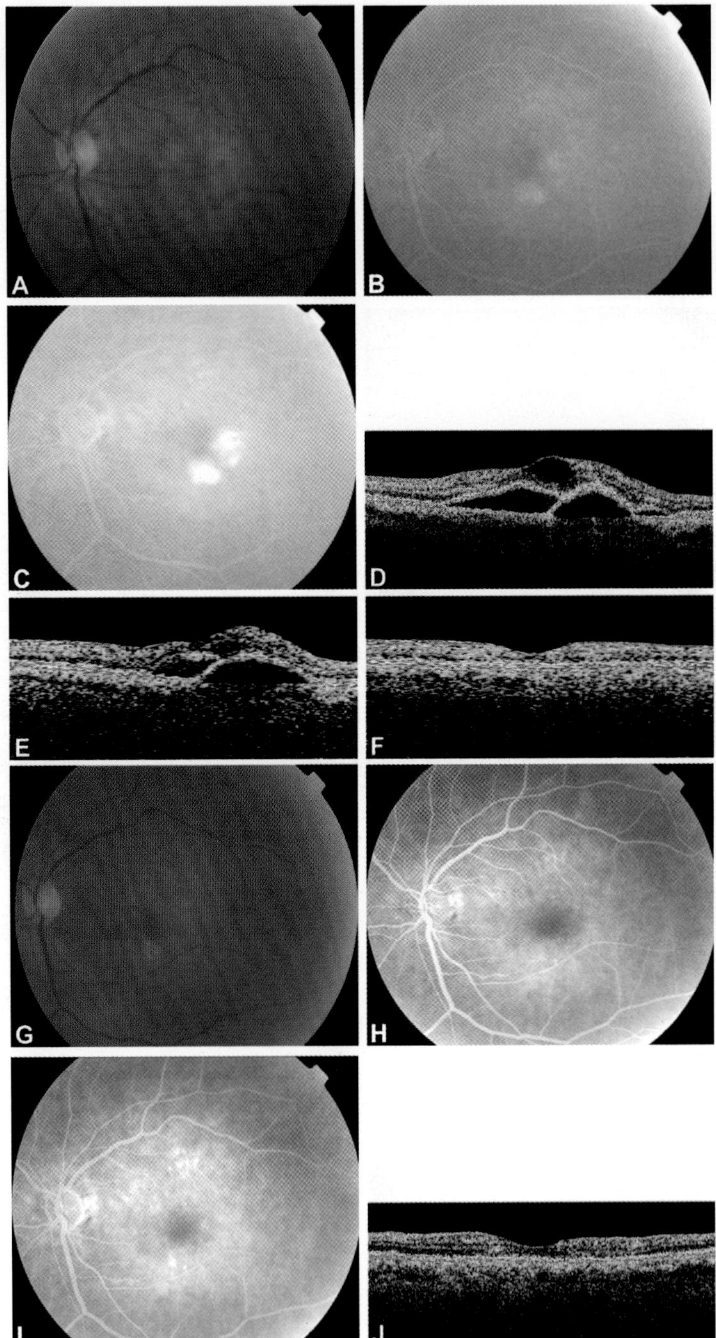

Figs 14A to J: (A to C) Fundus eye and FA (early and late phase) of a patient with occult subfoveal CNV associated to ARMD. (D and E) horizontal and vertical OCT previous treatment. F: OCT of a same patient after one Lucentis® intravitreal injection. (G to I) fundus eye and FA (early and late phase) of a same patient after three intravitreal injections of Lucentis®. (J) Final OCT after treatment

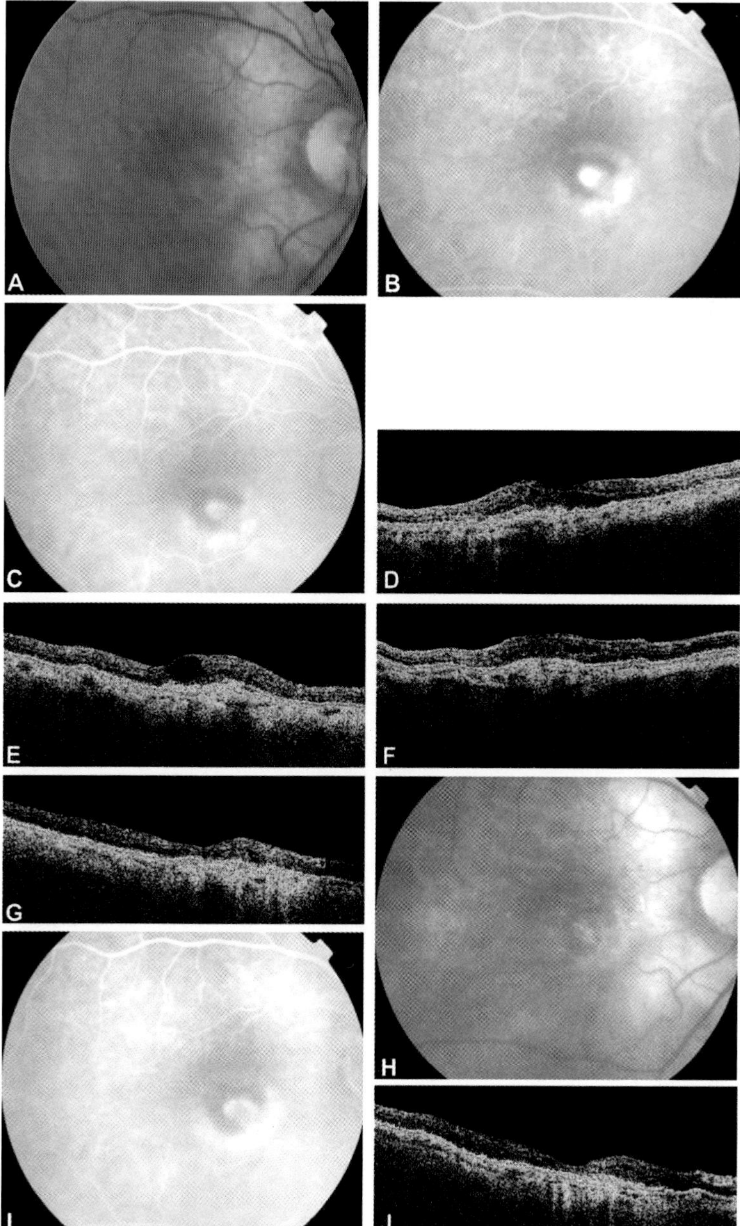

Figs 15A to J: (A to C) Fundus eye and FA (early and late phase) of a patient with minimally classic subfoveal CNV associated to ARMD. (D to G) OCT study during treatment with four Macugen® intravitreal injections. (H to J) FA (early and late phase) and OCT after treatment

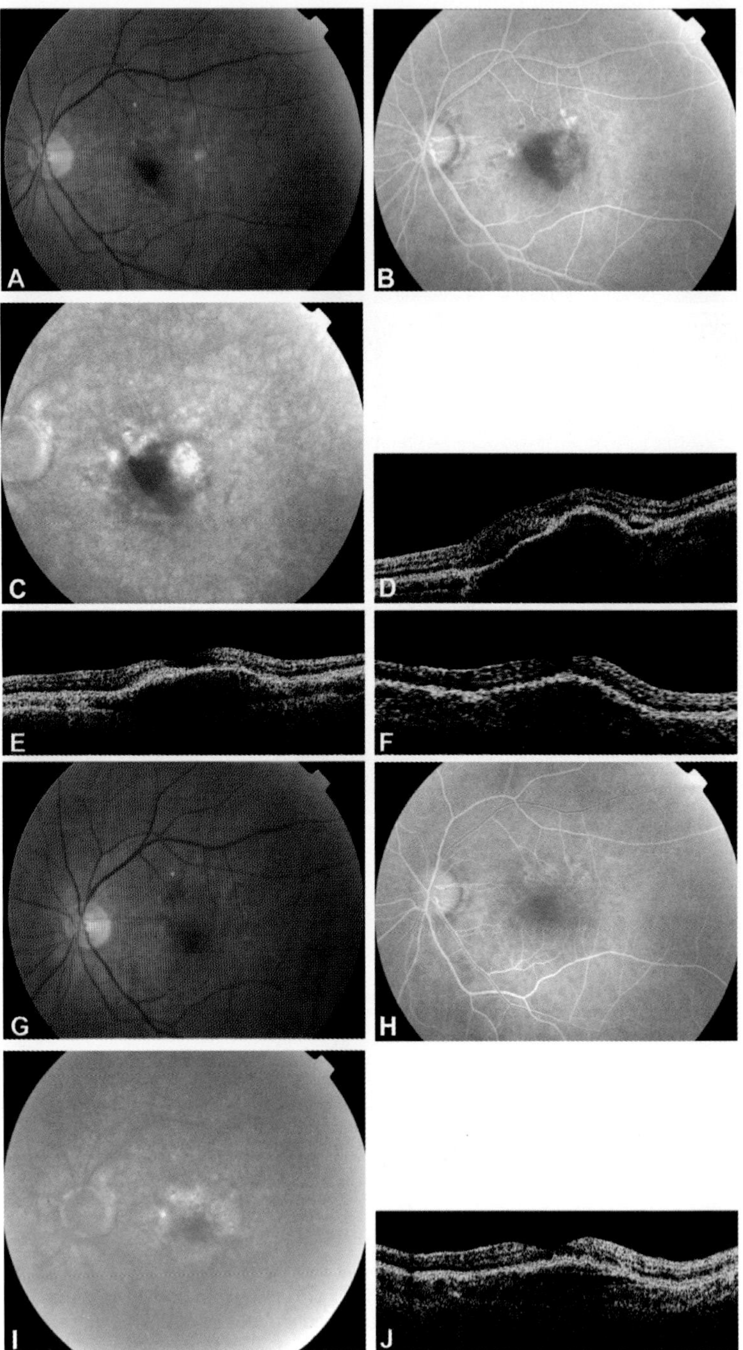

Figs 16A to J: (A to C) Fundus eye and FA (early and late phase) of a patient with occult subfoveal CNV associated to ARMD. (D) horizontal OCT previous treatment. (E and F) OCT study during treatment with three Avastin® intravitreal injections. (G to J) Fundus eye, FA (early and late phase) and OCT of a same patient after three intravitreal injections of Avastin®

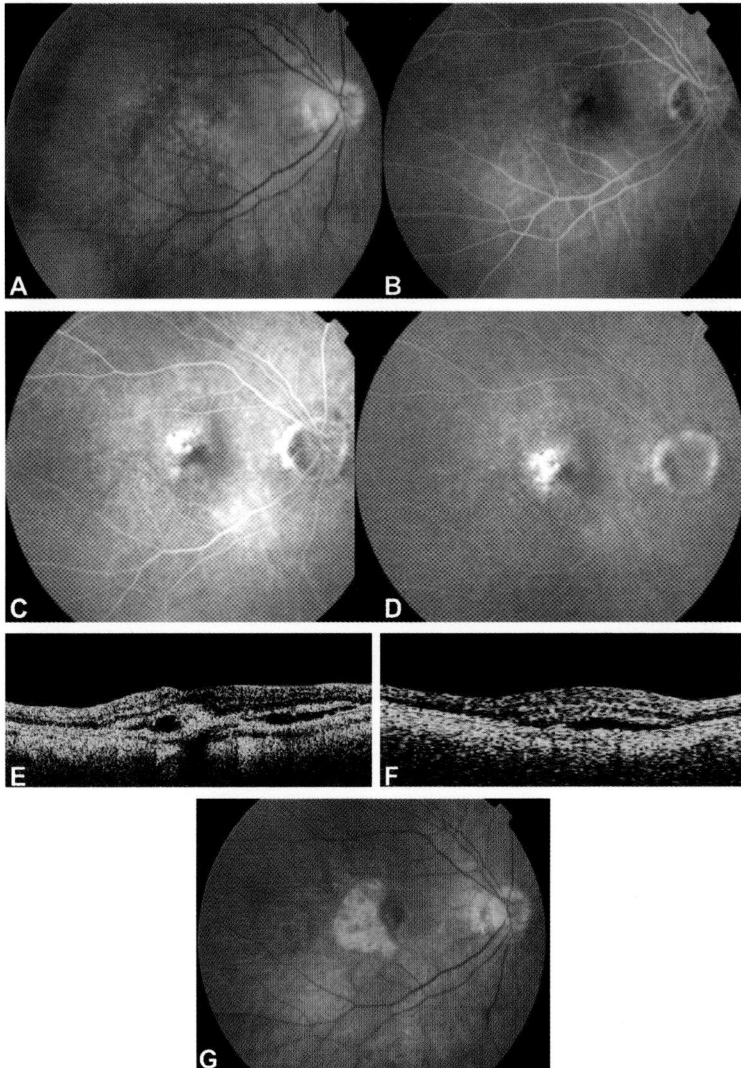

Figs 17A to G: (A to D) Fundus eye and FA (early, middle and late phase) of a patient with occult subfoveal CNV associated to ARMD. (E and F) Horizontal and vertical OCT previous treatment. (G) fundus photography of the same patient showing retinal pigmentary epithelium tear after one Lucentis® intravitreal injection

Age Related Macular Degeneration – II

T Mark Johnson (USA)

DRY AMD

INTRODUCTION

Prevalence

- Represents 80% of cases of AMD
- Increased prevalence with age
  - 6% of patients > 52 years
  - 20% > 75 years.

Risk Factors

- Family history
  - Precise genetics of AMD remain unclear
  - Y402H variant of complement factor H gene may account for significant amount of the risk of macular degeneration
- Light racial pigmentation
- Smoking
- Hypertension
- Cardiovascular disease.

CLINICAL SIGNS AND SYMPTOMS

Symptoms

- Asymptomatic
- Decreased vision
- Decreased contrast acuity
- Distortion.

Signs

- Drusen
  - Yellow subretinal deposits
  - Hard drusen : well defined yellow deposits
  - Soft drusen : ill defined deposits
    - Coalescence produces drusenoid RPE detachment
- Pigmentary hypertrophy

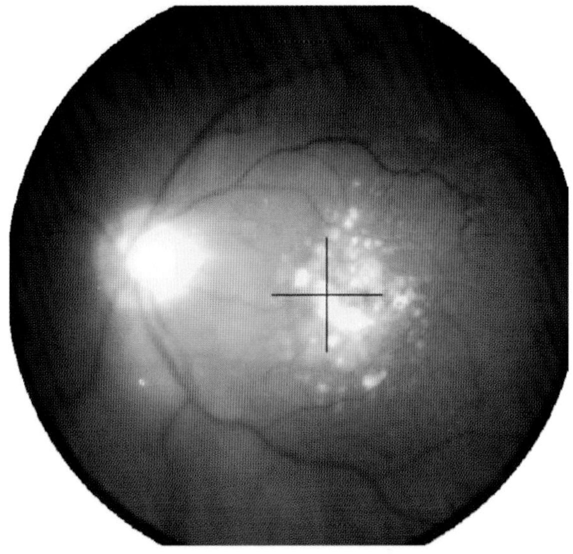

Fig. 1: Color photo of dry AMD with drusen and pigmentary changes

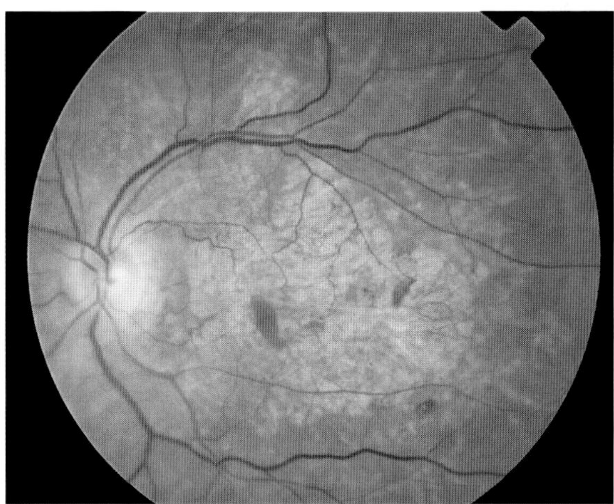

Fig. 2: Color photo of advanced dry AMD with extensive geographic atrophy

- Geographic atrophy
  - Well defined of the RPE and choriocapillaris leaving areas of visible deep choroids and sclera.

INVESTIGATIONS

Fluorescein Angiography

Indications

- Rule out evidence of CNVM.

Results

- Soft drusen have pooling of dye under the drusen resulting in late hyperfluorescence without leakage
- Areas of atrophy show well defined choroidal staining.

Macular Perimetry

Indications

- Evaluation of macular function.

Results

- Demonstrates significant macular dysfunction in dry AMD
- May be used to locate eccentric fixation points for visual rehabilitation.

DIFFERENTIAL DIAGNOSIS

- Congenital
  - Stargardt disease
  - Best disease
  - Central areolar choroidal atrophy.
- Acquired
  - Myopic degeneration
  - Drugs (example chloroquine)
  - Trauma
  - Posterior uveitis.

TREATMENT

Antioxidant Therapy

Indications

- Extensive intermediate (63-124 microns) drusen
- At least 1 large druse (>124 microns)
- Non central geographic atrophy
- CVNM in fellow eye.

Methods

- Supplementation with high dose beta carotene, vitamin C, vitamin E and zinc
- Smokers should receive zinc supplementation alone due to concerns about related lung cancers.

Results

- Age Related Eye Disease Study demonstrated a significant reduction in the risk of development of advanced macular degeneration
- Odds Ratio for developing advanced AMD in patients treated with antioxidants plus zinc 0.72 (0.52-0.98).

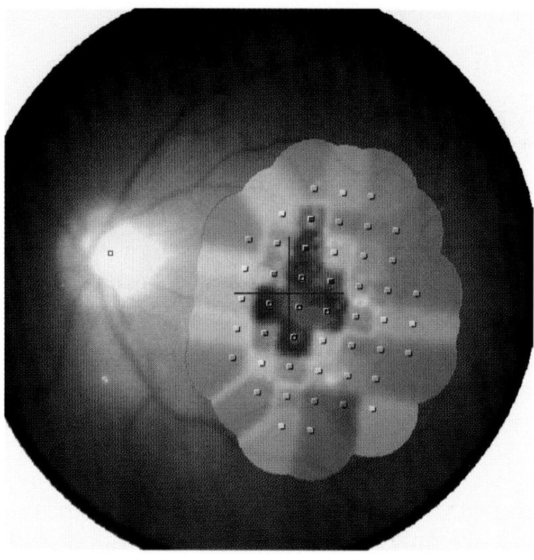

Fig. 3: Macular perimetry of patient with dry AMD showing depressed central retinal function

Laser

- Macular laser has been observed to reduce the number of drusen evident in the macula
- Initial clinical trials observed a reduction in drusen with a marginal visual benefit but possible increased risk of development of CNVM
- Currently considered investigational.

Inferences

- Dry AMD is the most common form of AMD
- 5 year incidence of development of CNV in patients with bilateral drusen is approximately 13%.

BIBLIOGRAPHY

1. AREDS Group. A randomized, placebo controlled clinical trial of high dose supplementation with vitamins C and E, beta carotene, and zinc for age-related macular degeneration and visual loss. Arch Ophth. 2001:119;1417-36.
2. Leibowitz HM, et al. The Framingham Eye Study Monograph VI. Surv Ophth. 1980:24(suppl);428-57.
3. Smiddy WE et al. Prognosis of patients with bilateral macular drusen. Ophth. 1984:91; 271-77.
4. The Choroidal Neovascularization Prevention Trial Research Group. Laser treatment in eyes with large drusen. Short term effects seen in a pilot randomized clinical trial. Ophth. 1998:105;11-23.
5. Zareparsi S, Branham KE, Shah S, et al. Strong association of the Y402H variant in complement factor H at 1q32 with susceptibility to age related macular degeneration. Am J Human Genetics. 2005:77;149-53.

EXUDATIVE AMD

INTRODUCTION

Prevalence

- 10% of macular degeneration
- Accounts for majority of legal blindness secondary to AMD
  - 80% of legal blindness secondary to AMD is due to exudative AMD
  - Prevalence of legal blindness in Caucasian population secondary to exudative AMD is 2.7/1000 persons.

Incidence

- 5 year incidence of CNVM in patients with bilateral drusen is about 13%
- 3 year incidence of CNVM in patients with unilateral CNVM is about 30%.

Risk Factors

- Family history
- Smoking
- Cardiovascular disease
- Hypertension.

CLINICAL SIGNS AND SYMPTOMS

Symptoms

- Decreased visual acuity
- Distortion.

Signs

- Subretinal fluid: Appears as turbid, grey elevation of retina
- Subretinal hemorrhage
- Lipid exudation: Typically at margins of extend of exudation
- Serous pigment epithelial detachment: Dome shaped elevation of RPE, may have a notch at the margin of the choroidal neovascular membrane
- Fibrovascular pigment epithelial detachment: Irregular elevation of RPE, may have associated fibrosis
- Subretinal fibrosis: Fibrotic tissue indicative of regressed choroidal neovascularization.

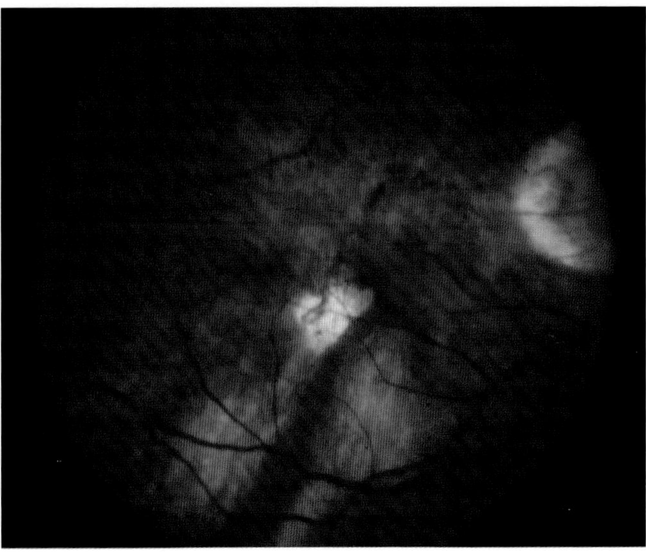

Fig. 4: Recurrent subfoveal CNVM at the margin of prior MPS laser treatment. Subretinal blood and fluid are present

INVESTIGATIONS

Fluorescein Angiography

Describes the pattern of the choroidal neovascularization.

Location

- Subfoveal: Located under the center of the fovea
- Juxtafoveal: 1-199 mm from fovea
- Extrafoveal: Greater than 200 mm from fovea.

Pattern of CNVM

- Classic: Well-defined early hyperfluorescence with late leakage
- Occult: Ill-defined early hyperfluorescence with late leakage or ill defined late leakage with an obvious early source.

ICG Angiography

Allows visualization of CNV through areas of blood, subretinal fluid or pigment epithelial detachment.

Plaque

Greater than 1 disc area of hyperfluorescence that is less intense than a hot spot.

Hot Spot

Bright hyperfluorescent lesion < 1 disc area, typically indicative of RAP lesion or polypoidal CNV (see below).

High Speed ICG Angiography

Utilize rapid capture of the early perfusion of the retina, phi motion produces a continuous motion of early vascular flow allowing visualization of arterial and venous flow of the CNVM.

OCT

Visualize intraretinal edema, subretinal fluid and PED.

DIFFERENTIAL DIAGNOSIS

- Myopic choroidal neovascularization
- Choroidal rupture
- Angioid streaks
- Idiopathic
- Presumed ocular histoplasmosis.

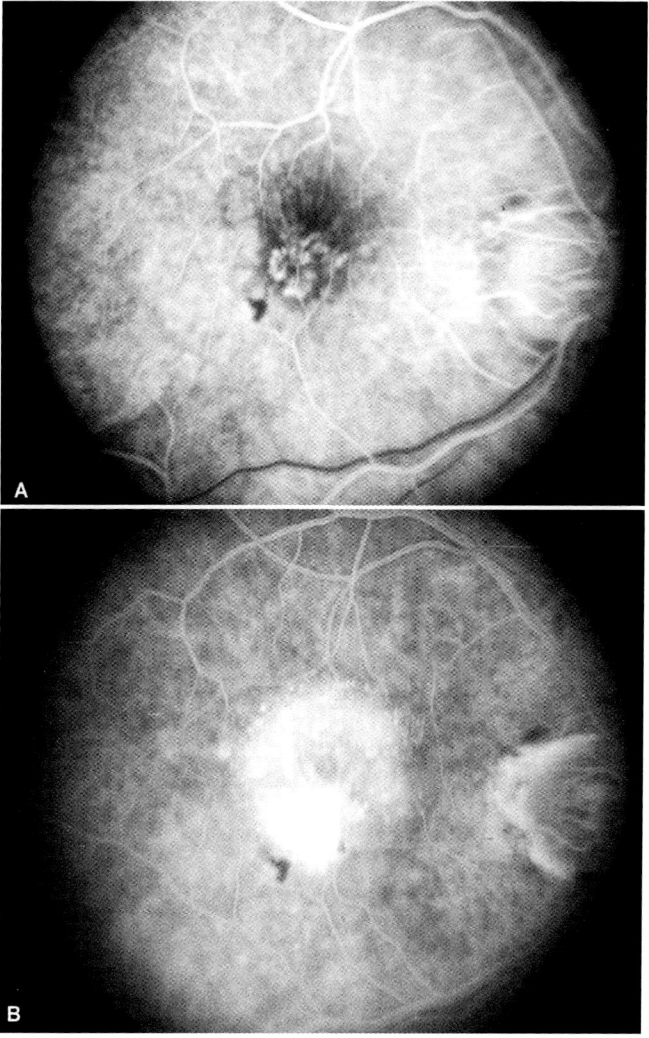

Figs 5A and B: Early and late fluorescein angiogram of patient with a well-defined choroidal neovascular membrane with late leakage

TREATMENT

Focal Laser.

Indications

- Extrafoveal CNVM
- Juxtafoveal: The scotoma generated by focal laser has led most practitioners to use alternative treatments
- ? Subfoveal CNVM.

Methods

- Confluent ablation of the entire CNV complex with treatment border of 100 microns beyond the CNV margin.

Results

- Treatment reduces the risk of severe visual loss (< 20/200)
- Treatment is associated with permanent scotoma
  - While subfoveal MPS trial showed better stabilization of vision with treatment the scotoma and immediate visual decline has led to alternative therapies
- Recurrence rates are high
  - Extrafoveal MPS had a 54% 5 year recurrence rate with the majority of recurrences extending into the fovea
  - Recurrence is associated with a greater risk of visual loss.

Photodynamic Therapy

Indications

- Subfoveal choroidal neovascularization
- Juxtafoveal choroidal neovascularization.

Methods

- Intravenous infusion of verteporfin dye
  - Administer 6 mg/m^2
- Application of 689 nm laser to lesion at 50 J/cm^2
  - Treatment is extended 300-500 microns beyond the border of the lesion.

Results

- PDT slows the rate of visual loss with exudative AMD
- CNVM with > 50% classic component may experience a greater benefit from treatment with PDT

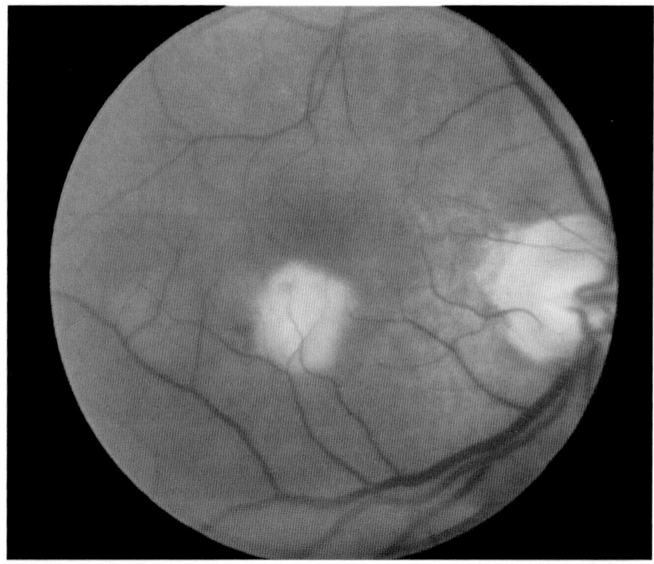

Fig. 6A: Color photo of patient immediately post laser photocoagulation

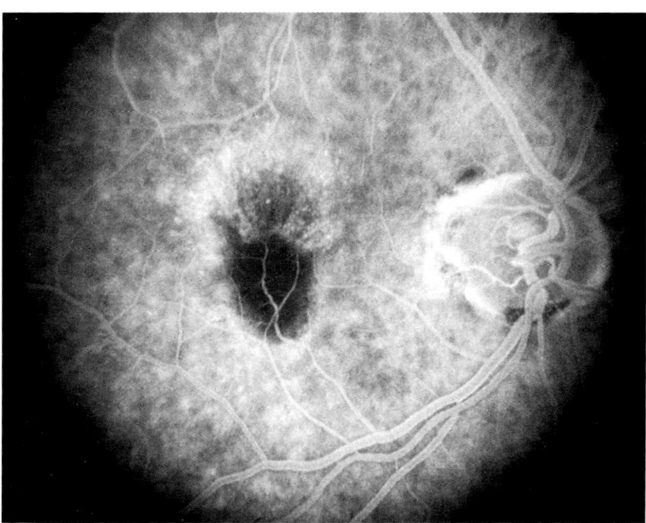

Fig. 6B: Postoperative fluorescein angiogram shows blockage of fluorescence with ablation of CNVM

Transpupillary Thermotherapy

Indications

- Subfoveal choroidal neovascularization.

Methods

- 810 nm diode laser applied to the entire choroidal neovascular membrane to obtain light grey burn to the entire neovascular complex.

Results

- Initial case series demonstrated promising results
- Randomized controlled trial failed to show significant benefit for TTT in patients with AMD.

Intravitreal Anti VEGF Therapy

Indications

- Monotherapy for choroidal neovascularization
- ? Role in combination therapy.

Methods

- Available Agents
  - Pegaptanib (Macugen)
  - Ranibizumab (Lucentis)
  - Bevacizumab (Avastin)
- Method of Administration
  - intravitreal injection
  - frequency of dosing varies with medication type.
- Complications
  - Endophthalmitis
  - Cataract
  - Retinal detachment
  - Uveitis.

Results

- Clinical trials demonstrate pegaptanib is effective at preventing visual loss
  - Clinical trials have demonstrated pegaptanib to be better than placebo at stabilizing visual loss
  - Repeated injections are required every 6 weeks
  - Limited subset of patients regains visual acuity.

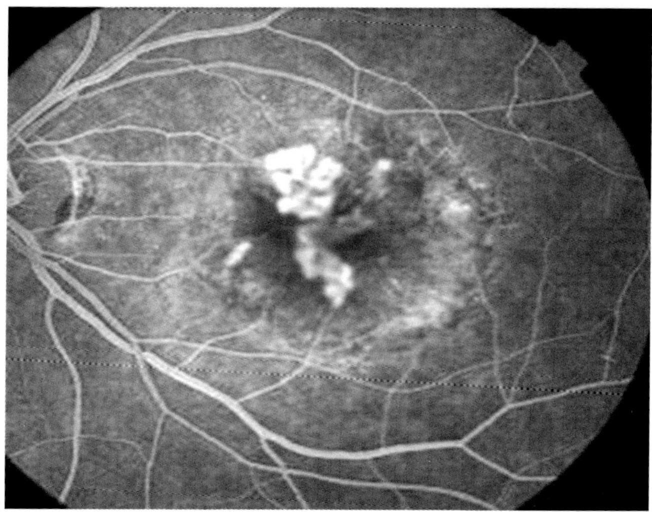

Fig. 7A: Patient with mixed classic and occult CNV prior to photodynamic therapy

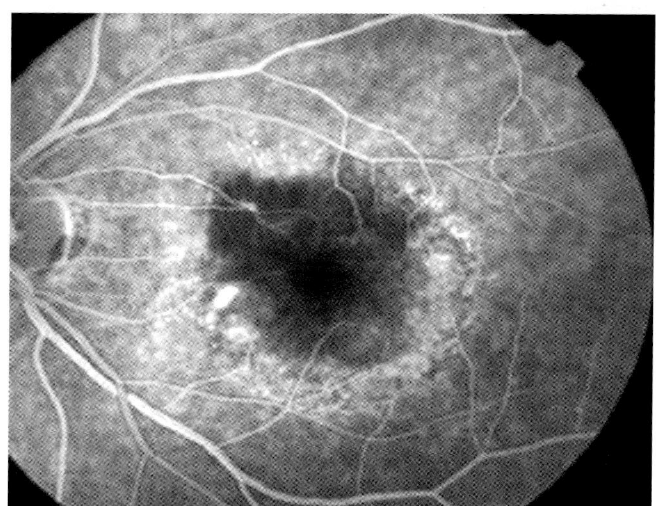

Fig. 7B: Same patient 2 weeks post photodynamic therapy with complete closure of neovascular complex

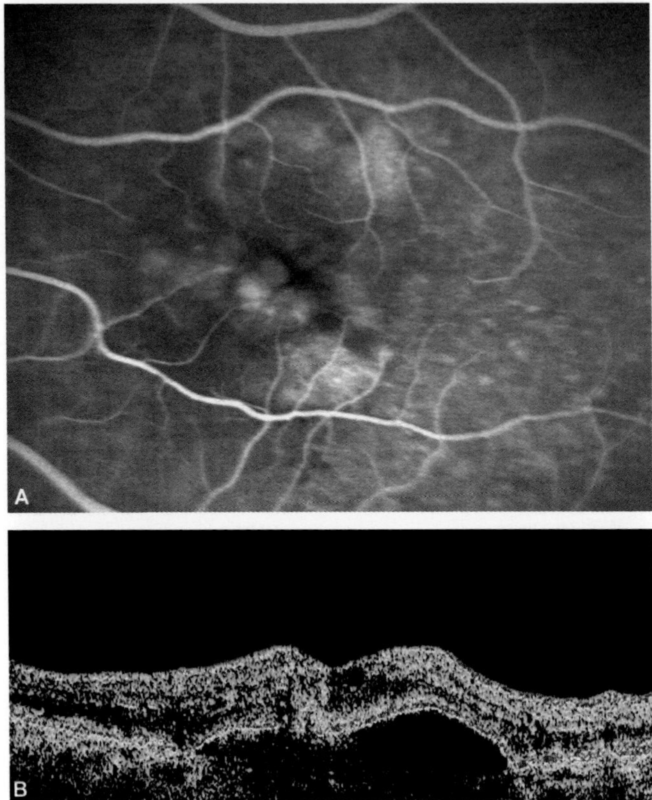

Figs 8A and B: Patient with choroidal neovascularization prior to therapy with occult leakage, pigment epithelial detachment and retinal edema. Visual acuity 20/125

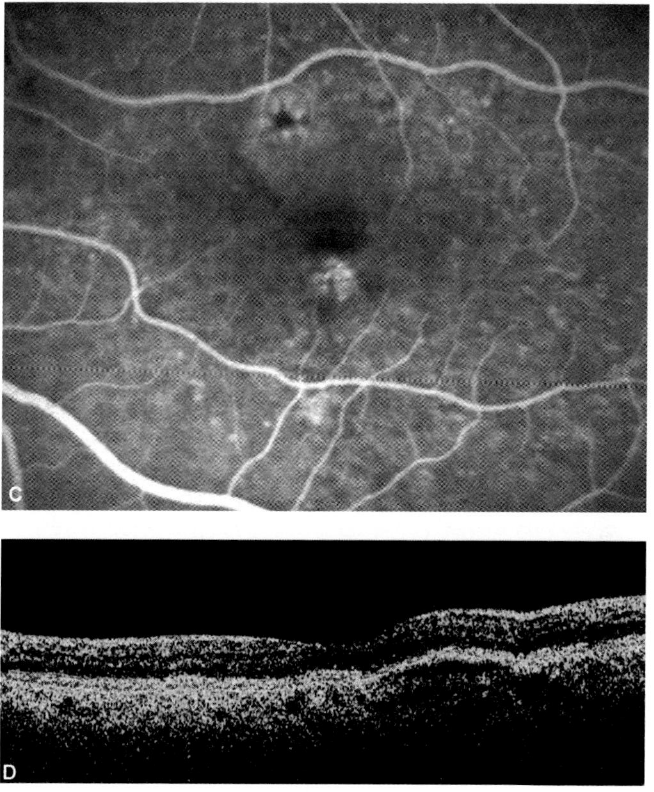

Figs 8C and D: Patient after 12 injections of ranibizumab. Visual acuity 20/25

- Clincal trials demonstrate benefit to ranibizumab therapy
  - MARINA Trial studied ranibizumab versus placebo in occult CNVM
    - 95% of treated eyes lost < 15 ETDRS letters
    - 25-34% gained > 15 ETDRS letters
  - ANCHOR Trial demonstrated ranibizumab to be superior to verteporfin for treatment of predominately classic CNVM
- Case series report significant success with intravitreal bevacizumab therapy
  - Direct trial comparing ranibizumab and bevacizumab is pending.

Intravitreal Steroids

Indications

- Monotherapy for occult CNVM
- Combination therapy with PDT, feeder vessel treatment.

Method

- Intravitreal injection.

Results

- Cases series describing combined use of triamcinolone with PDT suggest a prolonged treatment effect and possibly improved visual outcomes
- Use of triamcinolone as monotherapy is not well supported by published studies.

Submacular Surgery

Indications

- Unclear at present time
- ? Subfoveal CNVM in elderly patient without significant drusen.

Method

- Vitrectomy with removal of the subfoveal CNVM.

Result

- Submacular Surgery Trial did not show significant benefit to surgery compared with observation at 2 year follow up.

Macular Translocation

Indication

- Unclear at this time.

Methods

- 360 degree translocation
  - Vitrectomy followed by cutting the retina 360 degrees allowing a large degree of macular translocation
  - Secondary extraocular muscle surgery is required due to torsional diplopia
- Limited translocation
  - Vitrectomy with creation of localized macular detachment
  - Scleral imbrication allows small degree of macular translocation.

Result

- Case series described benefit in selected patients however no RCT has been conducted to date.

Inferences

- Poor untreated natural history
- Early recognition and treatment can lead to preservation of vision.

BIBLIOGRAPHY

1. Gragoudas ES, Adamis AP, Cunningham ET, et al. Pegaptanib for neovascular age-related macular degeneration. New Engl J Med. 2004;351:2805-16.
2. Guyer DR, Yannuzzi LA et al. Classification of choroidal neovascularization by digital indocyanine green video angiography. Ophth 1996;103:2054-60.
3. Hawkins BS, et al. Surgery for subfoveal choroidal neovascularization in age-related macular degeneration: ophthalmic findings. SST report no.11. Ophthalmology 2004:111;1967-80.
4. Macular Photocoagulation Study. Argon laser photocoagulation for neovascular maculopathy : 3 year results. Arch Ophth 1986;104:694-701.
5. Macular Photocoagulation Study. Krypton laser photocoagulation for neovascular lesions of age related macular degeneration. Arch Ophth 1990;108;816-24.
6. Macular Photocoagulation Study. Laser photocoagulation of subfoveal neovascular lesions in age related macular degeneration. Arch Ophth 1991;109:1220-31.
7. Rosenfeld PJ, Brown DM, Heier JS, et al. Ranibizumab for neovascular age related macular degeneration. New Engl J Med. 2006:355;1419-31.
8. TAP Group. Photodynamic therapy of subfoveal choroidal neovascularization in age related macular degeneration with verteporfin - one year results of 2 randomized clinical trials - TAP report 1. Arch Ophth. 1999;117:1329-45.

AMD VARIANTS

RETINAL ANGIOMATOUS PROLIFERATION

INTRODUCTION

- Variant of AMD believed to originate with intraretinal neovascularization rather than subretinal
- May account for up to 15% of wet AMD
- Female > Male
- Elderly.

Classification

- Stage I : neovascularization confined to the neurosensory retina
- Stage II : neovascularization extending from the retina into the subretinal space
- Stage III : neovascularization extending from the retina into the choroid.

CLINICAL SIGNS AND SYMPTOMS

- Symptoms of wet AMD
- Intraretinal hemorrhage (versus subretinal hemorrhage)
- Cystic intraretinal edema
- Pigment epithelial detachement
- Later development of subretinal neovascularization with retinal – choroidal anastamoses.

INVESTIGATIONS

Fluorescein Angiography

- Majority have occult CNVM.

ICG Angiography

- Focal Hot Spot: Intraretinal neovascularization
- Plaque: Associated subretinal neovascularization.

High Speed ICG

- Demonstrates the intraretinal and subretinal components of neovascularization.

OCT

- Intraretinal cystic edema
- Intraretinal neovascularization may be demonstrated in some cases.

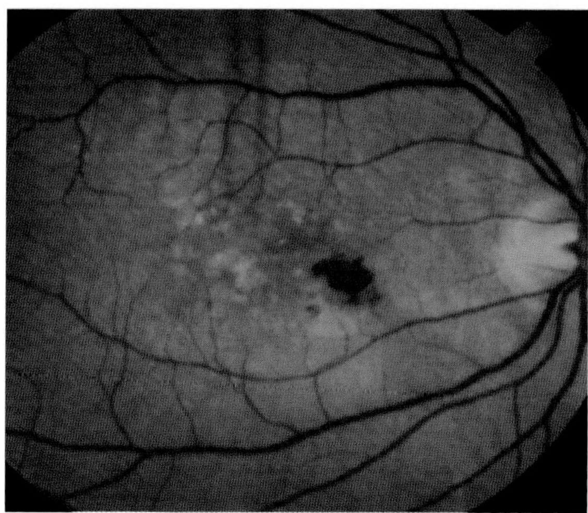

Fig. 9A: Color photo of patient with RAP lesion. Note the predominant intraretinal hemorrhage rather than subretinal hemorrhage

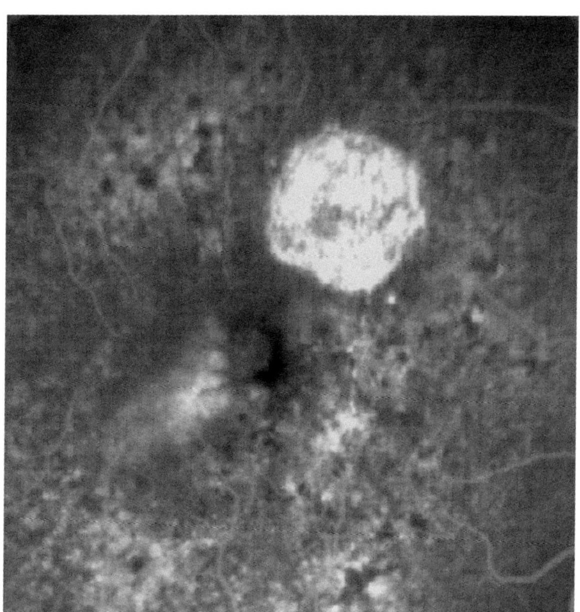

Fig. 9B: Fluorescein angiogram demonstrating occult leakage inferonasally with cystoid macular edema. Small flecks of intraretinal hemorrhage block fluorescence. Clinical features are typical for a RAP lesion. Geographic atrophy is noted superiorly

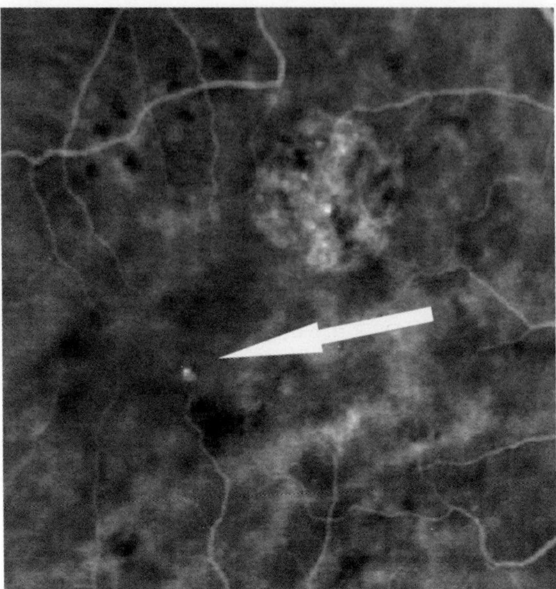

Fig. 9C: Single frame from high speed ICG angiogram demonstrates small focus of intraretinal neovascularization (RAP)

TREATMENT

Methods

- Focal Laser
- Photodynamic Therapy
- Anti VEGF injections.

Result

- To date no large trials have been conducted comparing treatment modalities.

INFERENCES

- Common variant form of wet AMD characterized by intraretinal neovascularization
- Natural history is poor
- High rate of bilateral disease
- Unclear what the optimal treatment modality is currently.

BIBLIOGRAPHY

1. Gross NE, et al. Nature and risk of neovascularization in the fellow eye of patients with unilateral retinal angiomatous proliferation. Retina 2005;25:713-18.
2. Yannuzzi LA, Negrao S, Iida T, et al. Retinal angiomatous proliferation in age-related macular degeneration. Retina 2001;21:416-34.

POLYPOIDAL CHOROIDAL VASCULOPATHY

INTRODUCTION

- Middle aged female
- More common in pigmented racial groups
- Association with hypertension.

CLINICAL SIGNS AND SYMPTOMS

- Large subretinal or sub RPE hemorrhages
- Lesions center on optic nerve rather than fovea.

INVESTIGATIONS

Fluorescein Angiography

- Mainly occult CNV.

ICG Angiography

- Focal Hot Spots in grape like clusters.

High Speed ICG

- Central feeder vessel supplying dilated vascular clusters.

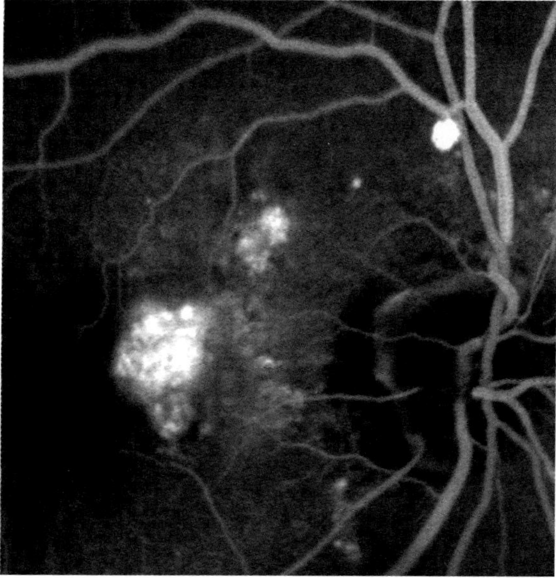

Fig. 10A: Fluorescein angiogram shows subretinal hemorrhage and ill-defined leakage of dye superior to the optic nerve. Window defects consistent with macular drusen are present centrally

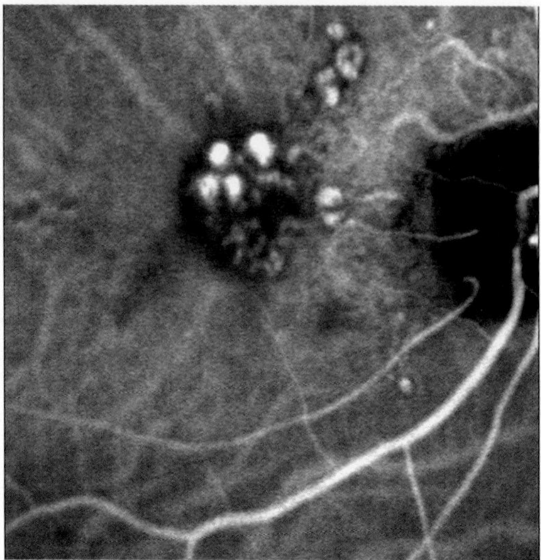

Fig. 10B: ICG angiogram shows multiple focal hot spots typical of polypoidal neovascularization

MANAGEMENT

Treatment Options

- Focal Laser
- Feeder Vessel Laser
- Photodynamic Therapy
- Anti VEGF therapy.

Result

- No comparative trials of therapy for polypoidal CNVM exist.

Inferences

- Variant of AMD with hemorrhage centered on optic nerve rather than fovea
- More common in non
- Caucasian populations
- Unclear natural history
- No comparative trials for therapy.

BIBLIOGRAPHY

1. Kleiner RC, Brucker AJ, Johnston RL. Posterior uveal bleeding syndrome. Ophth 1984;91(suppl 9):110.
2. Otani A, Sasahara M, Yodoi Y, et al. Indocyanine green angiography: guided photodynamic therapy for polypoidal choroidal vasculopathy. Am J Ophthalmol 2007;144;7-14.

CHAPTER TWO

MACULAR DISEASES

Pedro Amat – Peral, Jose M Ruiz Moreno,
Javier A Montero, Francisco L Lugo (Spain)

- Macular Hole
- Epiretinal Membrane (EM)
- Vitreomacular Traction Syndrome (VTS)
- Myopic Macular Schisis (MMS)

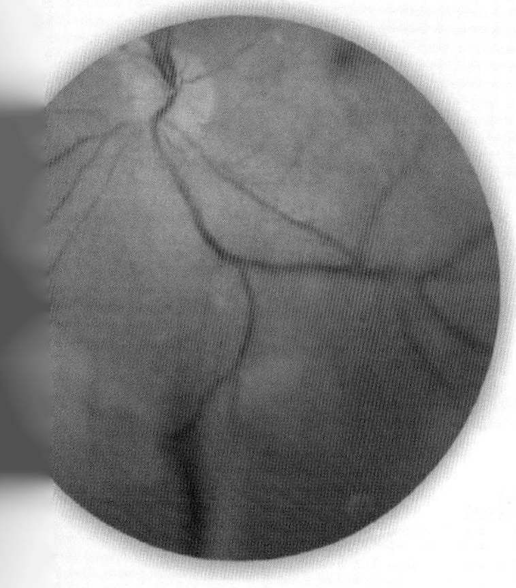

MACULAR HOLE

INTRODUCTION

Idiopathic macular hole (MH) is a full-thickness defect of the retina affecting the fovea producing loss of central visual acuity. MH appears mainly in the sixth and seventh decades. The classification for idiopathic macular holes was described by Gass. Spontaneus tangencial traction of the external part of the prefoveolar cortical vitreous detaches foveolar retina, creating an intraretinal yellow spot (stage 1A). The fovea rises to the level of the surrounding perifoveal retina transforming the yellow spot into a small donut-shaped yellow ring (stage 1B). In stage 2 vitreous traction progresses to a complete breakage of the fovea, visual symptoms get worse due to the production of a full-thickness hole. When the small hole becomes wider the yellow ring becomes grey or disappears creating an annular neurosensorial retina detachment. Stage 3 MH are full thickness holes 400 µm or wider. The existence of a tangential traction widens the hole and the edges are thickened and some times lifted without a complete posterior vitreous detachment. Posterior hyaloid is not completely detached. Stage 3 can be subdivided in (-3 A): posterior hyaloid not detached; (-3 B): posterior hyaloid adhered to one of the edges of the hole; (-3 C): posterior hyaloid detached on the foveal area but adhered to optical disk. Stage 4 holes are complete MH with retinal edema in the margins, complete posterior vitreous detachment and vitreous collapse.

MH is bilateral in 15-20%. There are other causes of MH related to contuse ocular trauma, high myopia, cystoid macular edema, ocular inflammation, solar retinopathy, evolution of the vitreomacular traction syndrome and traction from epiretinal membranes; secondary MH are 20% of all the cases of MH. Macular pseudoholes (epiretinal membrane, lamellar MH, subfoveal cyst and subfoveal retinal detachment) can be misdiagnosed as MH.

CLINICAL FINDINGS

Loss of visual acuity: blurred vision (mainly for near vision as reading), metamorphopsia and central scotoma. In stages 1A and 1B impeding macular holes, metamorphopsia and mild loss of central vision, are usually present and central scotoma is absent. In stage 2, the visual symptoms of the patients may be more severe; vision may initially improve due to a spontaneous partial vitreo-foveal separation. Stages 3 and 4 usually show moderate loss of central vision to 20/200. Central metamorphopsia is often severe, and some patients describe a symptomatic absolute central scotoma. A high correlation of central visual acuity to MH diameter has been reported. Central visual acuity has been correlated to the size of the neurosensory retinal detachment surrounding the MH. Hole size and neurosensory detachment size have been correlated to the durations of symptoms.

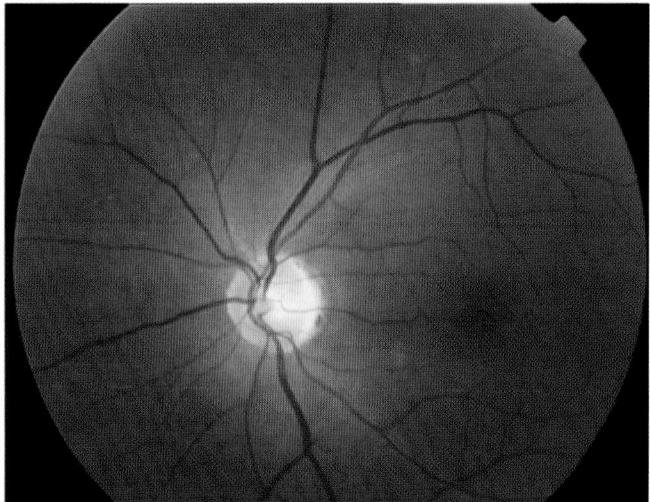

Fig. 1

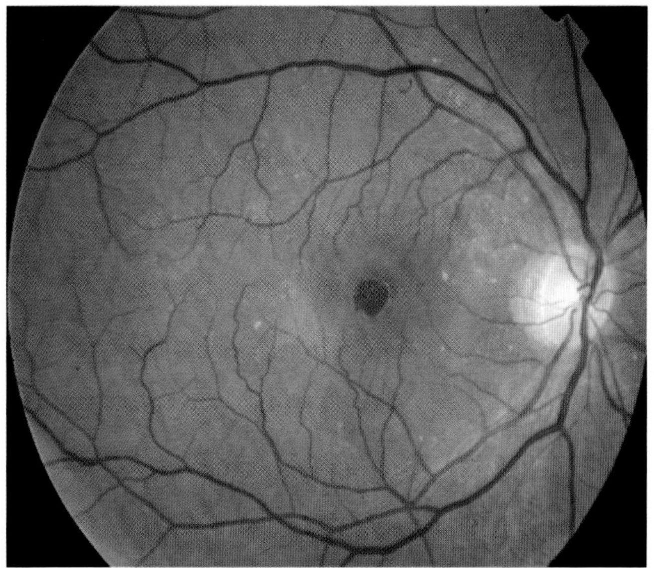

Fig. 2

Figs 1 and 2: Retinography of macular hole

DIAGNOSIS

Direct and indirect ophthalmoscopy and especially biomicroscopy. Green or blue filters can be used in order to intensify visualization of vitreous structures. Using a thin slit beam an absolute scotoma mat appear to the patient as a break in the beam when it is centered over larger holes (Watzke-Allen sign). When centered over smaller holes, or over the surrounding neurosensory retinal detachment in larger holes, the patient may experience only narrowing or distortion of the beam.

Fluorescein angiography usually demonstrates a window defect with early fluorescence.

B scan permits a complete evaluation of the posterior hyaloid. It is advisable to use high gain B scan (90 dB or more) to identify the posterior hyaloid.

Analysis of the MH by OCT has provided a better knowledge of MH geometry and features even when the hyaloid is not detached. The relationship between the posterior vitreous cortex and the macular area has been greatly enhanced by OCT. OCT has helped to establish the role of anterioposterior and tangential forces caused by contraction of the internal limiting membrane in MH development.

TREATMENT

Vitrectomy does not provide a benefit in the prevention of macular hole. Surgical adjunctive agents have been used with varying degrees of reported success: transforming growth factor-β2 (TGF-β2) autologous serum, platelets, plasma and fibrinogen have achieved limited success.

Surgery is considered in most eyes with moderate to large stage 3 or 4 holes with symptoms and visual acuity in the range of 20/60 to 20/400 or eyes with small but definite full-thickness, stage 2 or 3 symptomatic MH with visual acuity in the range between 20/40 and 20/60.

Posterior hyaloid detachment is induced and epiretinal membranes and internal limiting membrane are removed after staining with indocyanine green (0.125%, 1.25 mg/ml, 1 min). Fluid-air and air-gas exchange with 14% perfluoropropane is performed and face-down position is maintained for 1 week after surgery. Toxicity by ICG and atrophic changes in the RPE have been reported. Trypan blue offers an alternative. In order to minimize toxic effects on the retina dye should be used in concentrations as low as possible, avoiding repeated ICG injections onto bare retina and injecting dye far from the macular hole, reduce incubation time with ICG and keep the light pipe far from the retina.

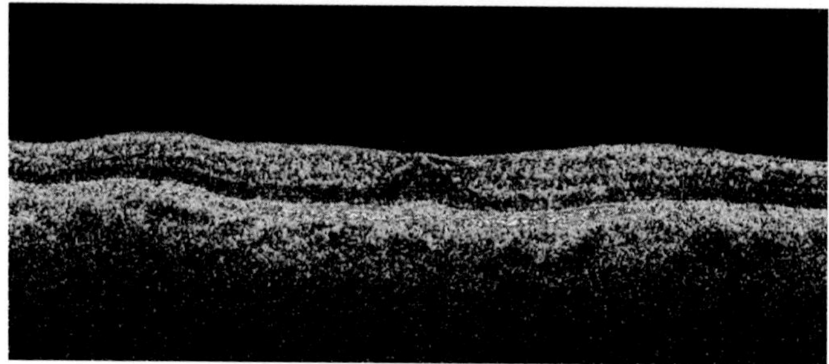

Fig. 3

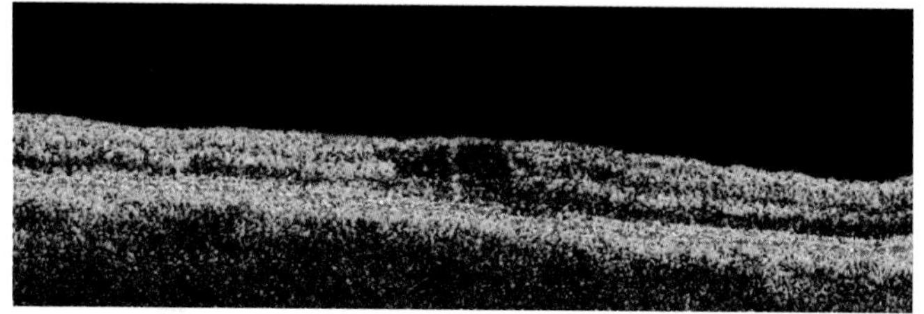

Fig. 4

Figs 3 and 4: OCT of macular holes stage 1-A

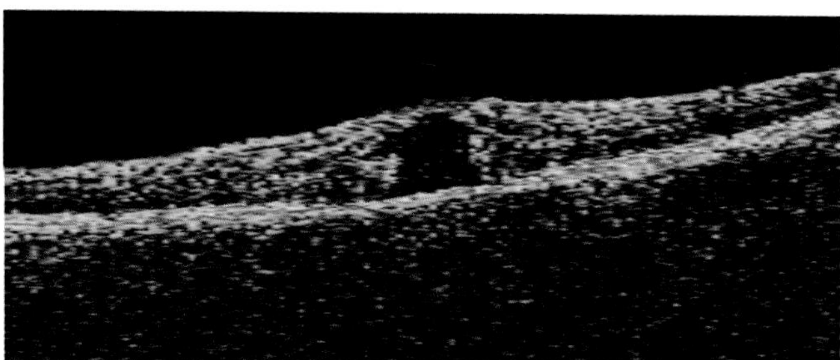

Fig. 5

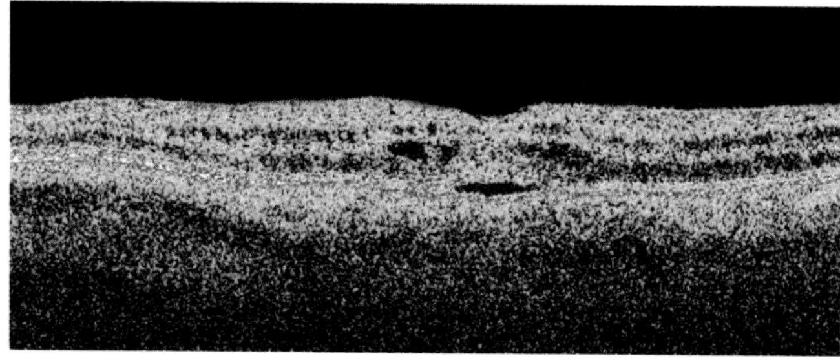

Fig. 6

Figs 5 and 6: OCT of macular holes stage 1-B

EPIRETINAL MEMBRANE (EM)

EM is an avascular fibrous tissue adhered to the internal layers of the retina in the macular area, which frequently appear in otherwise healthy eyes or be associated to vascular or inflammatory conditions. Idiopathic EM may be adhered to the maculaand induce retinal suffering with distortion of temporal vascular arcades and macular edema. EM is frequent and associated with age. EM has been related to posterior vitreous detachment (PVD).

CLINICAL FINDINGS

Most of the patients are asymptomatic. Symptomsmay range from metamorphopsia to marked decrease in visual acuity. The onset may be slow and almost imperceptible in some patients, or acute. Central diplopia, photopsia and macropsia may appear. 85% of patients have visual acuity of 20/70 or better. Once an EM is formed visionremains stable.

DIAGNOSIS

Biomicroscopy ranges from bright internal limiting membrane, without alteration of the vascular course or existence of edema to white-grayish EM affecting vessels causing retinal suffering.

FA shows vascular traction increasing vascular permeability and edema.

FA is useful in assessing the extent of retinal wrinkling caused by the membrane, foveal ectopia and vascular leakage.

B scan shows macular thickening.

OCT is the most important test to identify EM as flat separation from the retinal surface.

TREATMENT

EM may detach spontaneously from the retina. The membranes tend to remain stable and vision rarely improves or worsens dramatically. In most of eyes, once the membrane is present for several months, a significant loss of vision occurs seldom. If vision decreases, other ocular diseases should be considered. Vitreoretinal surgery removes epiretinal membranes causing significant vision loss.

The aim of surgery is to remove the traction secondary to the EM. Surgery is usually indicated in cases in which the vision has decreased to 20/60 or better if diplopia or incapacitating metamorphopsia are present.

The etiology of EM influences the final result. EMsecondary to retinal detachment have worse prognosis than idiopathic ones. The factors associated with a better postoperative vision are fine EM with non detached macula,

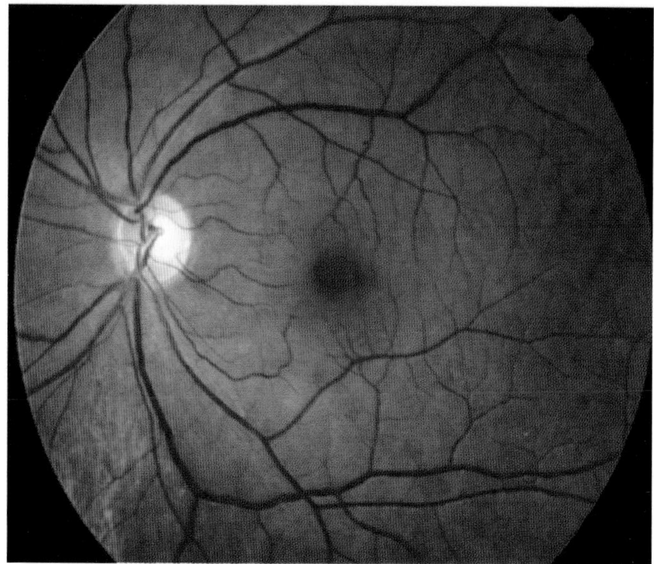

Fig. 7: Retinography of macular hole stage 1

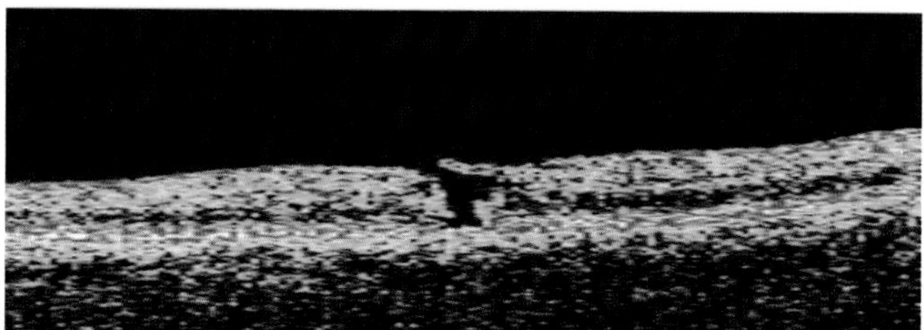

Fig. 8

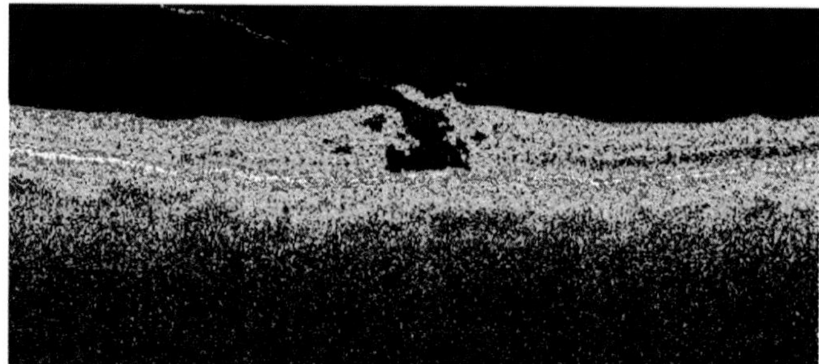

Fig. 9

Figs 8 and 9: OCT of macular holes stage 2

initial vision 20/60 or better, short duration of the symptoms of blurred vision. Eyes with transparent EM may respond better to the surgery than opaque membranes.

Detachment of the posterior hyaloid is performed and EM are removed after staining with trypan blue. Thick EM may be directly grasped with intraocular foreign body forceps. However, in most cases a barbed microvitreoretinal blade is used to engaged the membrane and lift it from the retinal surface.

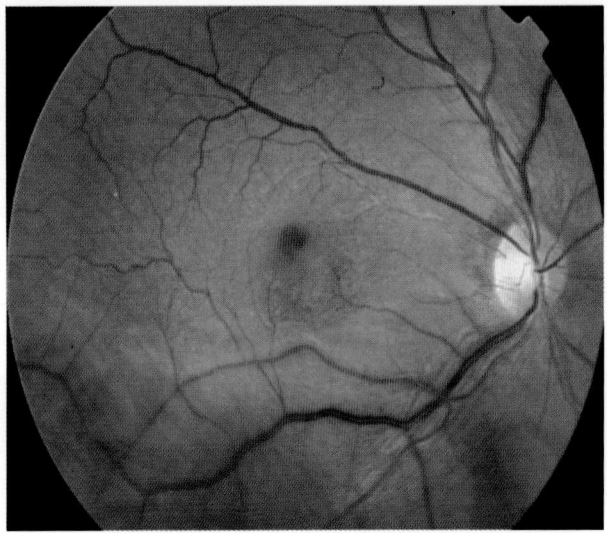

Fig. 10: Retinography of macular hole stage 2

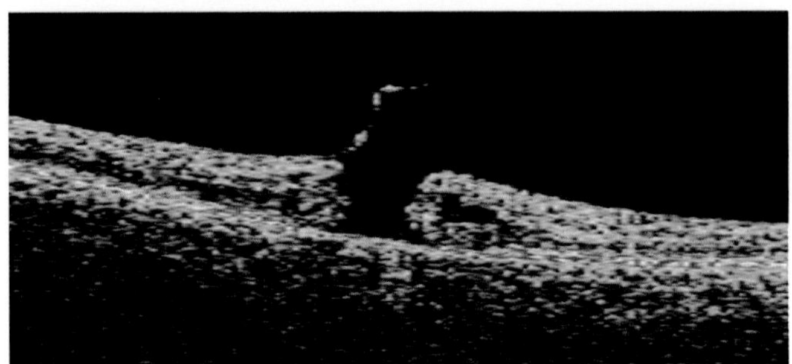

Fig. 11: OCT of macular holes stage 3-B

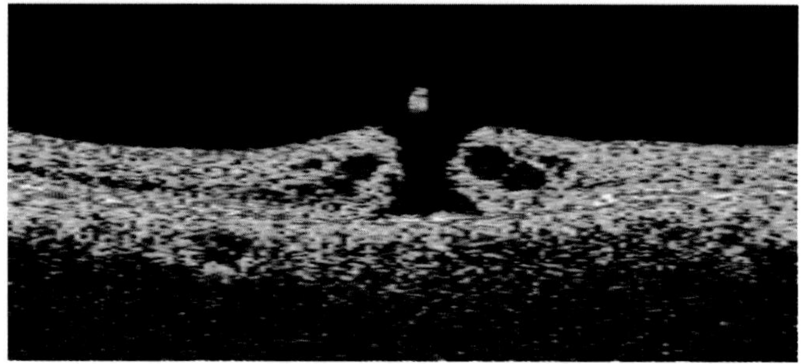

Fig. 12

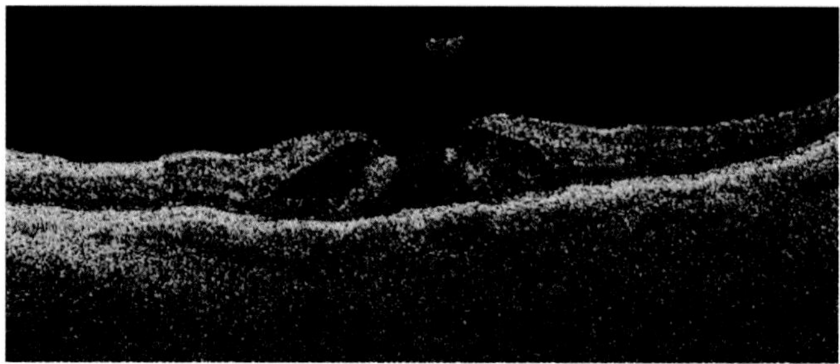

Fig. 13

Figs 12 and 13: OCT of macular holes stage 3-C

VITREOMACULAR TRACTION SYNDROME (VTS)

VTS represents those cases in which the traction on posterior hyaloid is demonstrated on the macular area with a peripheral hyaloid detachment. OCT has documented perfectly the existence of this pathology.

Two forms of OCT presentation have been reported, a V shaped detachment causing a foveal detachment with the possibility of a good visual recovery after vitrectomy; and a partial detachment of posterior hyaloid temporary to the fovea associated with cystoid macular edema, which can evolve to a full-thickness MH or to an atrophy of the retina after vitrectomy.

VTS can be idiopathic caused by a strong adhesion of the posterior hyaloid in the macular area or secondary to other pathological conditions such as uveitis or tractional macular edema.

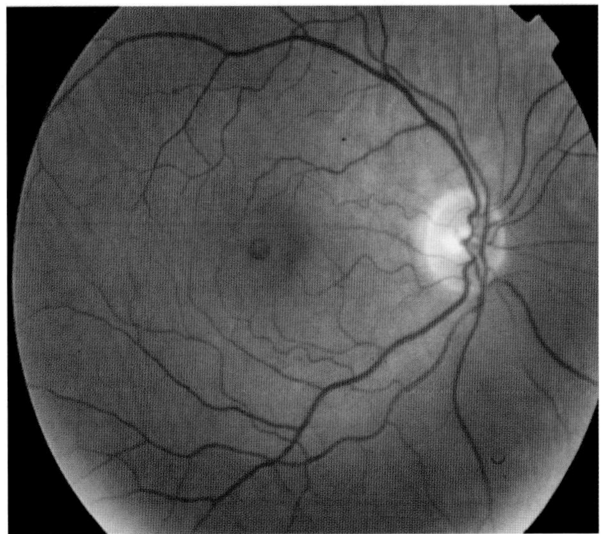

Fig. 14

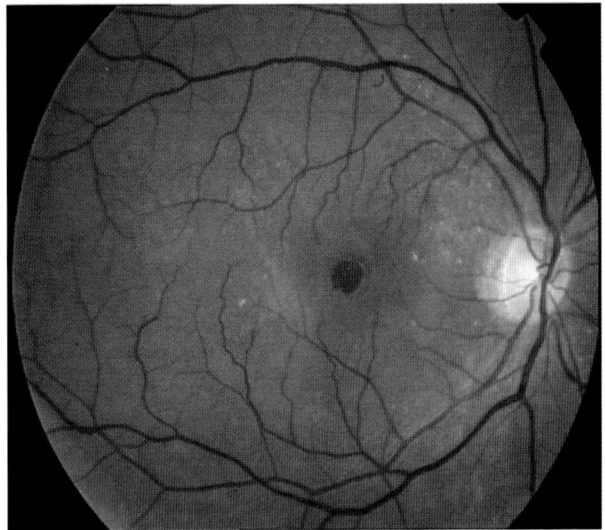

Fig. 15

Figs 14 and 15: Retinography of macular hole stage 3

MYOPIC MACULAR SCHISIS (MMS)

Several reports have been made about its pathogenia and treatment. This condition justifies loss of visual acuity in patients with high myopia in which other signs of the disease are not detected, or are not sufficiently advanced to justify the symptoms.

MMS is defined by the presence of the following signs:

- Retinal thickening in the area of posterior staphyloma
- Retinal traction secondary to EM or adhesion of posterior hyaloid
- Foveal detachment associated with foveal cysts
- Lamellar holes

Macular thickening can take place by a separation of fibers of Henle or the external plexiform layer.

The natural evolution of this entity is very variable: MSS may remain stable during many years or evolve rapidly decreasing vision when a subfoveal detachment exists in relation with the staphyloma or in those takes place in which the rupture of the roofs of the foveal cysts causes a secondary MH. Biomicroscopy does not detect easily all the cases of foveal cysts.

B scan is a very useful technique to detect the presence of a posterior staphyloma, macular thickening and foveal detachment. The vitreous may show adhesions to the posterior pole that can be implied in the appearance of this pathology.

OCT can be difficult to perform in these eyes.

TREATMENT

Treatment of this pathology is controverted. Vitrectomy is reserved for the cases of fast evolution with visual deterioration threatening vision. However, one of the great risks of vitrectomy is the evolution towards a full-thickness MH.

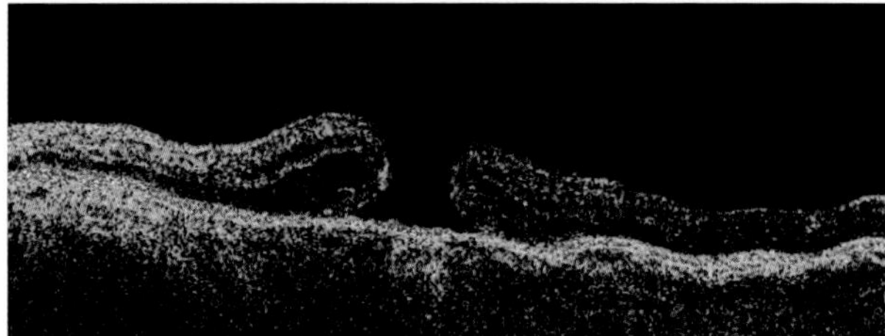

Fig. 16

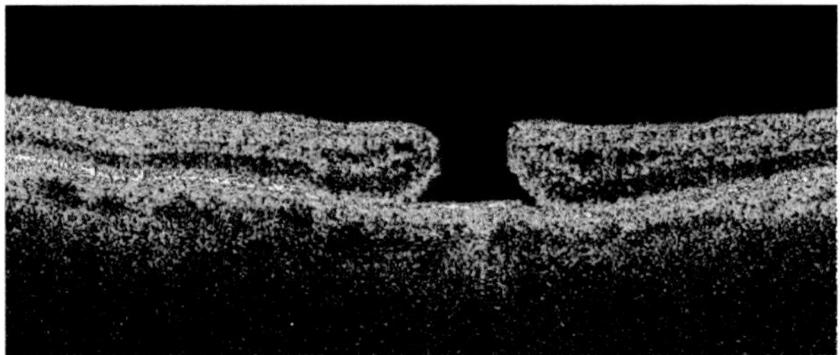

Fig. 17

Figs 16 and 17: OCT of macular holes stage 4

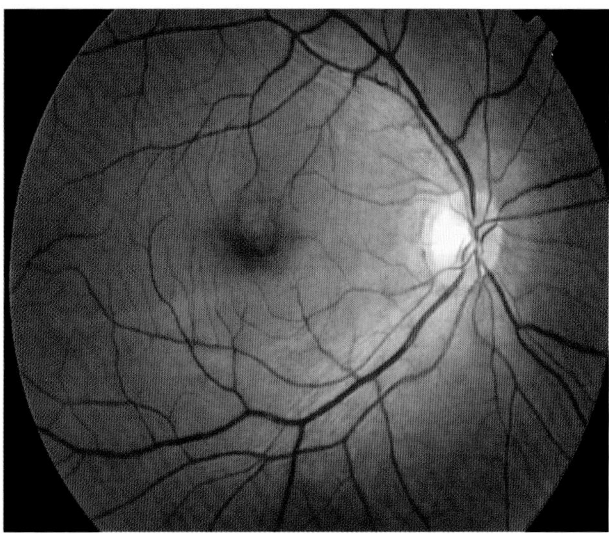

Fig. 18: Retinography of macular hole stage 4

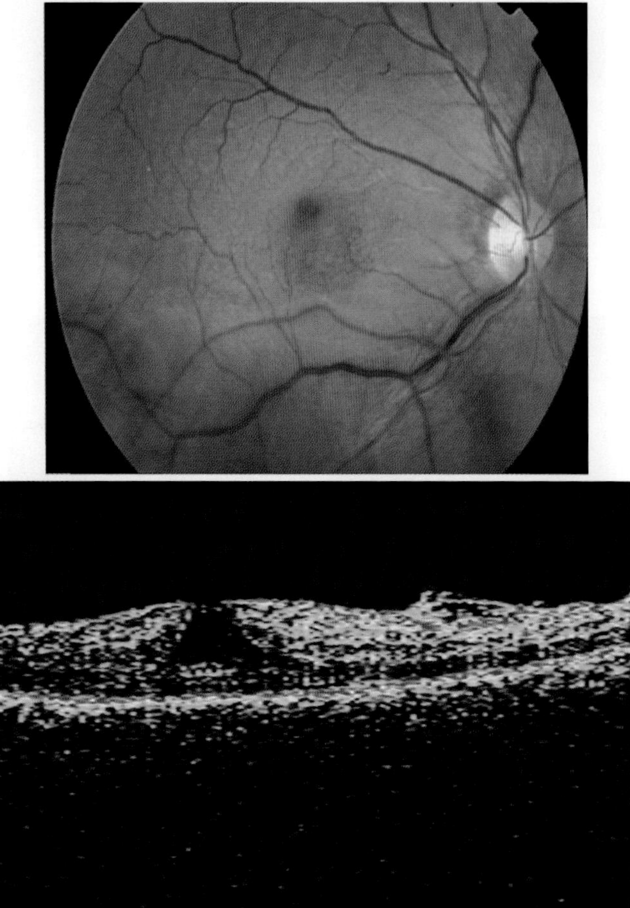

Fig. 19: Preoperative retinography and OCT stage 2

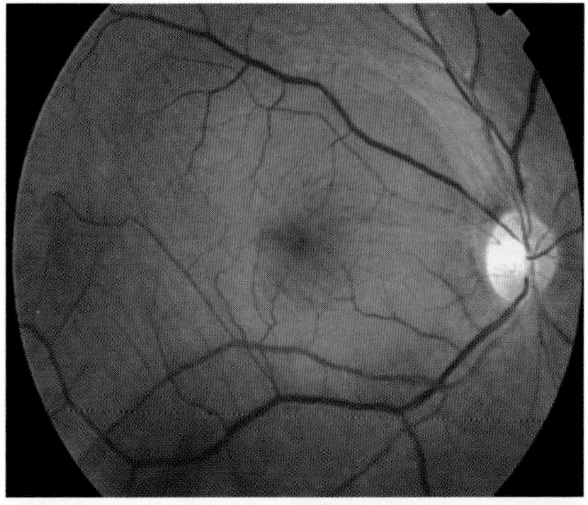

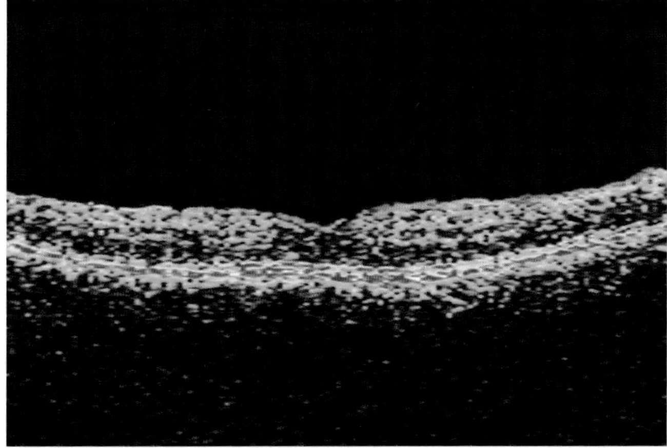

Fig. 20: Postoperative retinography and OCT stage 2

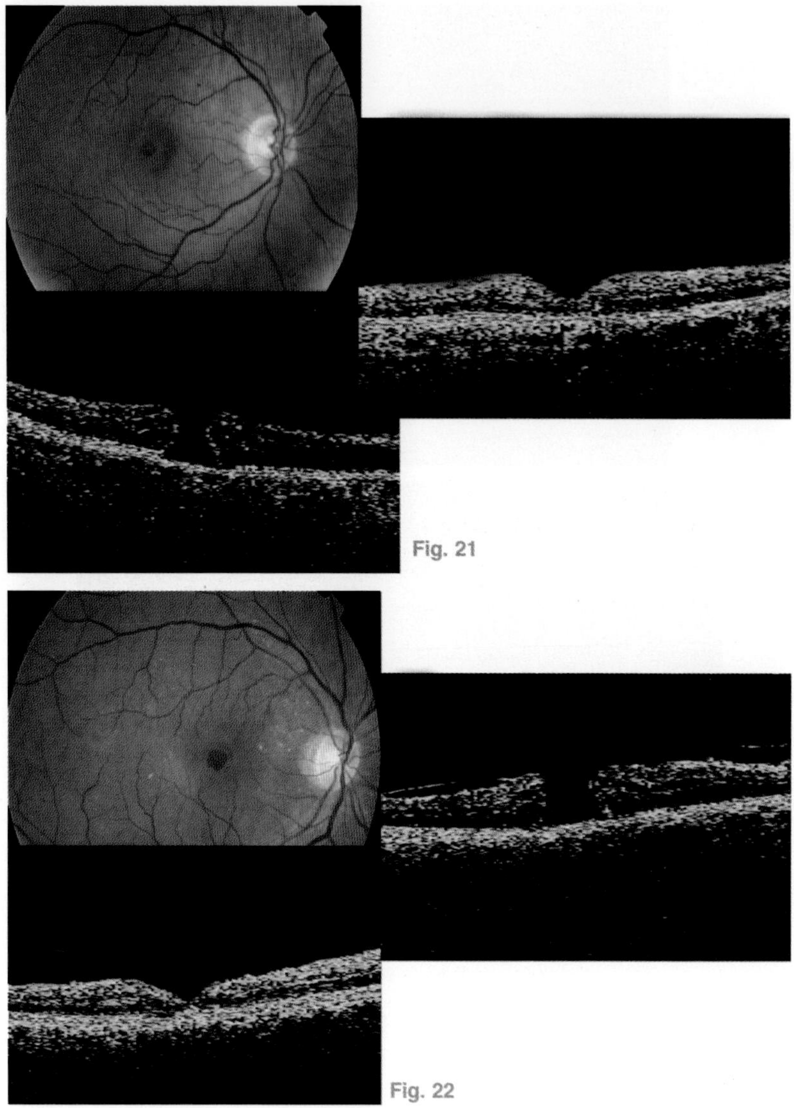

Figs 21 and 22: Preoperative OCT and retinography and postoperative OCT of patient with macular hole stage 3

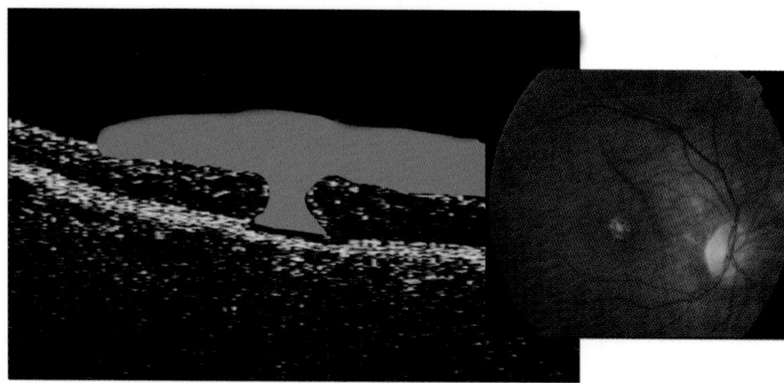

Fig. 23: Possibility of producing damage with ICG by contacting it with retinal pigmentary epithelium

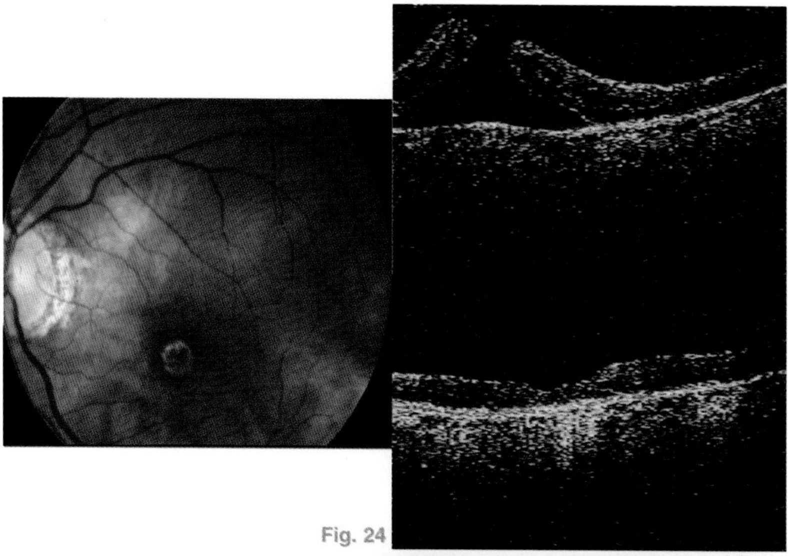

Fig. 24

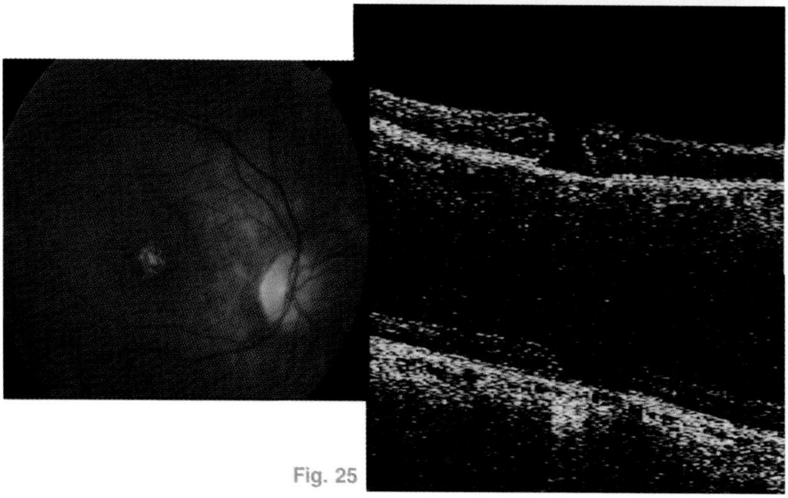

Fig. 25

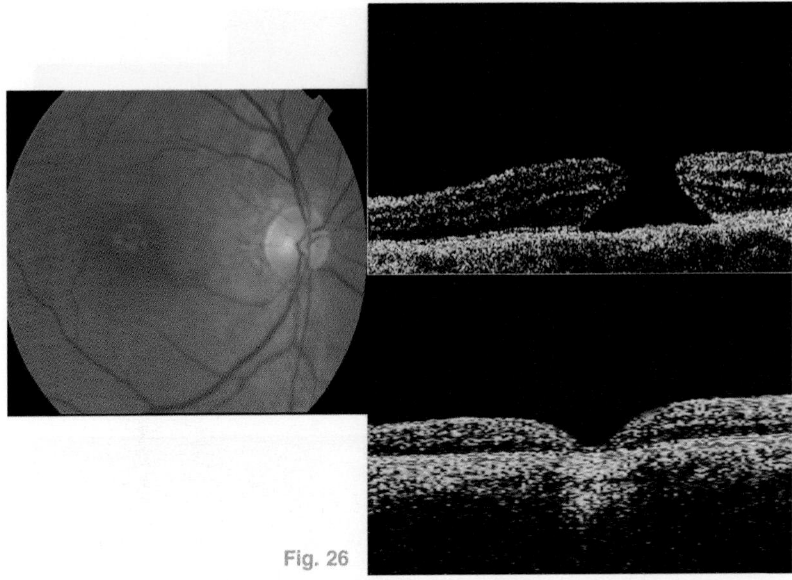

Fig. 26

Figs 24 to 26: Closure of macular hole using ICG. Preoperative OCT (above) and postoperative OCT (below) image shows closure of macular hole. Hyper and hyporeflectivity can be seen. Retinography of closed macular hole with hyper and hypopigmented areas corresponding to OCT image

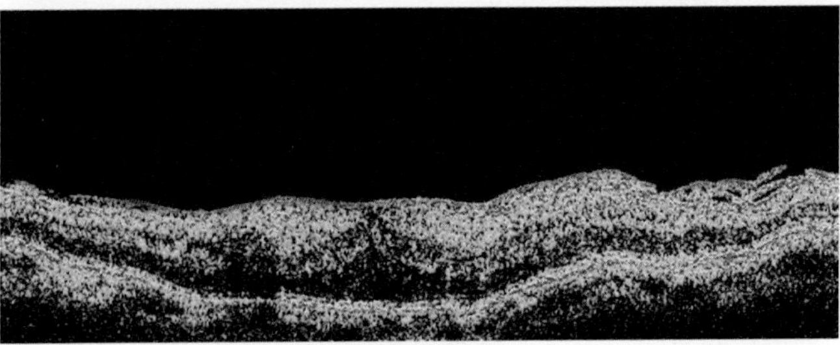

Fig. 27

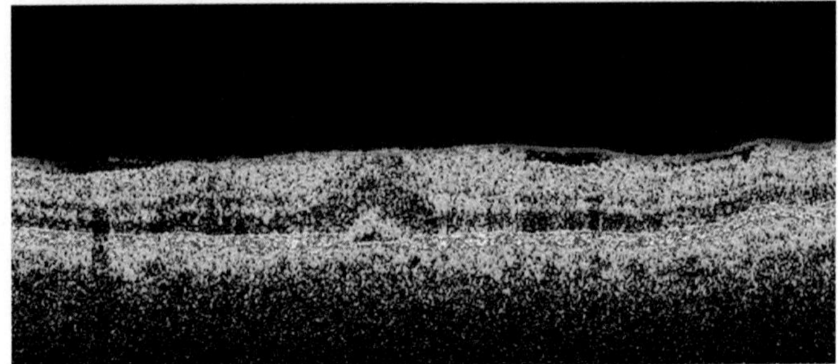

Fig. 28

Figs 27 and 28: OCT of epiretinal membrane

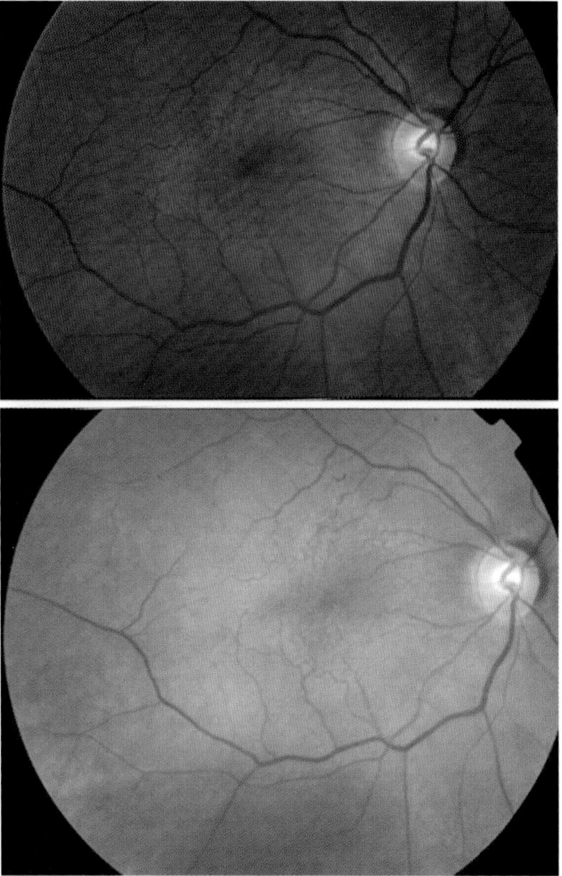

Fig. 29: Retinography and aneritre of epiretinal membrane

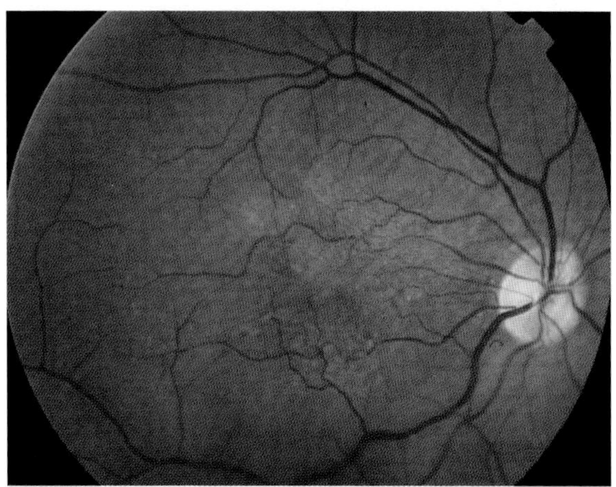

Fig. 30: Retinography showing the traction of vessels produced by epiretinal membrane

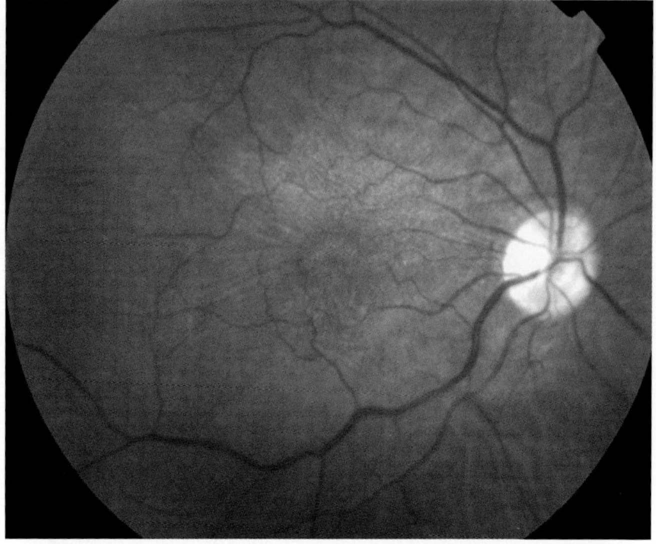

Fig. 31: Aneritre of epiretinal membrane

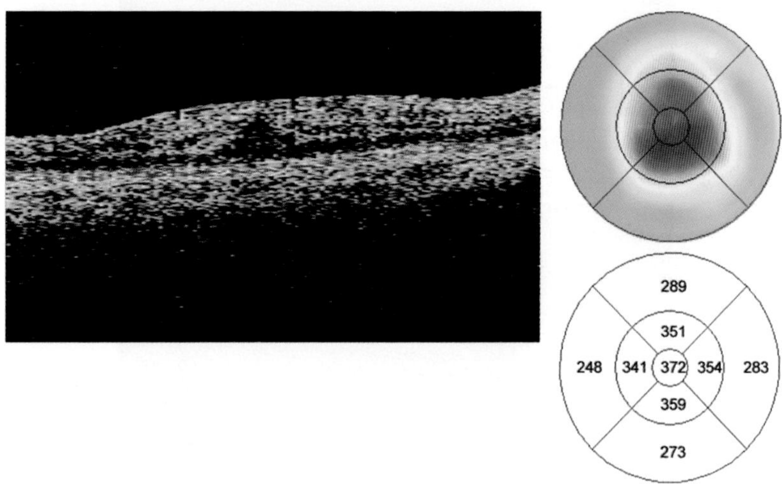

Fig. 32: OCT of epiretinal membrane and macular thickness map showing the elevation of this caused by epiretinal membrane

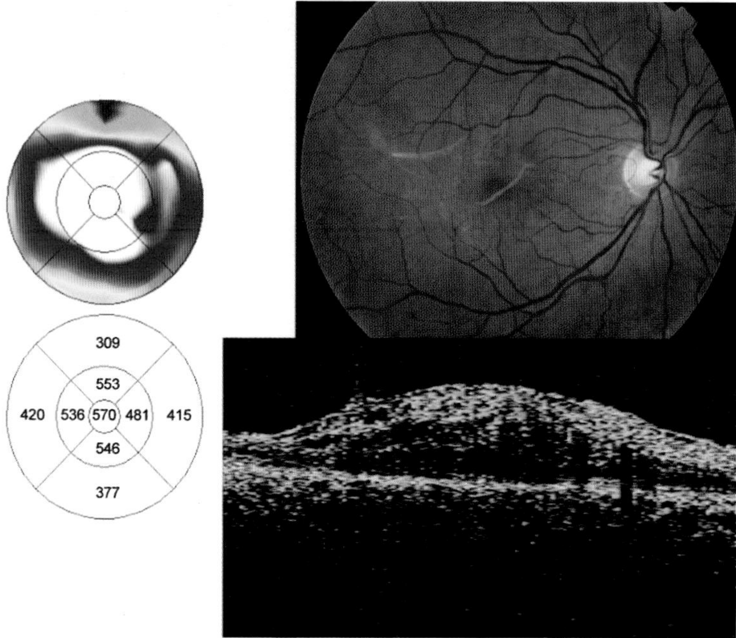

Fig. 33: Retinography and OCT of epiretinal membrane and macular thickness map showing the elevation of this caused by epiretinal membrane

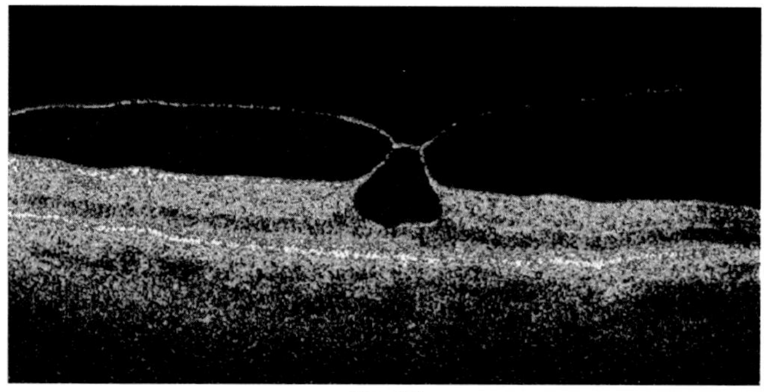

Fig. 34

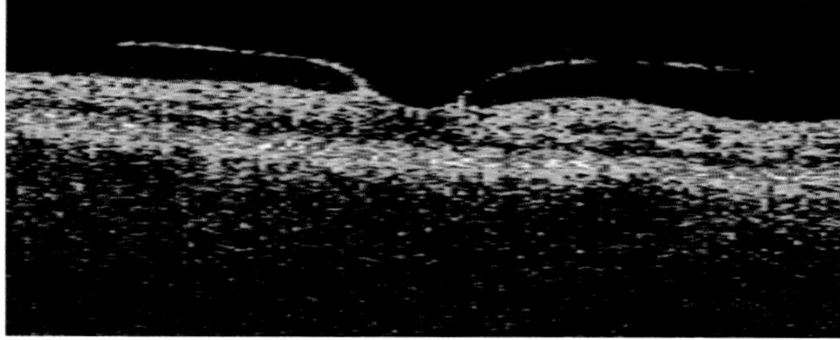

Fig. 35

Figs 34 and 35: OCT of vitreomacular traction syndrome showing the form of wings gulls

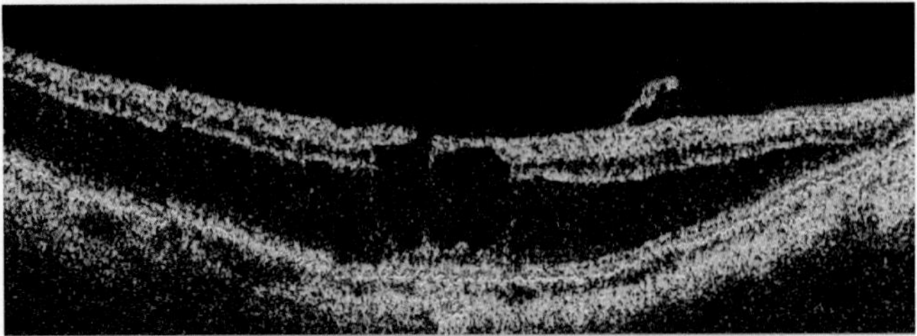

Fig. 36: OCT of myopic macular schisis

CHAPTER THREE

MACULAR DISORDERS

- **MACULAR DISORDERS**
  T Mark Johnson (USA)
  - Presumed Ocular Histoplasmosis
  - Central Serous Retinopathy
  - Epiretinal Membrane (ERM)
  - Vitreomacular Traction Syndromes
  - Macular Hole
  - Cystoid Macular Edema

- **CENTRAL SEROUS RETINOPATHY**
  Ashok Garg (India)

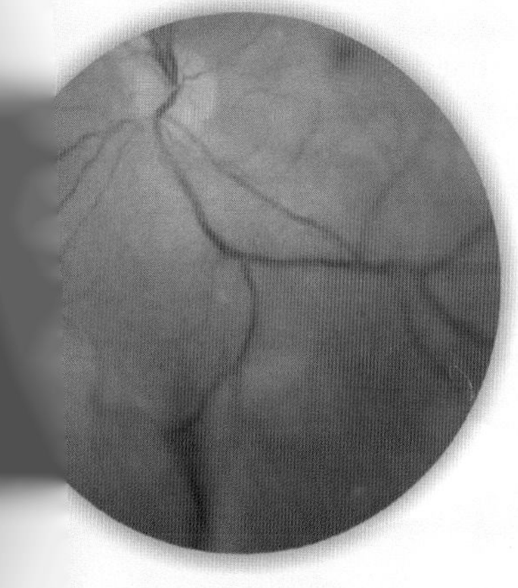

Macular Disorders

T Mark Johnson (USA)

PRESUMED OCULAR HISTOPLASMOSIS

INTRODUCTION

- Predominates in watershed areas of major river systems (i.e. Mississippi, Ohio)
- Approximately 2000/year in the United States lose central vision secondary to CVNM in POHS.

CLINICAL SIGNS AND SYMPTOMS

Symptoms

- Asymptomatic
- Symptomatic CNVM.

Signs

- Signs of CNVM : subretinal hemorrhage, fluid
- Bilateral, punched out midperipheral chorioretinal scars
- Peripapillary atrophy
- Linear areas of choroidal atrophy
- No vitreous cells.

INVESTIGATIONS

Fluorescein Angiography

- Peripheral chorioretinal scars show late staining
- CNVM evident in macula.

High Speed ICG

- Typically feeder vessel arises in area of prior chorio-retinal scarring.

DIFFERENTIAL DIAGNOSIS

- Multifocal choroiditis with secondary choroidal neovascularization
- Myopic degeneration
- Angioid streaks
- Idiopathic.

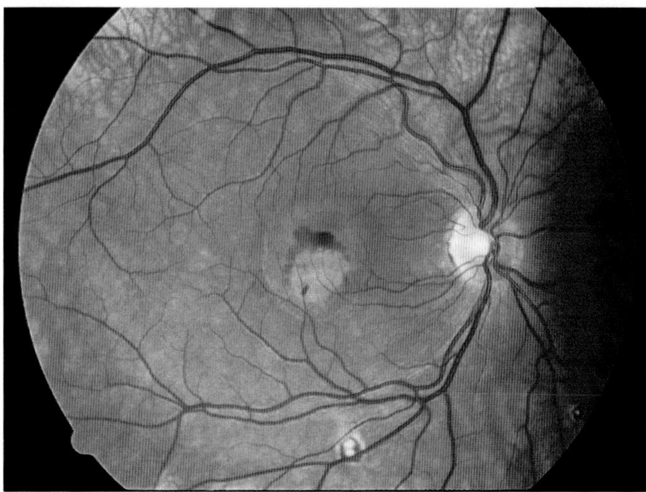

Fig. 1: Subretinal hemorrhage secondary to CNV. Midperipheral circumscribed chorioretinal scars are evident inferiorly typical of POHS

TREATMENT

Focal Laser Ablation

Indications

- Extrafoveal CNVM
- Juxtafoveal CNVM.

Methods

- Complete ablation of CNVM complex.

Results

- Laser ablation of CNVM prevents significant visual loss compared with observation
- 30 % recurrence rate
  - Recurrences occur under fovea associated with more significant visual loss.

Photodynamic Therapy

Indications

- Subfoveal CNVM .

Results

- No large trials exist
- Median visual acuity and leakage seems to improve 2 years after PDT therapy with approximately 4 treatments.

Submacular Surgery

Indications

- Subfoveal CNVM.

Methods

- Small guage retinotomy with complete removal of CNVM complex.

Results

- Multiple case series suggest benefit to removal
- Recurrent neovascularization occurs
- RCT suggested possible benefit to surgery in patients with subfoveal CNVM and VA < 20/100.

Anti-VEGF Therapy

- Limited data to date on the role of anti-VEGF therapy for CNVM secondary to POHS.

Inferences

- POHS is commonly noted in river valleys in United States
- Major complication is secondary choroidal neovascularization.

BIBLIOGRAPHY

1. Hawkins BS, et al. Surgical removal vs observation for subfoveal choroidal neovascularization, either associated with the ocular histoplasmosis syndrome or idiopathic: I. Ophthalmic findings from a randomized clinical trial: Submacular Surgery Trials (SST) Group H Trial: SST Report No. 9. Arch Ophth. 2004:122;1597-1611.
2. Rosenfeld PJ, et al. Photodynamic therapy with verteporfin in ocular histoplasmosis: uncontrolled, open label 2 year study. Ophth. 2004:111;1725-33.

CENTRAL SEROUS RETINOPATHY

INTRODUCTION

- Risk Factors
  - Type A Personality
  - Male > Female (9:1)
  - Young to middle age
  - Corticosteroids
  - Mild hyperopia.

CLINICAL SIGNS AND SYMPTOMS

Symptoms

- Decreased vision
  - Usually mild (50% better than 20/30)
- Decreased color perception
- Micropsia
- Distortion.

Signs

- Localized round or oval area of subretinal fluid
- Subretinal yellow precipitates
- Pigment epithelial detachment
- Pigmentary atrophy with previous episodes.

INVESTIGATIONS

Fluorescein Angiography

- Focal hyperfluorescence with expanding late leakage
- "Smokestack" leak is classic finding in CSR and is present in 15% of cases.

Optical Coherence Tomography

- Localized subretinal fluid
- Frequent pigment epithelial detachment.

DIFFERENTIAL DIAGNOSIS

- Choroidal neovascularization
- Vitreo macular traction
- Myopic foveo-schisis
- Macular hole

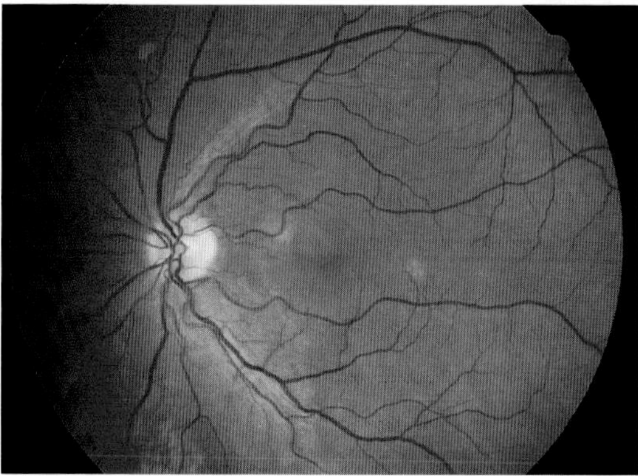

Fig. 2A: Color photo of patient with central serous retinopathy. Blister of subretinal fluid is present in the macula. Temporal RPE depigmentation suggestive of previous episodes of CSR

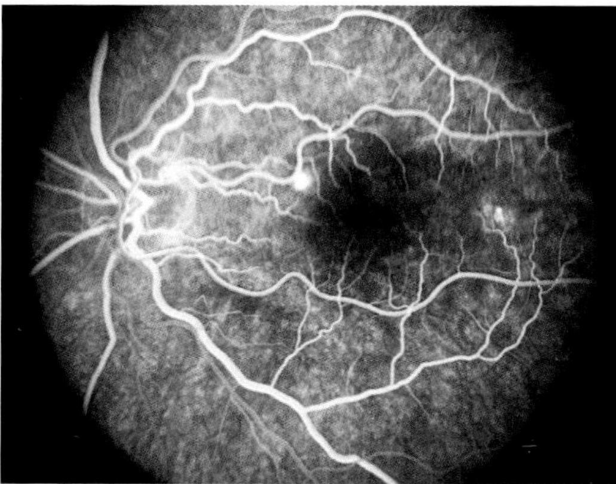

Fig. 2B: Early fluorescein angiogram frame shows hyperfluorescence superonasally. Window defects are present temporally at prior site of CSR leakage

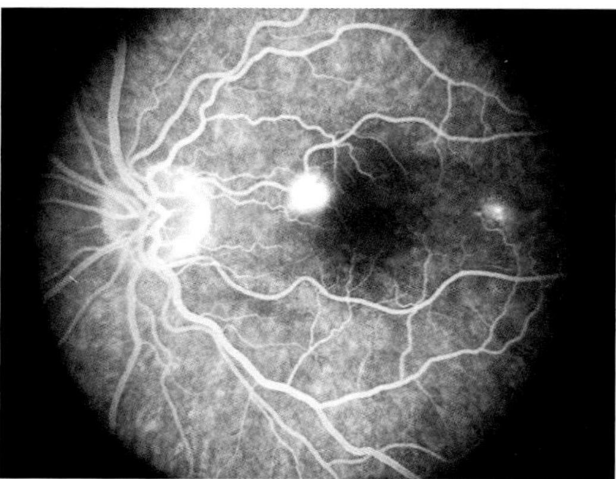

Fig. 2C: Late fluorescein angiogram frame shows progressive leakage superonasally

- Retinal detachment
- Optic pit with serous macular detachment
- Choroidal hemangioma
- Chorioretinitis.

TREATMENT

Observation

- Majority of cases will resolve spontaneously in 12-16 weeks
- Recurrence occurs in 30–50% of cases.

Focal Laser

Indications

- Prolonged CSR (greater than 16 weeks) with well defined leakage point
- Professional incapacity.

Methods

- Focal laser over the area of leakage
- 100–200 micron spot, long duration low intensity application
- Mild gray burn over the leak site.

Photodynamic Therapy

Indications

- Prolonged CSR with well defined leakage

Methods

- PDT applied to site of RPE leaks.

INFERENCES

- CSR is typically observed in young males
- Most cases resolve spontaneously
- No comparative trials exist for therapy of cases that do not resolve spontaneously.

BIBLIOGRAPHY

1. Burumcek E, et al. Laser photocoagulation for persistent central serous retinopathy. Ophth. 1997:104;616-22.
2. Klein ML, et al. Experience with nontreatment of central serous choroidopathy. Arch Ophth. 1974:91;247-50.

EPIRETINAL MEMBRANES (ERM)

INTRODUCTION

Incidence

- Prevalence is 4-11% of population
- Five year incidence of ERM was 5% in Blue Mountains Eye Study.

Etiology

- Idiopathic
- Branch/central retinal vein occlusion
- Uveitis
- Trauma
- Proliferative vitreo-retinopathy.

CLINICAL SIGNS AND SYMPTOMS

Symptoms

- Decreased vision
- Metamorphopsia

Signs

- Glistening sheen over macula with associated retinal vascular distortion
- Retinal edema
- Cystoid retinal changes
- Pseudohole is a gap in the ERM.

INVESTIGATIONS

Fluorescein Angiography

- Retinal vascular distortion
- Late intraretinal leakage.

OCT

- ERM is demonstrated on retinal surface
- Associated intraretinal edema and distortion
- Pseudohole appears as abrupt break in ERM

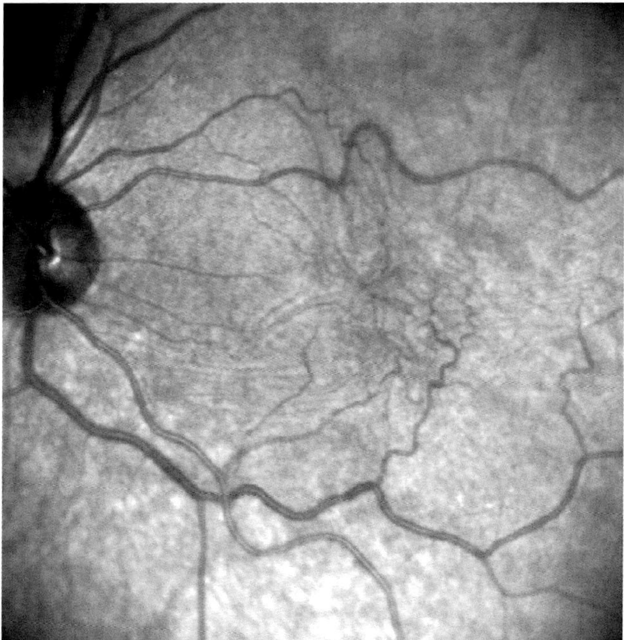

Fig. 3A: Infrared photo of patient with epiretinal membrane demonstrates retinal striae secondary to contracture of membrane

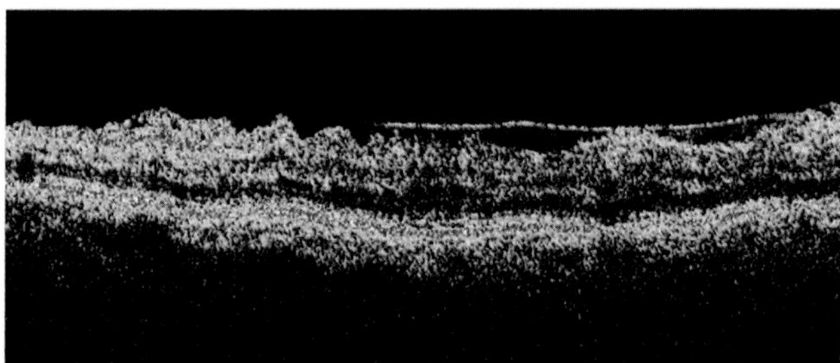

Fig. 3B: Horizontal OCT of same patient shows distortion of retina with visible ERM

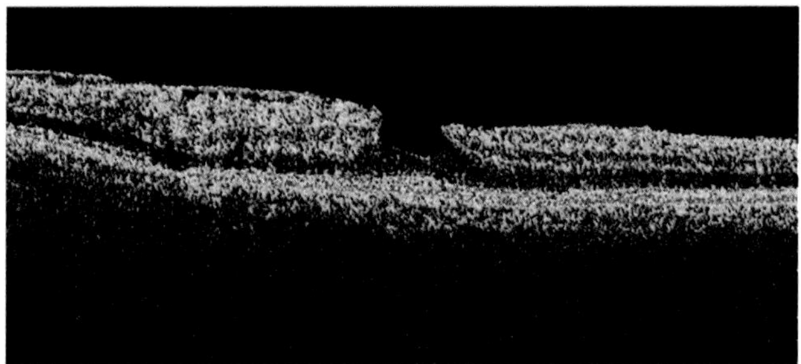

Fig. 3C: Horizontal OCT in a patient with an ERM and pseudohole. Note the abrupt break in the ERM with a right angled contour

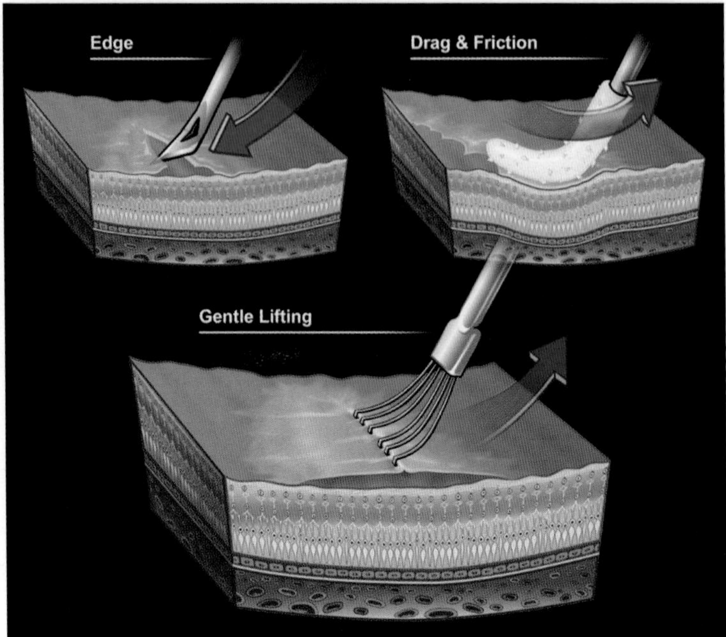

Fig. 3D: Diagram of multiple methods of removal of ERM

DIFFERENTIAL DIAGNOSIS

- Macular hole
- Retinal detachment
- Posterior uveitis
- Choroidal folds
- Combined hamartoma of RPE and retina.

TREATMENT

Observation

Indications

- Non-visually significant ERM

Results

- 10-25% of ERM show no progression of visual symptoms over time.

Vitrectomy

Indications

- Symptomatic decreased vision with ERM.

Methods

- Pars plana vitrectomy with stripping of ERM complex
- Controversy whether removal of internal limiting membrane influences outcome
- Dyes such as ICG and trypan blue may be utilized to visualized ERM intraoperatively.

Results

- 87% have improved visual acuity
- Better visual outcome with:
  - Pre Op VA > 20/100
  - Thin ERM
  - Absence of Traction Retinal Detachment
  - Shorter symptom duration

INFERENCES

- Most ERM are asymptomatic and non-progressive
- Progressive visual loss associated with ERM is treatable with vitrectomy
- Recovery of visual acuity following vitrectomy is significant, however, it is often incomplete
- Following ERM removal persistent cystoid macular edema is not uncommon.

BIBLIOGRAPHY

1. Bovey EH. Uffer S. Achache F. Surgery for epimacular membrane: impact of retinal internal limiting membrane removal on functional outcome. Retina. 2004;24(5):728-35.
2. de Bustros S. Thompson JT. Michels RG. Rice TA. Glaser BM. Vitrectomy for idiopathic epiretinal membranes causing macular pucker. British Journal of Ophthalmology 1988;72(9):692-5.
3. Haritoglou C, Eibl K, Schaumberger M, Mueller AJ, Priglinger S, Alge C, Kampik A. Functional outcome after trypan blue-assisted vitrectomy for macular pucker: a prospective, randomized, comparative trial. American Journal of Ophthalmology 2004;138(1):1-5.
4. Mitchell P, Smith W, Chey T, et al. Prevalence and association of epiretinal membranes—The Blue Mountains Eye Study, Australia. Ophthalmology 1997;104:1033–44.

VITREOMACULAR TRACTION SYNDROMES

INTRODUCTION

Epidemiology

- No large epidemiologic surveys of the prevalence and incidence of VMT.

Etiology

- Idiopathic
- Uveitis
- Diabetic retinopathy.

CLINICAL SIGNS AND SYMPTOMS

Signs

- Decreased vision
- Distortion.

SYMPTOMS

- Incomplete PVD
- ERM in 50% of cases
- Tractional detachment of fovea.

INVESTIGATIONS

OCT

- Demonstrates persistent vitreous adhesion to macula with associated traction on fovea
- May have associated retinal detachment.

DIFFERENTIAL DIAGNOSIS

- Macular hole
- Epiretinal membrane
- Central serous retinopathy
- Myopic foveo-schisis.

TREATMENT

Vitrectomy

Indications

- Symptomatic VMT

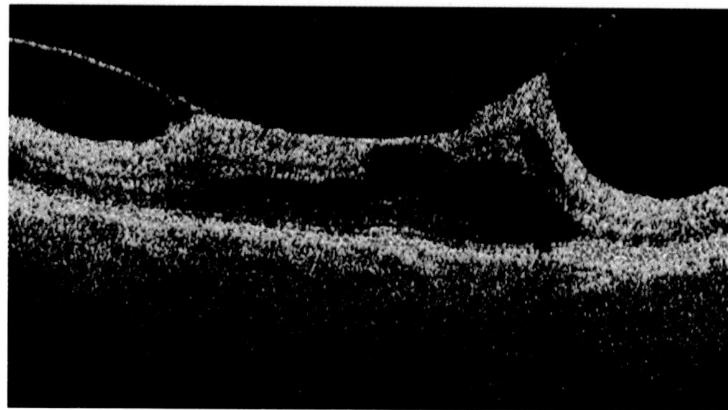

Fig. 4A: OCT demonstrating extensive vitreomacular traction with cystoid retinal edema

Methods

- Pars plana vitrectomy with complete removal of posterior hyaloid and ERM.

Results

- Separation of vitreous traction leads to resolution of edema and improved visual acuity.

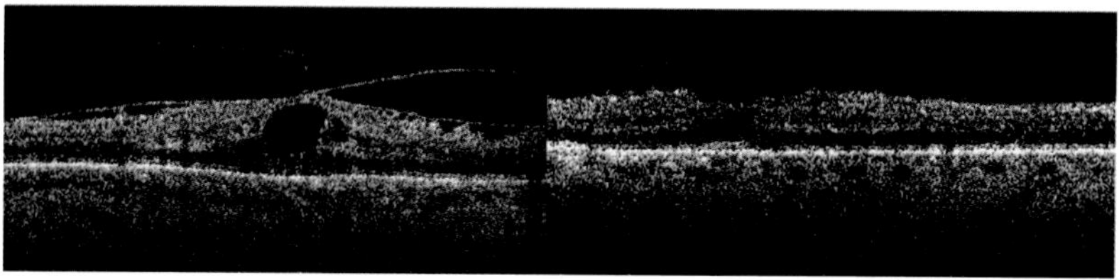

Fig. 4B: Pre- and post vitrectomy OCT of patient with ERM and vitreomacular traction syndrome. Note preoperative cystoid macular edema and insertion of posterior hyaloid into the ERM complex

INFERENCES

- Incomplete separation of posterior hyaloid produces retinal edema and visual dysfunction
- Vitrectomy is beneficial in visually significant cases.

BIBLIOGRAPHY

1. Gandorfer A, Rohleder M, Kampik A. Epiretinal pathology of vitreomacular traction syndrome. Br J Ophth. 2002:86;902-9.
2. Smiddy WE, Michels RG, Glaser BM, deBustros S. Vitrectomy for macular traction caused by incomplete vitreous separation. Archives of Ophthalmology 1988;106(5):624-8.

MACULAR HOLE

INTRODUCTION

Prevalence

- < 1% population.

Risk Factors

- Female > Male
- About 10% of cases are bilateral.

Etiology

- Idiopathic
  - May represent an advanced form of vitreo-macular traction
- Trauma
- High myopia.

CLINICAL SIGNS AND SYMPTOMS

Symptoms

- Decreased vision
  - Correlates with the size of the hole
- Distortion.

Signs

- Full thickness defect in the macula with central yellow deposits in the base of the hole
- Watzke Allen Sign
  - A thin slit lamp beam placed across the hole is perceived as having a gap
  - Commonly patients perceive a narrowing of the beam rather than a complete gap
  - Cuff of retinal edema or subretinal fluid
  - Associated ERM.

Classification

- Stage 1: Central yellow spot or ring with flattening of the foveal depression
- Stage 2: Eccentric, oval full thickness hole
- Stage 3: Complete, round full thickness hole without PVD
- Stage 4: Full thickness hole with PVD.

INVESTIGATIONS

Autofluorescence Imaging

- Increased autofluorescence due to absence of macular xanthophyl.

Fluorescein Angiography

- Window defect at base of hole.

OCT

- Complete gap in retina with associated intraretinal edema and subretinal fluid at margin.

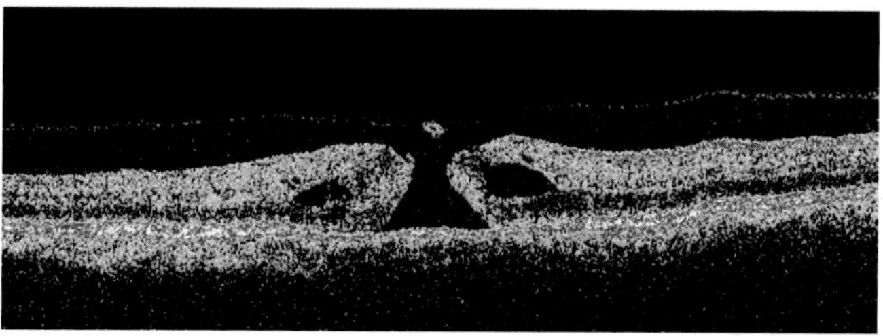

Fig. 5A: Horizontal OCT shows full thickness macular hole with perifoveal vitreous separation. Centrally there is vitreous condensation consistent with clinically observed pseudo-operculum

DIFFERENTIAL DIAGNOSIS

- Epiretinal membrane with pseudohole
- Vitreomacular traction
- Myopic degeneration
- Geographic atrophy
- Cystoid macular edema.

TREATMENT

Vitrectomy

Indications

- Stage 2, 3 or 4 hole.

Methods

- Pars plana vitrectomy with removal of posterior hyaloid and epiretinal membrane
- Removal of internal limiting membrane appears to increase success rate but may delay visual recovery
- Gas tamponade with face down positioning.

Results

- 80-90% single procedure macular hole closure rate reported
- Predictors of anatomic success and visual improvement
  - Shorter duration hole (< 6 months)
  - Smaller diameter hole (< 400 microns)

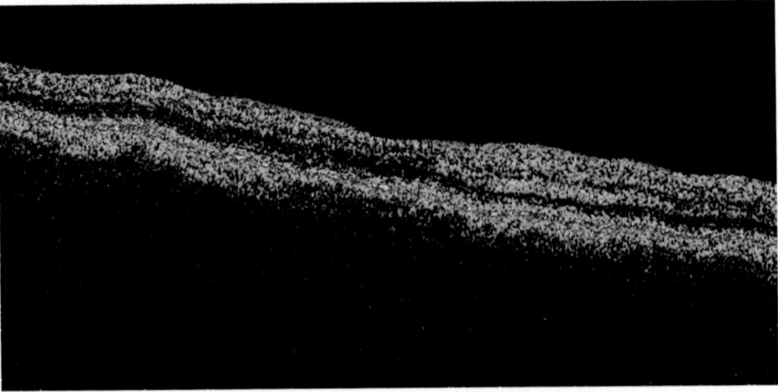

Fig. 5B: Post vitrectomy OCT shows complete closure of macular hole

INFERENCES

- Macular holes typically develop in middle aged females
- The untreated natural history has poor visual results
- Vitrectomy has a high success rate for achieving closure
- Visual outcomes are better with smaller and more recent onset holes.

BIBLIOGRAPHY

1. Gass DJM. Reappraisal of biomicroscopic classification of stages of development of a macular hole. Am J Ophth 1995;119:752-9.
2. Freeman WR, et al. Vitrectomy for the treatment of full thickness stage 3 or 4 macular holes. Arch Ophth 1997;115:11-21.
3. Burk SE, Mata AP, Snyder ME, et al. Indocyanine green assisted peeling of the retinal internal membrane. Ophth 2000;107:2010-14.

CYSTOID MACULAR EDEMA

INTRODUCTION

Prevalence

- Varies with the underlying cause and definition
  - Intermediate uveitis : 30%
  - Post-cataract angiographic CME : 50%
  - Post-cataract CME with VA <20/40 : 8%.

Etiology

Congenital

- Retinitis pigmentosa
- Autosomal dominant CME
- Familial exudative vitreoretinopathy.

Acquired

- Central/branch retinal vein occlusion
- Diabetic retinopathy
- Perifoveal telangiectasis
- Uveitis
- Post surgical
- Epiretinal membrane/vitreo macular traction
- Drugs
  - Nicotinic acid
  - Prostaglandin analogues
  - Topical epinephrine.

CLINICAL SIGNS AND SYMPTOMS

Symptoms

- Decreased vision
- Micropsia.

Signs

- Visible cystic changes in macula.

INVESTIGATIONS

Fluorescein Angiography

- Late fluorescein leakage into cystic intraretinal spaces.

OCT

- Demonstrates intraretinal cystoid spaces
- Able to demonstrate vitreomacular traction.

TREATMENT

Observation

- Many cases of post cataract CME will resolve without treatment
- Treatment is indicated with prolonged CME with visual impairment

Topical Non-Steroidal Anti-Inflammatory Drugs (NSAIDs)

- Demonstrated to be beneficial in prolonged postoperative CME
- Typically given as 3 to 6 week course of treatment
- Longer courses may be required in chronic cases of CME.

Topical Steroids

- Often combined with topical NSAID
- Traditional experience suggests benefit, however, no comparative trials have been conducted.

Injectable Steroids

- Used in cases of prolonged CME
- Can be administered as subtenon or intravitreal injection.

Laser

- Nd-YAG vitreolysis can be performed to divide vitreous strands in anterior chamber.

Surgery

- Vitrectomy with meticulous removal of vitreous incarceration in anterior segment
- Multicentered prospective trial demonstrated benefit in aphakic patients with chronic CME (> 6 months) and vitreous incarceration
- Case series demonstrate benefit in pseudophakic CME with anterior prolapsed vitreous.

INFERENCES

- The causes of cystoid macular edema are varied
- Therapy is directed at the underlying cause.

Central Serous Retinopathy

Ashok Garg (India)

INTRODUCTION

- Central Serous Retinopathy (CSR) is known as serous detachment of retina due to leaking of serum from the choroidal circulation through a break in the diffusion barrier which is located at the level of tight junction around the RPE cells.
- It is common in males with age group of 25-50 age and about 30% cases are unilateral.

Pathophysiology

- The pathological changes are seen at the level of choriocapillaries or Bruch's membrane where a focal abnormality allows serous fluid to accumulate under the retina resulting in a localized separation of retina from the pigment epithelium CSR is also defined as a Localized Retinal Detachment.
- Four theories known Gass's theory, Watzke's theory, Behrendt's theory and Friedman's theory have been advocated to explain the pathogenesis of CSR.
- Etiological factors for CSR include.
- Mechanical (After Cataract or Glaucoma operation).
- Infective (Due to virus, Allergic or vasomotor instability).

CLINICAL SIGNS AND SYMPTOMS

- History of Premonitory transient attacks of Blurred vision.
- When the lesion develops, there is a positive scotoma.
- Decreased visual acuity.
- Central serous retinopathy is divided into six stages.

- **Stage I** : Acute—(Multifocal areas of epithelial junction are involved. Patients are asymptomatic as there is no break in diffusion barrier.
- **Stage II** : Subacute—As the acute stage of disease progresses some patients develop focal breaks in the tight junction around the diseased RPE cells. This stage usually resolves in three months.
- **Stage III**: Chronic—The leaking through the break of tight junction becomes chronic, a field defect will develop which often involves fovea resulting marked decrease in visual acuity.

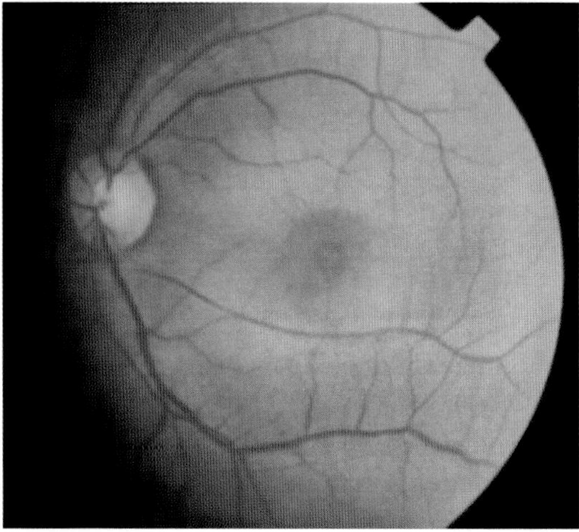

Fig. 1: Central serous retinopathy (Serous detachment of retina at the macula)

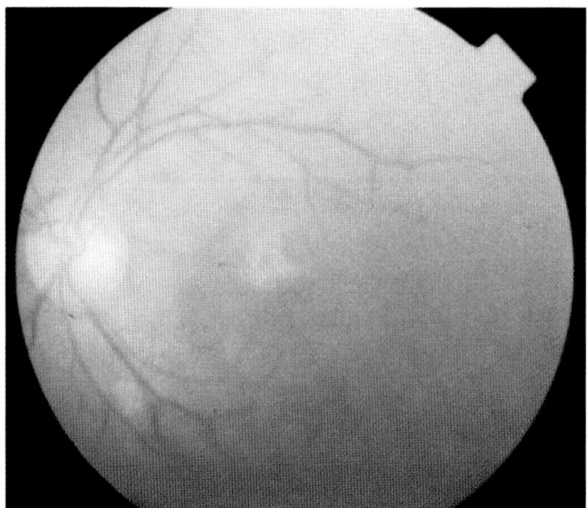

Fig. 2: Central serous retinopathy (circumscribed swelling)

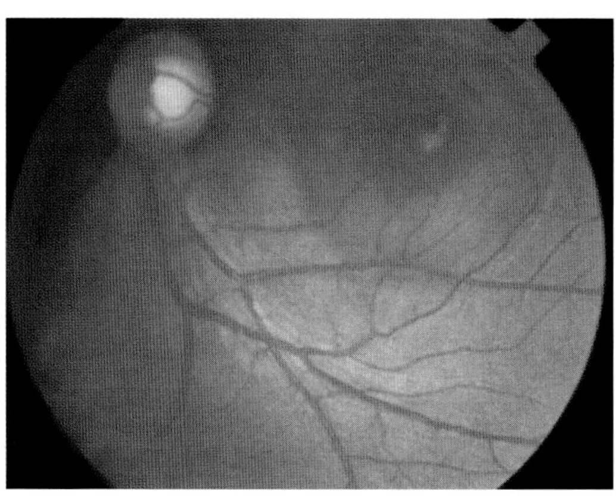

Fig. 3: Central serous retinopathy

- **Stage IV**: Inactive—Most of the patients in this stage have no history of previous eye problem. They had asymptomatic stage and spontaneously improve.
- **Stage V**: Late complications.

RPE decompensation occurs: This late complication is seen 5-10 years after the first diagnosis of CSR.

Stage VI: Late complications

Subretinal neovascularization develops which are of two types:
- Typical (one or two leaking areas are seen on FA)
- Atypical (Multiple leaks are seen)
- Circumscribed macular swelling usually clearly delimited from the surrounding retina is seen.
- The optic disc color is variable but in most of cases it is darkish red and yellowish white spots are visible on the surface.
- Foveal reflex is distorted or absent and is characteristic feature on ophthalmoscopic examination.

INVESTIGATIONS

Fluorescein Angiography

On FA different patterns are seen
- Smoke stack sign (in this leakage of Fluorescein starts as a small spot which increases and spread upwards filling the subretinal space and looks like umberella.
- Odd spot (Inkblot): In this pattern initial hyperfluorescent spool increases gradually in size till entire subretinal space is occupied.
- Multiple leaks (Multiple leaks are seen in atypical type of CSR).

Amsler's Grid Pattern

- In this patient is examined for any distortion of lines or scotomas.

ERG which is subnormal in CSR

Visual Field Examination

An inverted pear shaped field defect occurs.

Slit Lamp Examination

It reveals a diffuse retinal edema and a displacement of the rounded contour of the internal limiting membrane or a macular whole.

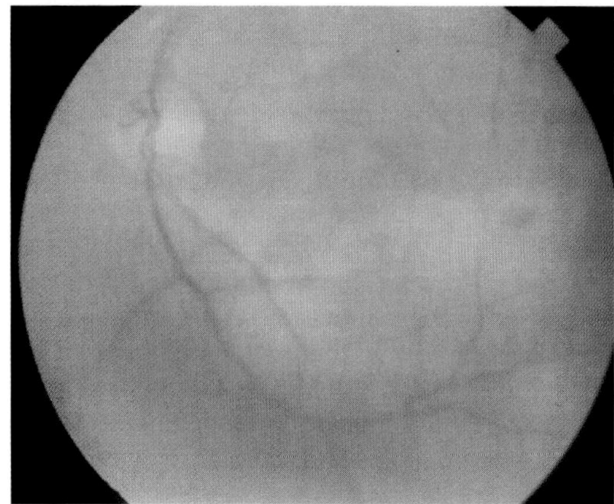

Fig. 4: Atypical central serous retinopathy

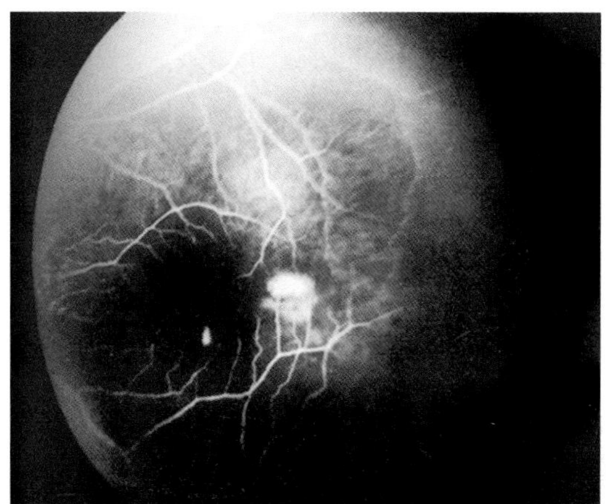

Fig. 5

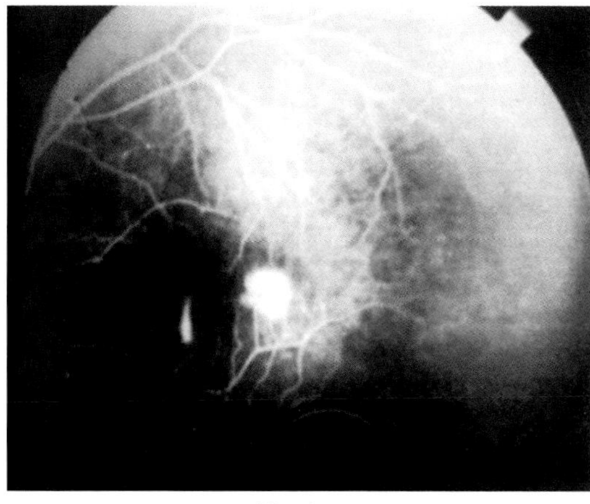

Fig. 6

DIFFERENTIAL DIAGNOSIS

- Optic disc pit
- Coat's disease
- Detached pigment epithelium
- Hollenhorst syndrome
- Incontinentia pigmenti
- Subpigment epithelium hemorrhage
- von Hippel-Lindau disease
- Post-neovascularization of vitreous
- Viral retinitis
- Vitreous degeneration.

TREATMENT

- In stage I (Acute) and stage II (sub acute) patient is usually asymptomatic and shall require no treatment.
- However, Stage II-VI require Argon Laser Photocoagulation (ALP) depending upon the condition. If CSR does not resolve after 6 weeks, Laser treatment is done. In recurrent CSR, immediate laser is done.

  In ALP Laser shot is given at leakage seen on Fluorescein angiography. The spot size used is 150 microns with the exposure time of 0.1 second and power at 200 watts.
- Local cycloplegics instillation is also recommended.
- In atypical cases of CSR systemic anti-tubercular drugs are also prescribed.

PROGNOSIS

- In chronic and later stages of CSR prompt Laser photocoagulation is advocated for the preservation of visual acuity.
- Patient should be vigilant and regular consultation with Retinal surgeon is required for proper follow-up otherwise CSR can be serious vision threatening condition.

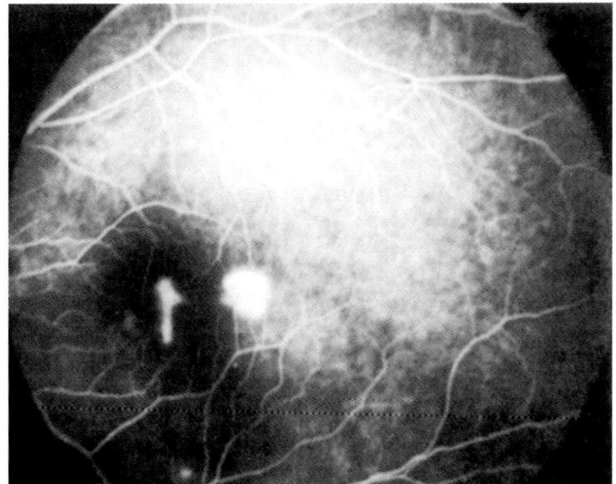

Fig. 7

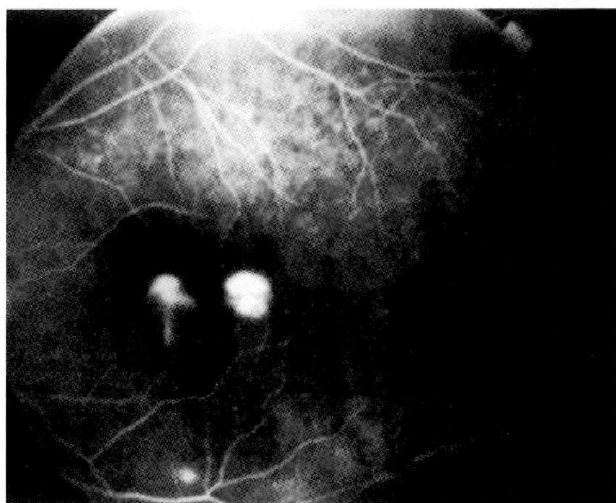

Fig. 8

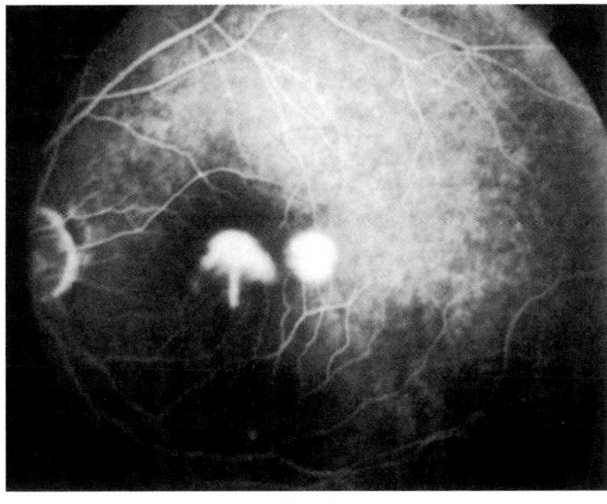

Fig. 9

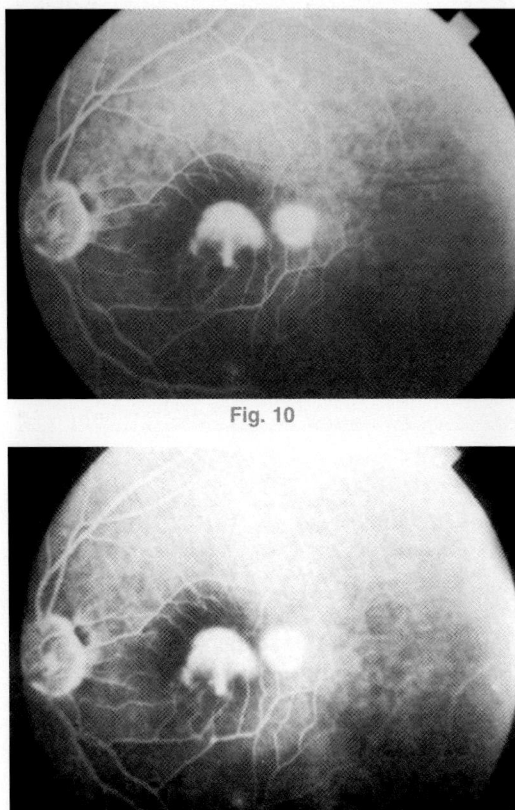

Fig. 10

Fig. 11

Figs 5 to 11: FFA in central serous retinopathy (smoke stack sign) leakage increasing and spreading upward

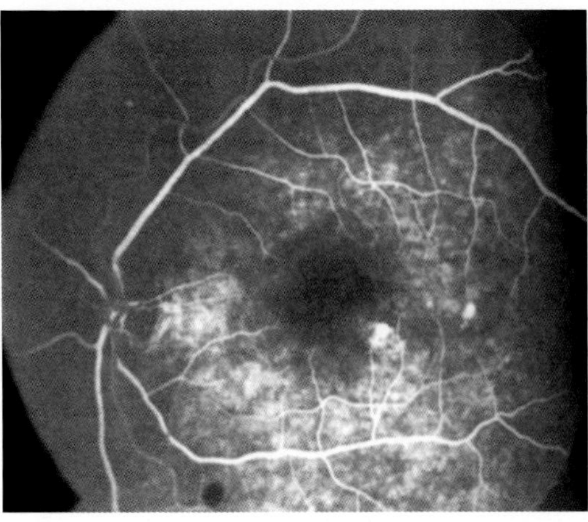

Fig. 12

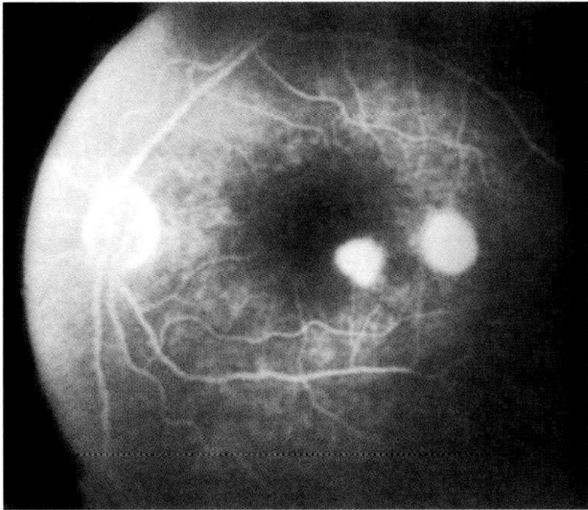

Fig. 13

Figs 12 and 13: FFA in central serous retinopathy (odd spot sign) spot of hyper-fluorescence increasing in size

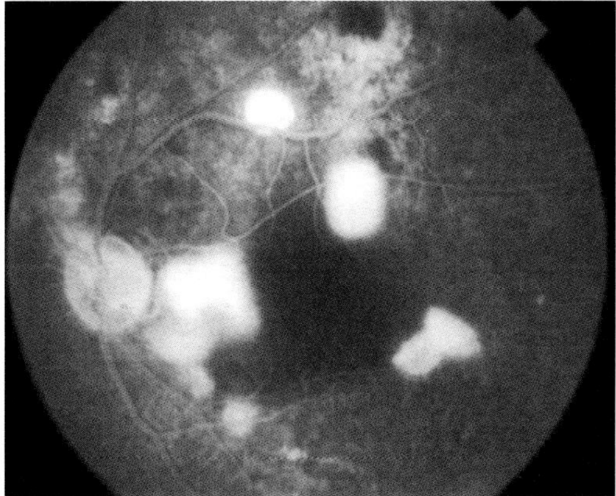

Fig. 14: Multiple leaks as seen in Atypical Central Serous Retinopathy

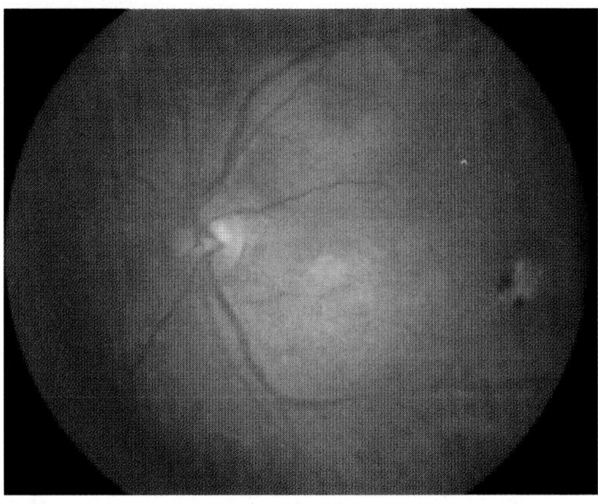

Fig. 15: Post Photocoagulation Central Serous Retinopathy case (Marks on the retina)

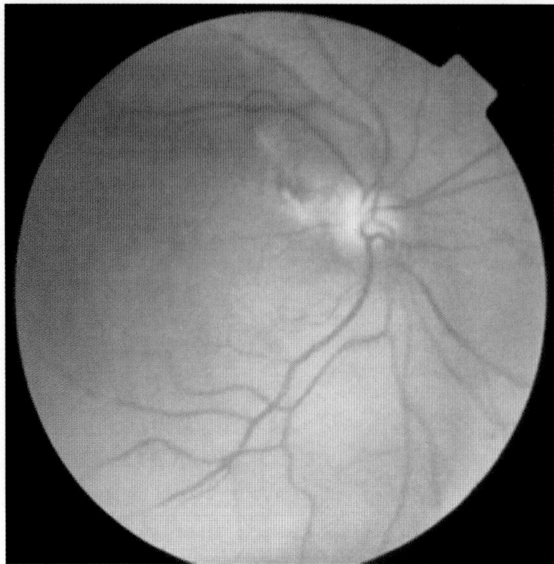

Fig. 16: Post photocoagulation central serous retinopathy

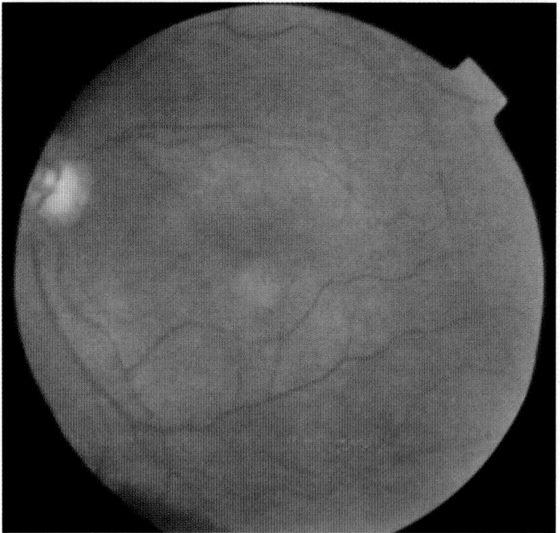

Fig. 17: Post-photocoagulation central serous retinopathy (vision restored to 20/20)

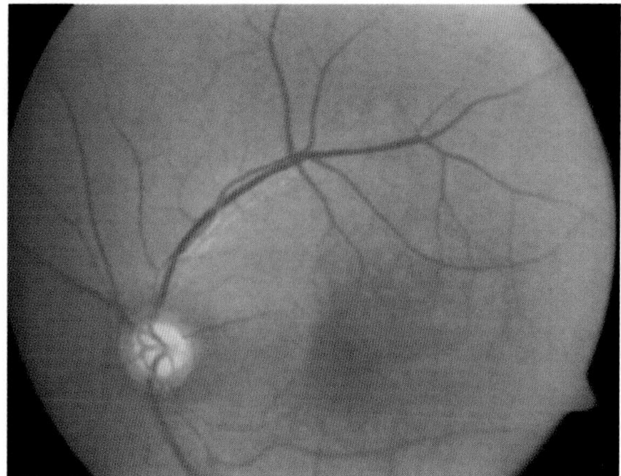

Fig. 18A: Central serous retinopathy

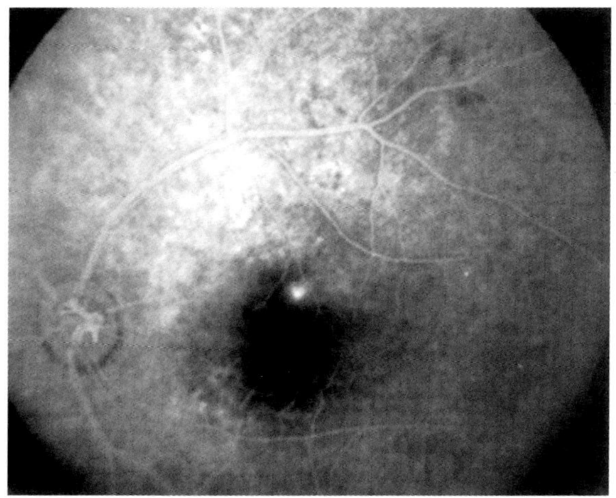

Fig. 18B: FFA of central serous retinopathy patient of Fig. 18A

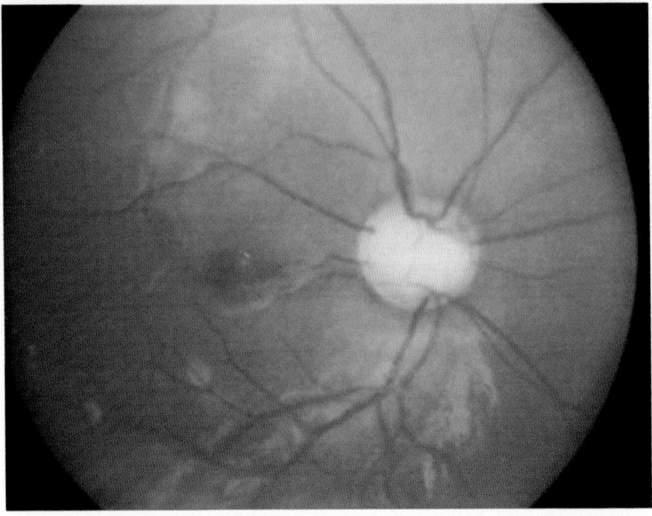

Fig. 19A: Optic disk pit with central serous retinopathy

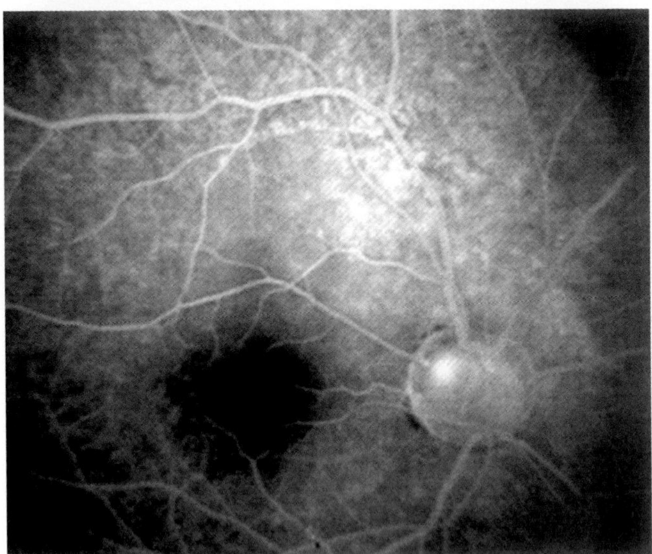

Fig.19B: FFA of optic disc pit with central serous retinopathy

CHAPTER FOUR

VASCULAR DISORDERS

- **VASCULAR DISORDERS**
  Francisco L Lugo, Jose M Ruiz Moreno, Javier A Montero, Pedro Amat Peral (Spain)
  - Venous Occlusive Disease
  - Branch Retinal Vein Occlusion
  - Central Retinal Vein Occlusion
  - Arterial Occlusive Disease
  - Central Retinal Artery Obstruction
  - Branch Retinal Artery Obstruction
  - Hypertensive Retinopathy
  - Hypertensive Choroidopathy
  - Hypertensive Neuropathy
  - Retinal Arterial Macroaneurysms
- **BRANCH RETINAL VEIN OCCLUSION**
  Emanuel Rosen (UK)
- **MALIGNANT HYPERTENSION RETINOPATHY**
  Emanuel Rosen (UK)
- **SUBHYALOID HEMORRHAGE**
  Shaifali Singla, Lalit Verma, Avnindra Gupta, Madhu Karna, Dinesh Talwar, HK Tewari (India)

Vascular Disorders

Francisco L Lugo, José M Ruiz-Moereno,
Javier A Montero, Pedro Amat-Peral (Spain)

Retinal vascular disorders are among the most frequent conditions causing visual loss in adults which in many cases may be permanent. Since the retinal vasculature can be examined *"in vivo"* by diagnostic techniques such as fluorescein angiography (FA) and the optical coherence tomography (OCT), the mechanisms of most of these disorders can be studied. Retinal vascular disorder may represent a true reflection of the systemic circulatory conditions.

VENOUS OCCLUSIVE DISEASE
BRANCH RETINAL VEIN OCCLUSION

INTRODUCTION

Branch retinal vein occlusion (BRVO) is an important cause of visual impairment in middle-aged and elderly individuals. BRVO is caused by an obstruction of one retinal vein branch, usually temporal to the optic disc.

PATHOGENESIS AND ETIOLOGY

BRVO usually occurs at arteriovenous crossings. The retinal artery and vein share a common adventitial sheath at the crossing site. Hypertension and arteriosclerosis increase the rigidity of the artery, causing turbulent venous blood flow, endothelial cell injury, and thrombotic venous occlusion. Risk factors include systemic hypertension, cardiovascular disease, increased body mass at 20 years of age, glaucoma, elevated serum levels of alpha-2-globulin, and a shorter axial lengths.

CLINICAL CHARACTERISTICS

Misty or distorted vision with sudden visual acuity loss and campimetric defects. Biomicroscopy shows dilated, tortuous veins, superficial hemorrhages, retinal edema, and cotton-wool spots in a sector of retinal drained by the affected vein.

INVESTIGATION

Primary and secondary (following laser photocoagulation) intravitreal triamcinolone acetonide (TA) injection reduces macular edema and serous

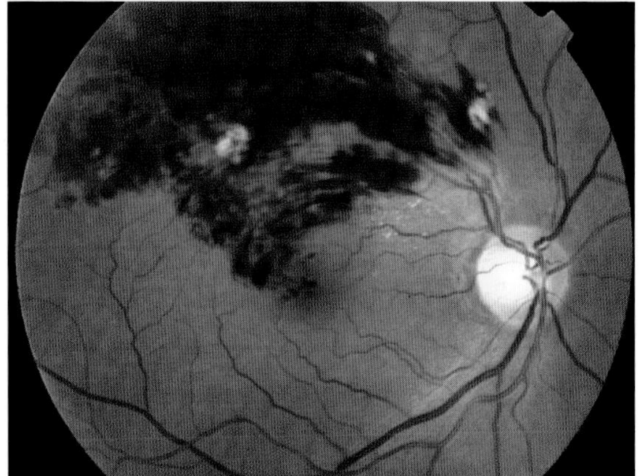

Fig. 1

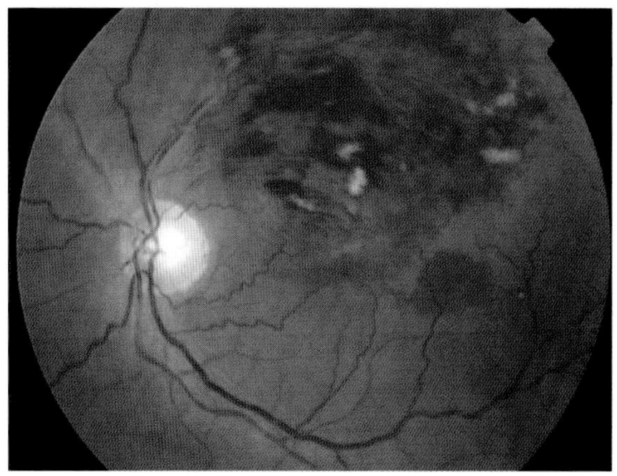

Fig. 2

Figs 1 and 2: BRVO

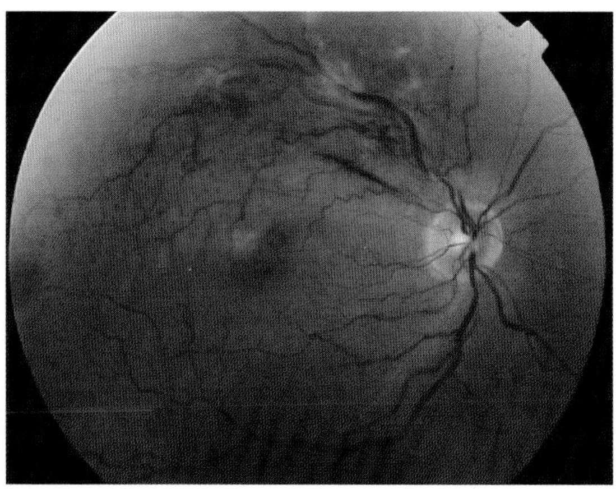

Fig. 3

macular detachment, increasing visual acuity. Good results may not be permanent and repeated injections may be necessary.

Initial reports showed a significant reduction of central retinal thickness and improved visual acuity after bevacizumab injections in macular edema secondary to BRVO. Multiple injections are needed for continued control of macular edema and preservation of visual acuity. Frequent OCT examinations every 3 to 6 weeks may help for judging the appropriate timing for re-injections.

DIFFERENTIAL DIAGNOSIS

Diabetic retinopathy and hypertensive retinopathy.

Treatment: For the underlying systemic disorders. Laser photocoagulation is useful in the treatment of chronic macular edema and posterior segment neovascularization. Macular photocoagulation may be delayed 3 to 6 months to permit spontaneous resolution of the edema; treat with vision in the 20/40 to 20/200 range if the perifoveal retinal capillaries are intact. Laser treatment reduces the rate of neovascularization and the risk of vitreous hemorrhage, improving visual outcome.

Vitreoretinal Surgery is indicated for complications such as retinal detachment, nonclearing vitreous hemorrhage and macular edema. Pars plana vitrectomy with arterovenous sheathotomy may improve visual acuity.

PROGNOSIS

Is related to the extent of capillary damage and retinal ischemia. Macular edema may persist and be responsible for permanently decreased vision. Extensive retinal ischemia results in neovascularization. Permanent visual loss may be related to macular ischemia and edema, subretinal fibrosis, epiretinal membrane, pigmentary macular alteration.

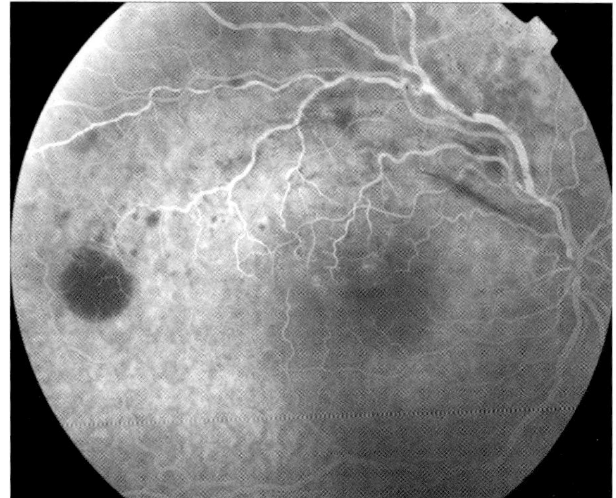

Fig. 4

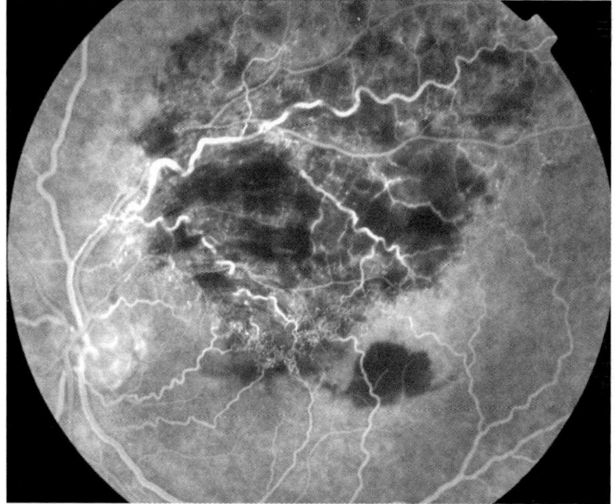

Fig. 5

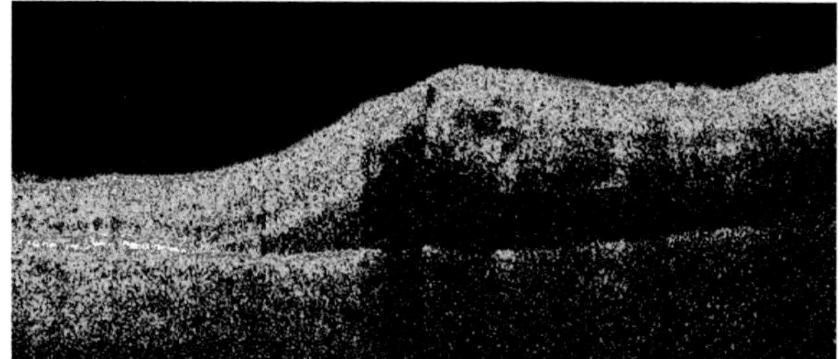

Fig. 6

Figs 3 to 6: BRVO with retinal edema and extension into the macula

CENTRAL RETINAL VEIN OCCLUSION (CRVO)

The pathogenesis of CRVO consists of a physical blockage at the lamina cribrosa, and hemodynamic factors obstructing blood flow.

ETIOLOGY

The most common risk factors are age over 50 years, systemic hypertension, diabetes mellitus and open-angle glaucoma. Oral contraceptives, diuretics, blood dyscrasias, dysproteinemias, sarcoidosis, systemic erythematous lupus may increase the risk.

CLINICAL CHARACTERISTICS

Non-ischemic Central Retinal Vein Occlusion

It is much milder and more variable than ischemic CRVO. Patients are 5 years younger than those with ischemic vein occlusion. Visual acuity may range from normal to counting fingers, but most of patients have an initial visual acuity of 20/50 or better. Mild dilation and tortuosity of all branches of the central retinal vein, with dot and flame hemorrhages in all quadrants of the retina; optic disc edema may be present and cotton-wool spots are rare. FA shows prolongation of retinal circulation time with capillary permeability breakdown. Capillary nonperfusion is not a significant feature and anterior segment neovascularization is rare.

PROGNOSIS

The natural course is relatively benign, except in cases developing additional ischemia, resolving over several months. Cystoid macular edema, pigmentary changes, or residual microvascular abnormalities may persist. Most of patients have a final visual acuity of 20/40 or better.

ISCHEMIC CENTRAL RETINAL VEIN OCCLUSION

Patients with ischemic occlusion have an average age of 68.5 years and usually report a sudden, painless decrease in visual acuity ranging from 20/400 to hand movements. Retinal edema, cotton-wool patches and extensive hemorrhage in the posterior pole are common. FA shows a delayed filling of the veins, capillary and venous dilatation and extensive fluorescein leakage with capillary nonperfusion. Microaneurysms may appear. Early electroretinogram (ERG) may correlate strongly with visual prognosis and be a good indicator of retinal perfusion. The most reliable tests, in differentiation between ischemic and non-ischemic CRVO are relative afferent pupil defect,

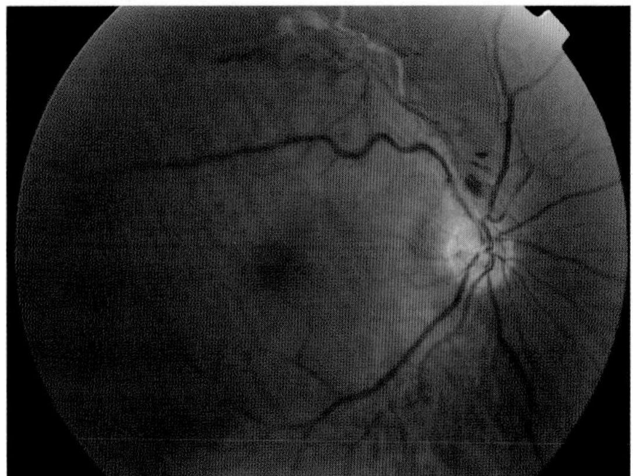

Fig. 7

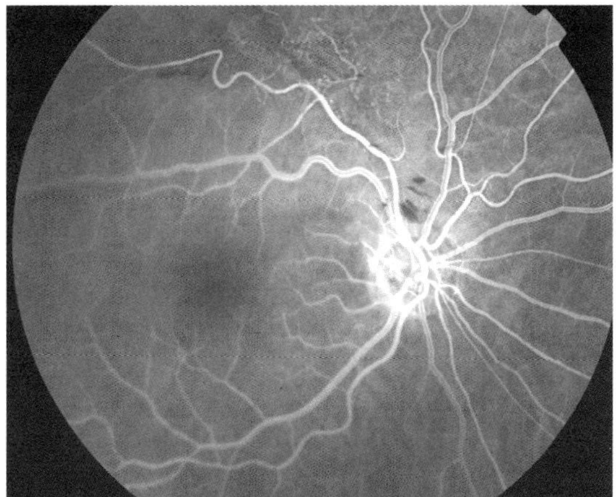

Fig. 8

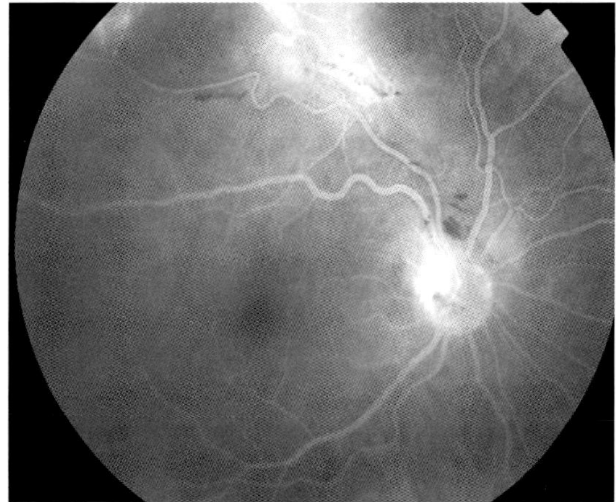

Fig. 9

Figs 7 to 9: Retinal neovascularization in BRVO

the electroretinogram, perimetry, visual acuity, fluorescein angiography, and ophthalmoscopy.

DIFFERENTIAL DIAGNOSIS

Ocular ischemic syndrome, diabetic retinopathy, papilloedema.

PROGNOSIS

It is generally poor, 10% of eyes with vision better than 20/400. Retinal edema usually subsides except in the macula. The most serious complication of central retinal vein occlusion is neovascularization (35 to 45%) which usually occurs in the first 3 months.

TREATMENT

Treatment of systemic conditions though indicated, seldom reverses vein occlusion but may prevent vascular occlusions in the fellow eye. Anticoagulants, fibrinolytic agents, corticosteroids, inhibitors of platelet aggregation and others have not proved their efficacy. No therapy is known to be effective against nonischemic CRVO. Photocoagulation does not affect the final visual acuity outcome, but is effective in the prevention and the regression of neovascularization. Prophylactic panretinal photocoagulation (PRP) has no significant advantage over treatment applied at the first sign of anterior segment neovascularization.

Intravitreal TA (4 mg in 0.1 ml) is effective for the treatment of macular edema secondary to CRVO and BRVO reducing central macular thickness and may increase visual acuity. Nonischemic CRVO may respond more favorably than ischemic CRVO. The risk of glaucoma and cataract induction is significant.

Intravitreal Bevacizumab appears to be safe and effective in improving visual acuity and reducing central macular thickness.

Vitreoretinal surgery is indicated in CRVO for complications such as nonclearing vitreous hemorrhages and/or traction retinal detachment. Surgical decompression (radial optic neurotomy) is associated with rapid reperfusion of the retina and resolution of the intraretinal hemorrhage improving visual acuity.

ARTERIAL OCCLUSIVE DISEASE

Retinal ischemia results from disease affecting the afferent vessels.

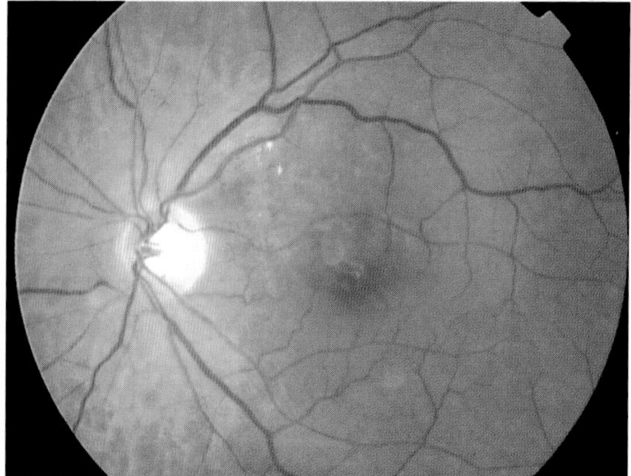

Fig. 10

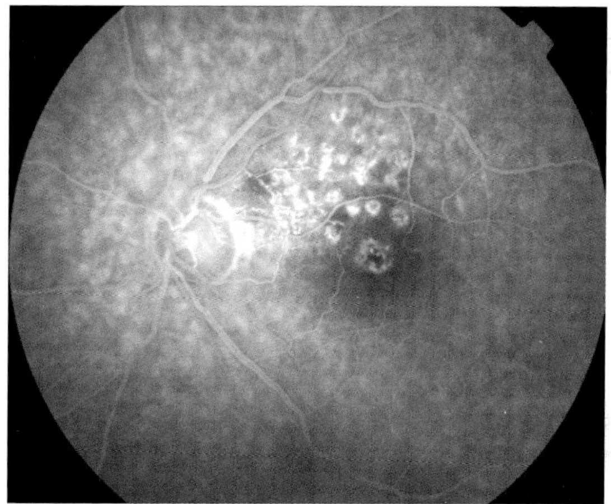

Fig. 11

Figs 10 and 11: Pigmentary macular alteration in BRVO

CENTRAL RETINAL ARTERY OBSTRUCTION (CRAO)

Usually occurs in patients who are in the fifth or sixth decades of life. Arteriosclerosis is the most commonly associated systemic condition.

ETIOLOGY

Migraine, coagulant disorders, intraocular abnormalities, and trauma (patients under 30 years of age), systemic arterial hypertension, atherosclerotic disease, diabetes mellitus (patients over 40).

CLINICAL CHARACTERISTICS

Sudden, severe and painless loss of vision with opaque and edematous retina. The appearance of a cherry-red spot in the fundus indicates preservation of choroidal circulation. Arteries are narrow and irregular; segmentation of the blood column is frequent. The retinal opacity decreases leaving an atrophic optic nerve with thin arteries and veins and loss of foveolar light reflex. FA segmentation is well defined and venous filling is usually slow. Abnormal choroidal filling reflects posterior circulation obstruction.

PROGNOSIS

66% of eyes have final vision worse than 20/400, and 18% had a vision 20/40 or better (in presence of a cilioretinal artery). Neovascularization is probably the most serious complication.

DIFFERENTIAL DIAGNOSIS

Ophthalmic artery occlusion, arteritic ischemic optic neuropathy.

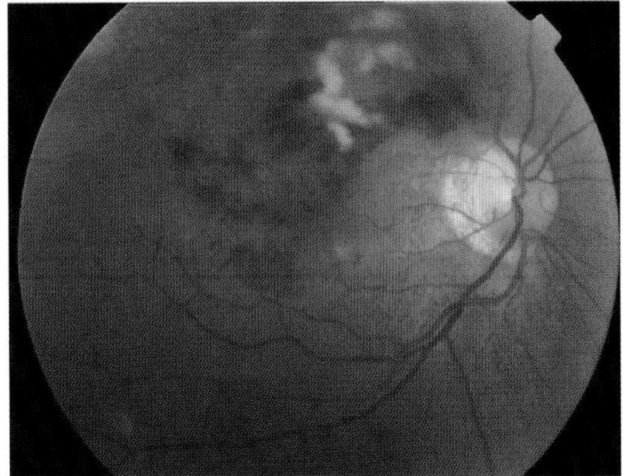

Fig. 12

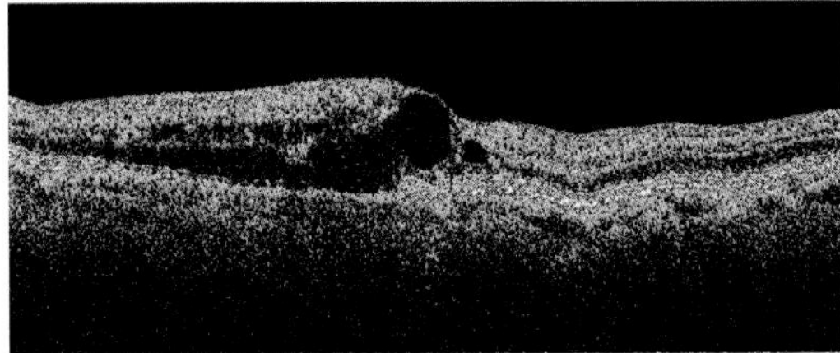

Fig. 13

Figs 12 and 13: BRVO before laser photocoagulation and intravitreal triamcinolone injections

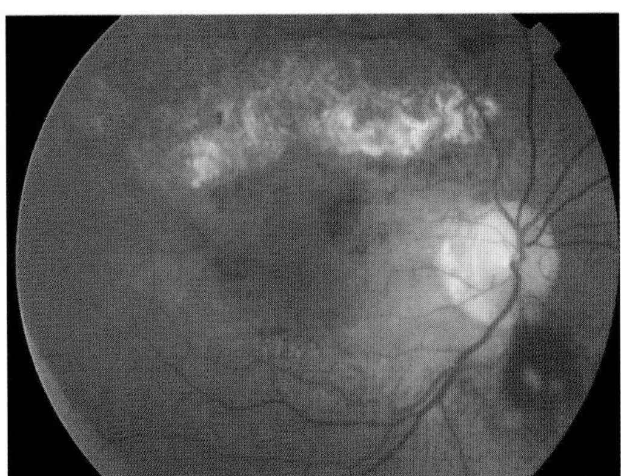

Fig. 14

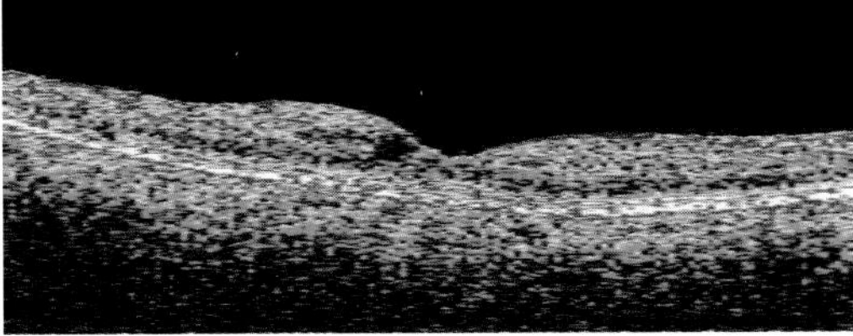

Fig. 15

Figs 14 and 15: BRVO after laser photocoagulation and intravitreal triamcinolone injections

BRANCH RETINAL ARTERY OBSTRUCTION (BRAO)

Usually occurs at bifurcations, its etiology is similar to that of CRAO. Three varieties of emboli are recognized: Cholesterol emboli (Hollenhorst plaques) arising in the carotid arteries, platelet-fibrin emboli associated with large-vessel arteriosclerosis and calcium emboli from heart valves. Others causes include cardiac mixoma, fat emboli from bone fractures, septic emboli, etc.

CLINICAL CHARACTERISTICS

Sudden loss of vision or a visual field defect depending on the affected area. May not be initially apparent, though it leads to edematous opacification of the retina and field defects.

TREATMENT

Systemic etiology factors. In presence of neovascularization the treatment is scatter photocoagulation to the ischemic retina. Conservative treatment (reduction in IOP) to dislodge an embolus from a large central vessel toward a more peripheral location. Hyperbaric oxygen, intravenous recombinant tissue plasminogen activator (rTPA) may improve visual outcome.

Invasive treatment: Selective ophthalmic artery catheterization and ophthalmic artery infusion of urokinase, with controversial results.

PROGNOSIS

Prognosis is poor. A systematic protocol including ocular massage, sublingual isosorbide dinitrate, intravenous acetazolamide, intravenous, manitol or oral glycerol, paracentesis, intravenous methylprednisolone, streptokinase and retrobulbar tolazoline may improve visual outcome.

HYPERTENSIVE RETINOPATHY

The ocular effects of hypertension can be observed with ophthalmoscopy and angiography as hypertensive retinopathy, hypertensive choroidopathy, and hypertensive optic neuropathy.

PATHOGENESIS AND CLINICAL CHARACTERISTICS

Arteriosclerosis leads to endothelial damage and necrosis of the muscular layer of the vessel walls causing exudative leakage into the retina.

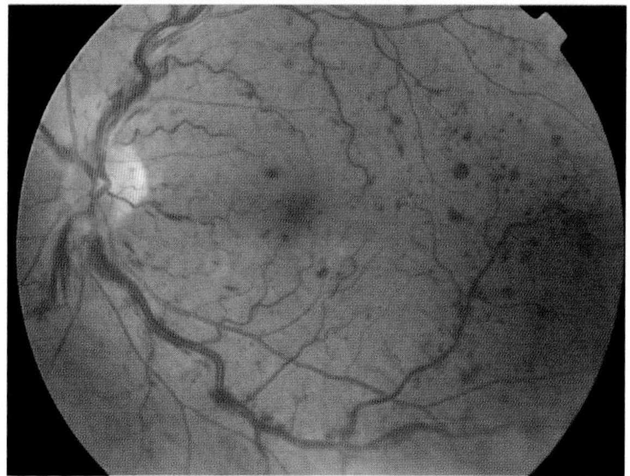

Fig. 16: CRVO nonischemic

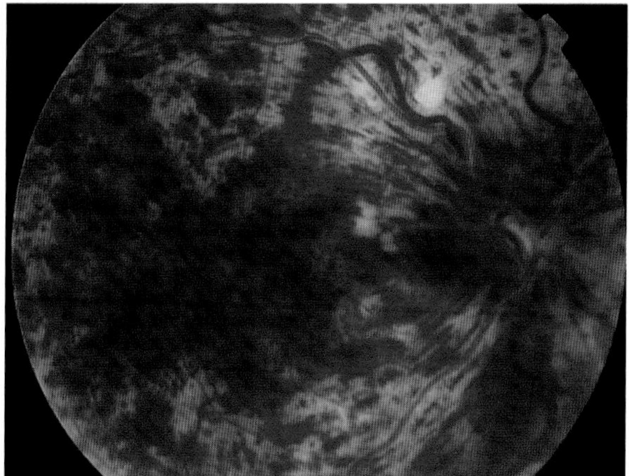

Fig. 17: CRVO ischemic

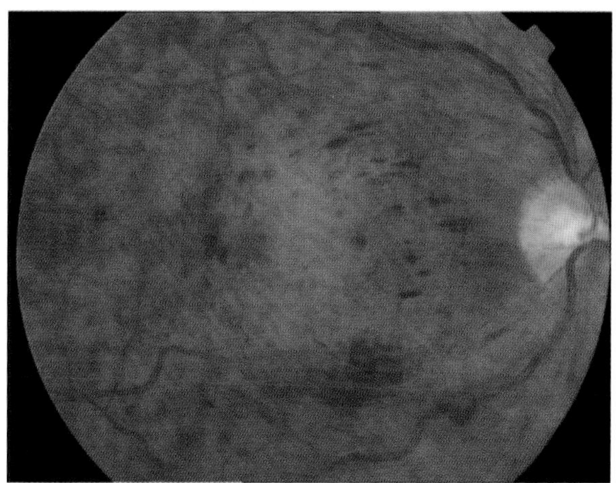

Fig. 18: CRVO nonischemic

CLINICAL FINDINGS

Include arteriolar narrowing, arteriovenous crossing changes, arterial sclerosis, arterial tortuosity, increased branching angles, hemorrhages, retinal and macular edema, edema residues (hard exudates), inner retinal ischemic spots (cotton-wool spots), nerve fiber layer loss and focal intraretinal periarteriolar transudates. Hypertensive retinopathy is associated with complications such as: CRAO or BRAO, CRVO or BRVO, macroaneurysms, epiretinal membrane, retinal neovascularization, vitreous hemorrhage and cystoid macular edema.

HYPERTENSIVE CHOROIDOPATHY

Occurs in young patients with acute hypertension. The clinical features include Elschnig's spots (ischemic infarcts of the RPE) and Siegrist's streaks (ischemic infarcts at the equator), subretinal exudates, serous retinal detachments, RPE depigmentation and choroidal sclerosis.

FA shows irregular choroidal filling pattern with areas of hypofluorescence caused by hypoperfusion. Chronic cases reveal a hyperfluorescent pattern corresponding to the RPE window defects.

HYPERTENSIVE NEUROPATHY

Hypertensive optic neuropathy appears in patients with severe or malignant hypertension. Clinically they appear as optic nerve head swelling with linear flame-shaped hemorrhages at the margin of the optic disk, blurring of the disc margins, congestion of associated retinal veins, disk edema and secondary macular exudates. Treatment of systemic arterial hypertension is essential. Advanced cases may show optic disk pallor and atrophy resulting from chronic ischemia.

DIFFERENTIAL DIAGNOSIS

Anterior ischemic optic neuropathy, radiation retinopathy, acute macular neuroretinitis and diabetic papillopathy.

RETINAL ARTERIAL MACROANEURYSMS

Arterial macroaneurysms are acquired round dilatations of the arterial walls, most common along the temporal arcades. Loss of the muscular layer and thinning and fibrosis result in decreased elasticity and increased dilation from intraluminal pressure. They are associated with systemic arterial hypertension in two thirds of cases and are frequently multiple.

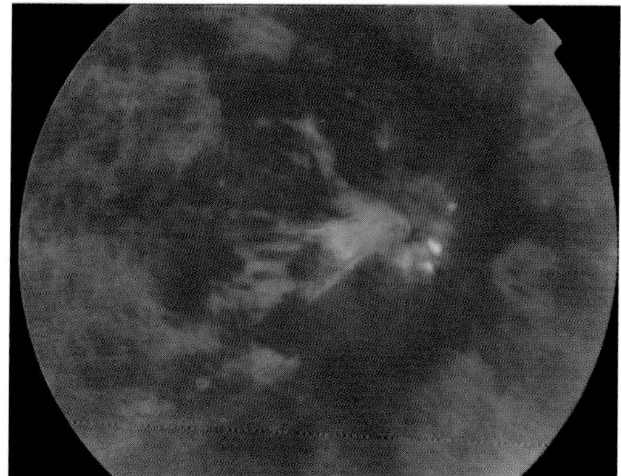

Fig. 19

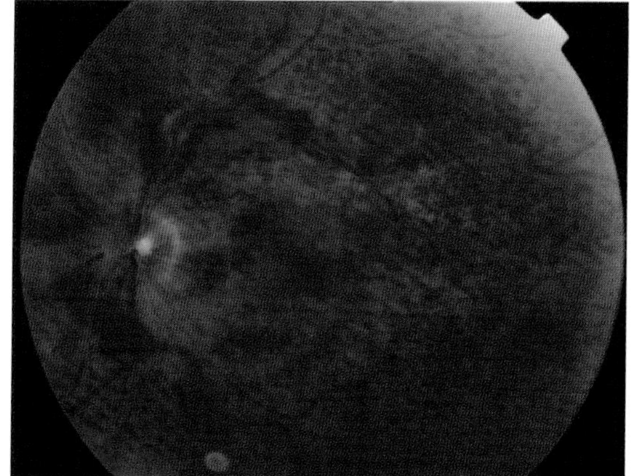

Fig. 20

Figs 19 and 20: CRVO ischemic

CLINICAL CHARACTERISTICS

Hemorrhages and intraretinal circinate or diffuse exudates are frequent; arteriolar emboli, capillary telangiectasia and vascular occlusions may also appear. Fluorescein leakage from the aneurysm or the proximal artery wall is frequent. Visual loss from hemorrhage, edema and exudates involving the macula or vitreous hemorrhage is the most common presenting symptom, or may remain asymptomatic. Most of macroaneurysms eventually involute spontaneously.

PROGNOSIS

For vision depends on the location of the hemorrhage and exudate as well as on the severity and duration of macular involvement.

DIFFERENTIAL DIAGNOSIS

Includes retinal telangiectasia, diabetic retinopathy, venous macroaneurysms, retinal cavernous hemangioma, choroidal melanoma, and age-related macular degeneration.

TREATMENT

Patients with good vision and no macular involvement should be observed. Laser photocoagulation may be considered if visual function is menaced by edema or hemorrhage. Treatment modalities include direct and indirect photocoagulation of the lesion.

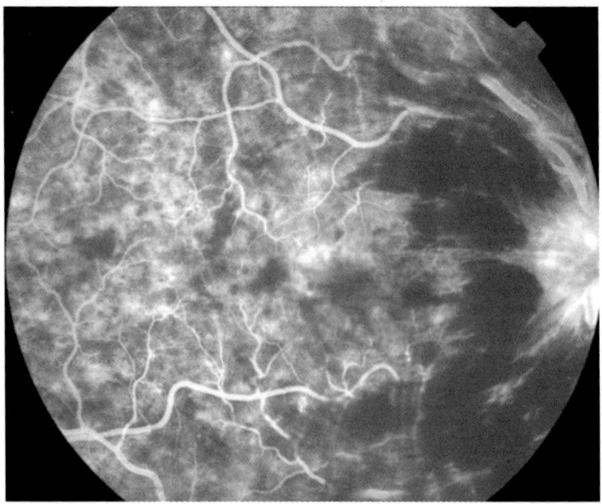

Fig. 21

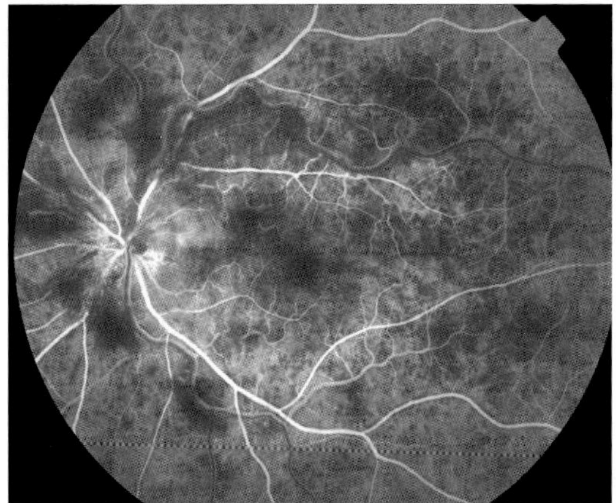

Fig. 22

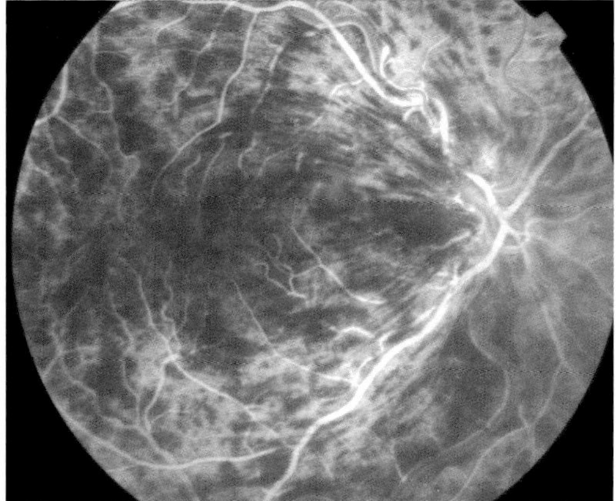

Fig. 23

Figs 21 to 23: Fluorescein angiography in CRVO ischemic

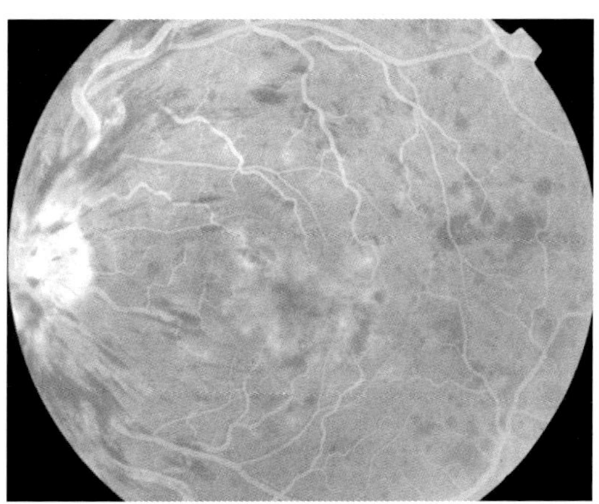

Fig. 24: Leakage of fluorescein in macula in CRVO

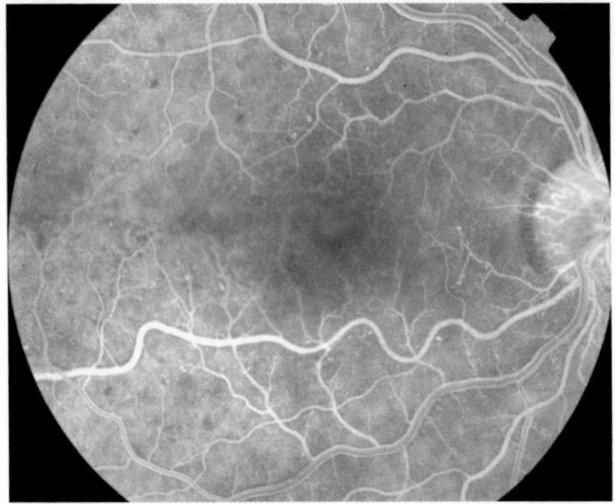

Fig. 25: Microaneurysms in CRVO

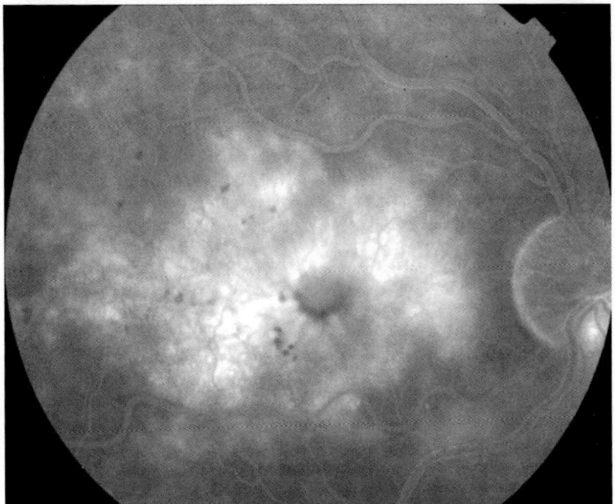

Fig. 26

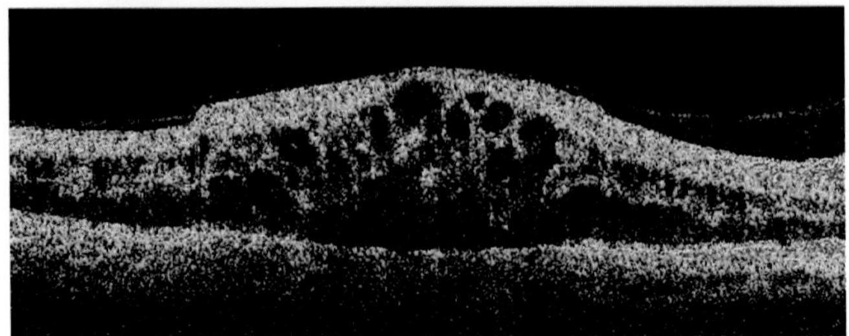

Fig. 27

Figs 26 and 27: Cystoids macular edema in CRVO

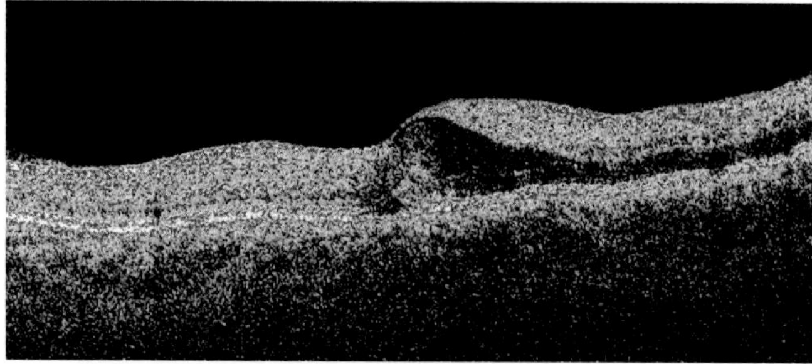

Fig. 28

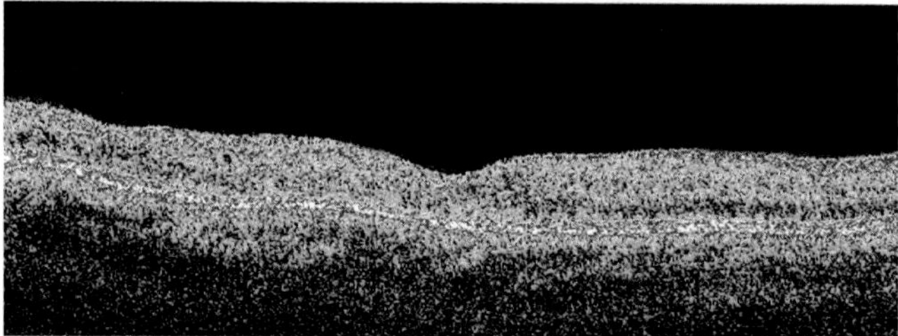

Fig. 29

Figs 28 and 29: OCT-macular area in CRVO before and after triamcinolone injections

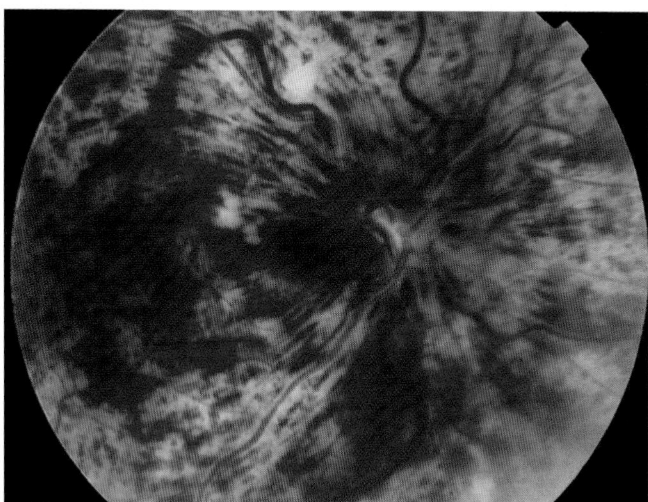

Fig. 30

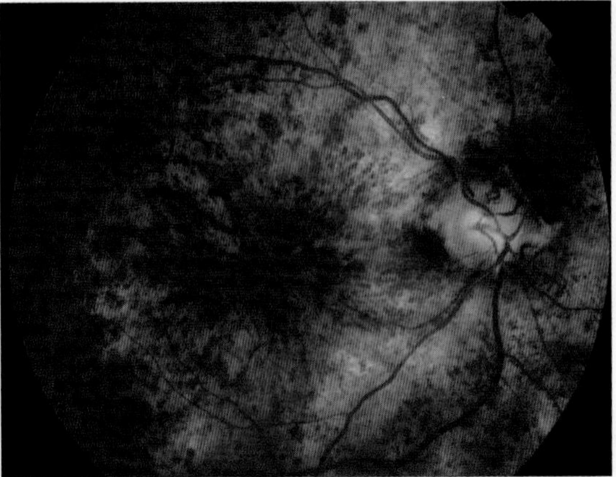

Fig. 31

Figs 30 and 31: CRVO before and after radial optic neurotomy

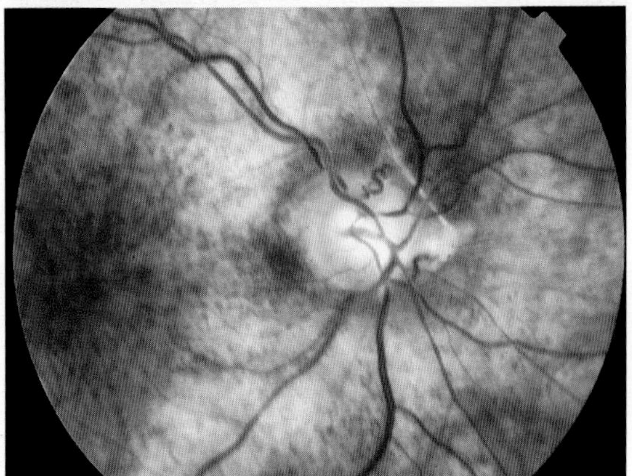

Fig. 32

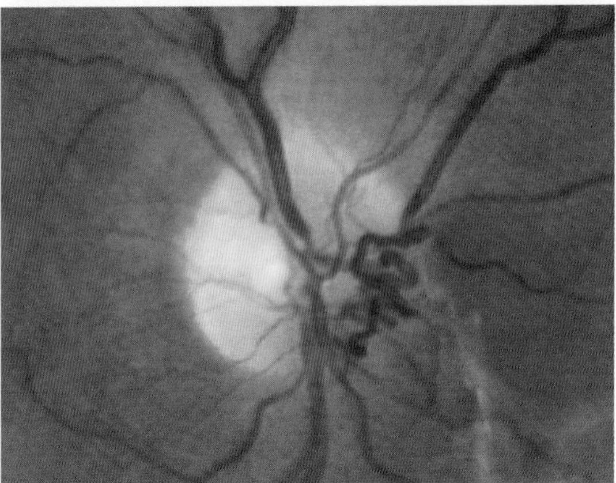

Fig. 33

Figs 32 and 33: Chorioretinal shunts after radial optic neurotomy

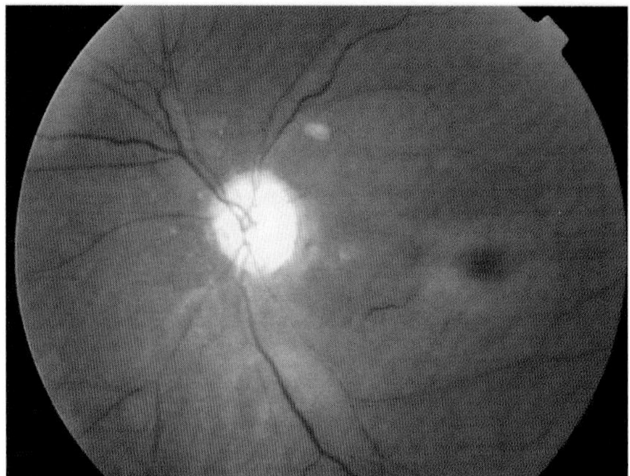

Fig. 34: CRAO

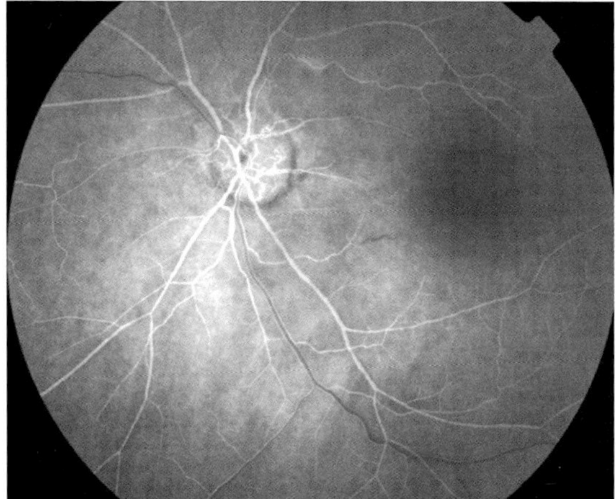

Fig. 35: Fluorescein angiography in CRAO

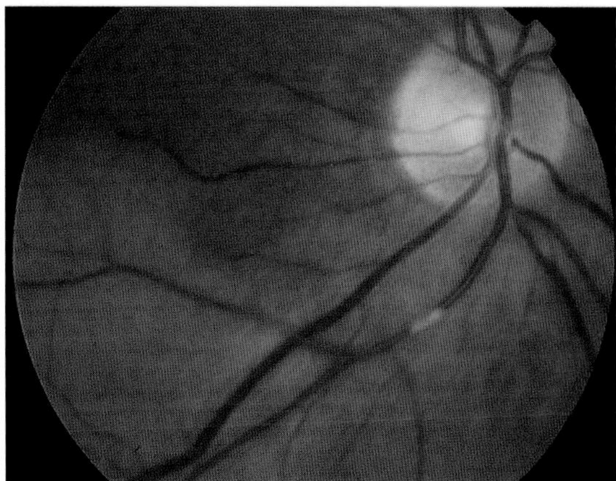

Fig. 36: Platelet-fibrin emboli

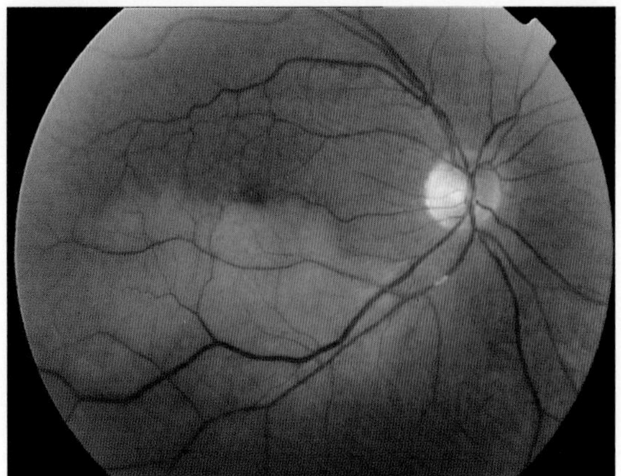

Fig. 37: BRAO

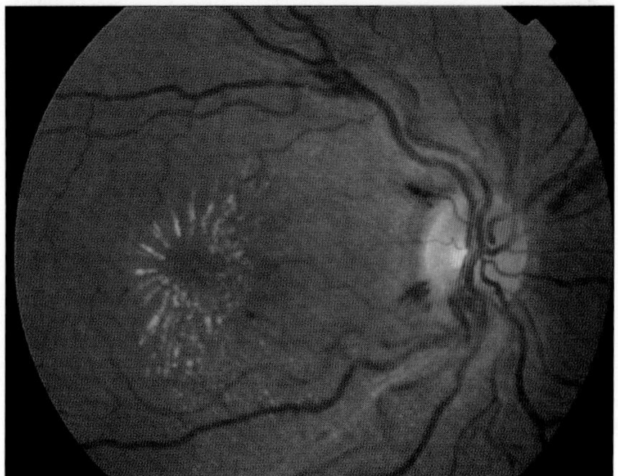

Fig. 38

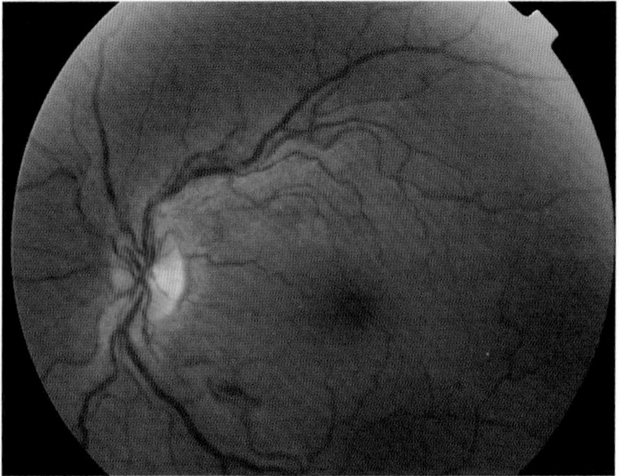

Fig. 39

Figs 38 and 39: Hypertensive retinopathy

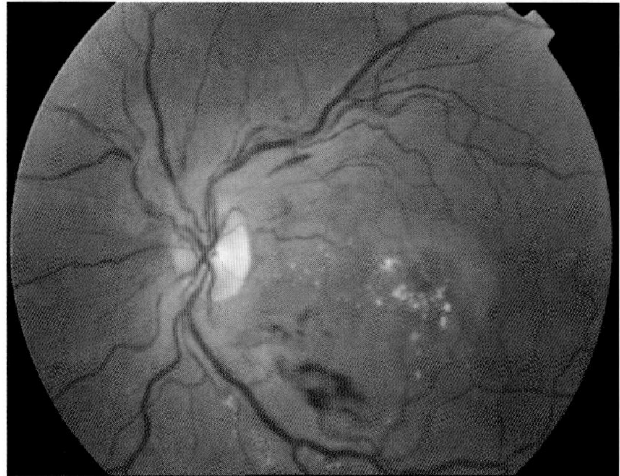

Fig. 40

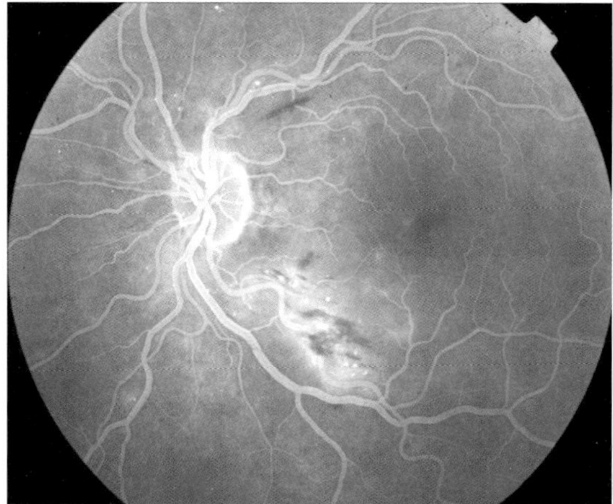

Fig. 41

Figs 40 and 41: BRVO in hypertensive retinopathy

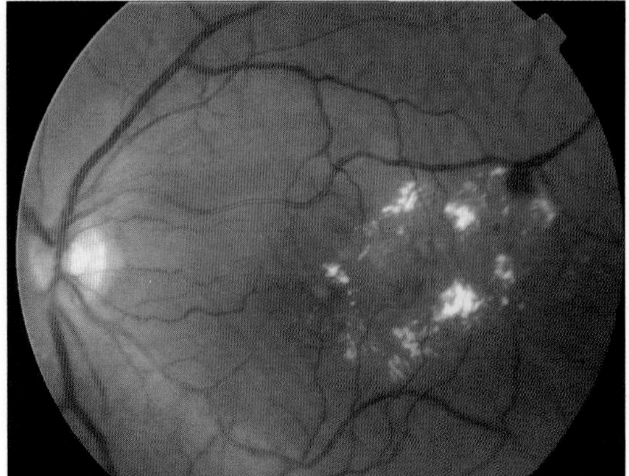

Fig. 42

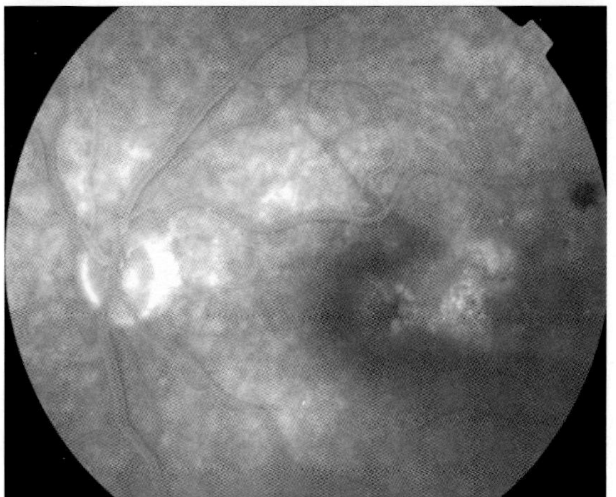

Fig. 43

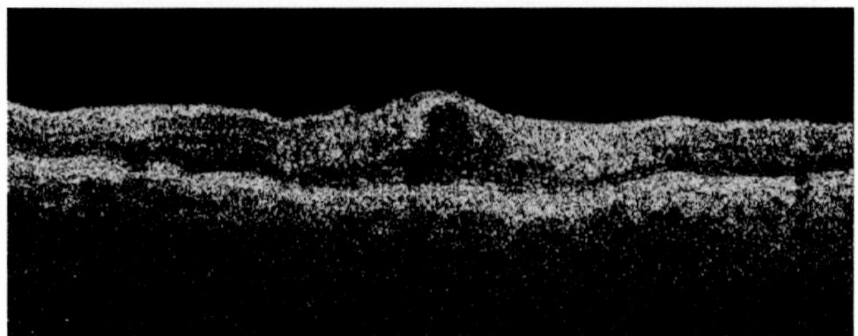

Fig. 44

Figs 42 to 44: Retinal arterial macroaneurysms

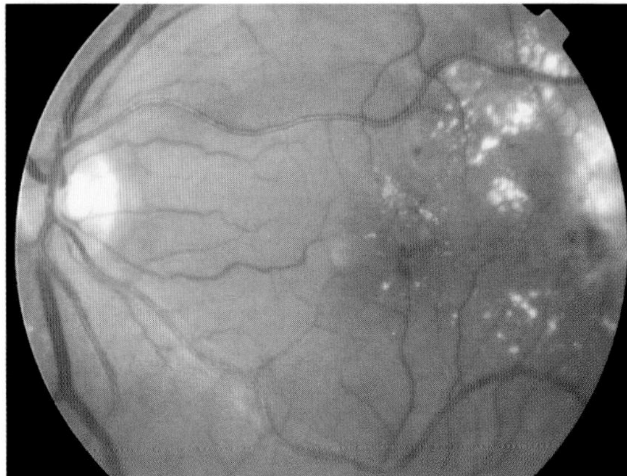

Fig. 45

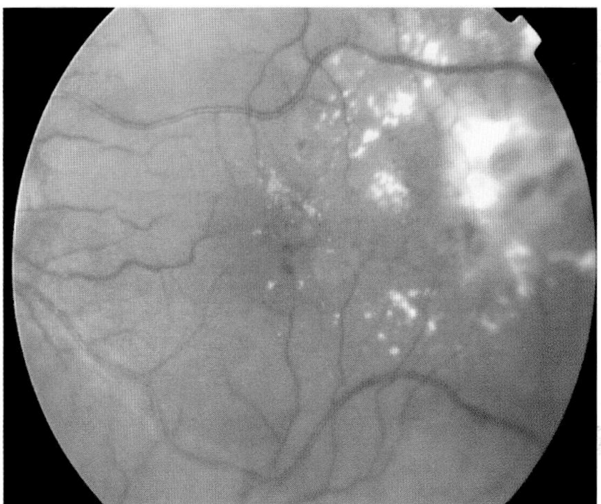

Fig. 46

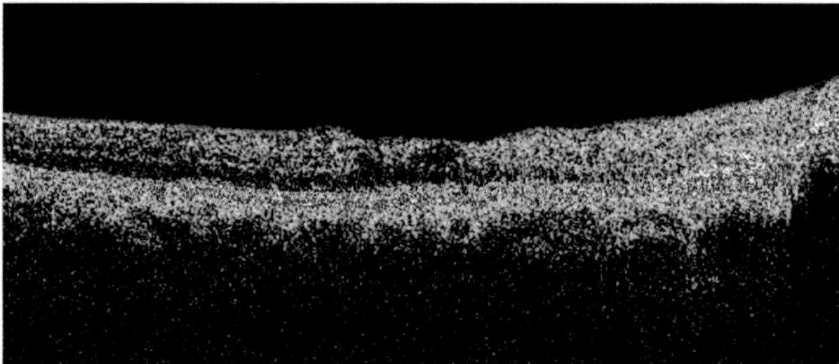

Fig. 47

Figs 45 to 47: Retinal arterial macroaneurysms after laser photocoagulation

Branch Retinal Vein Occlusion

Emanuel Rosen (UK)

INTRODUCTION

Retinal vascular occlusive disease usually seen in patient's with systemic hypertension. Arterial thickening may slow blood flow through compromised associated retinal vein to cause vascular stasis and therefore venous occlusion.

CLINICAL SIGNS AND SYMPTOMS

- Wedge shaped area of retinal haemorrhage, retinal edema, with apex invariably at an arterial venous crossing site (cotton wool spots - early in evolution)
- Superotemporal branch of central retinal vein most commonly involved
- Vein distal to the obstruction is invariably dilated, tortuous and darker in appearance
- Macular edema and haemorrhage are probable. Cystoid maculopathy eventuates in chronic cases
- With the passage of time collateral channels develop at the temporal edges of the site of the occlusion
- Symptoms of blurring or distortion dependent on macular involvement and degree of macular edema
- Visual loss may be sudden if the macula is involved
- Scotoma relative to occlusion
- Overall visual acuity of 6/60 or worse in 30%.

COMPLICATIONS

- Cystoid macular edema
- Macular hole
- Macular pucker
- Retinal neovascularization
- NVD new vessels at optic nerve head
- Vitreous hemorrhage
- Anterior segment neovascularization occurs in 1-2% eyes.

PATHOGENESIS

- Constriction of venous wall by arterial crossing resulting in thrombin formation and occlusion

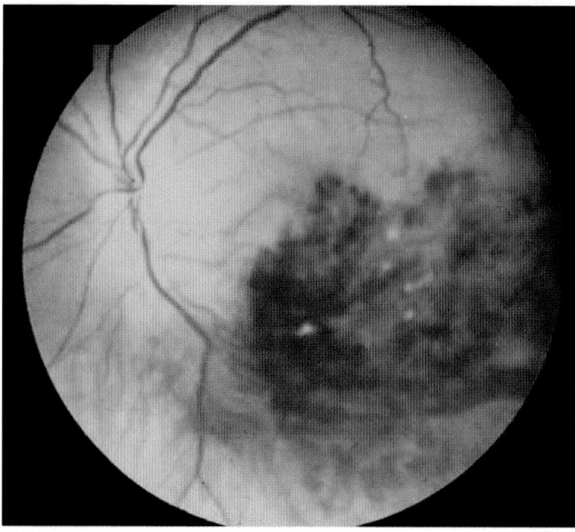

Fig. 1: Inferior temporal BRVO wedge shaped hemorrhagic pattern

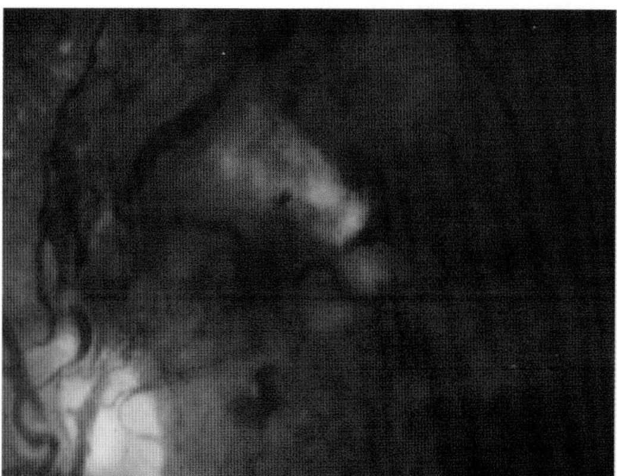

Fig. 2A: Superior temporal BRVO vein occluded at A-V crossing. Resolving CWS Ischemic central retina and NV response at optic disc

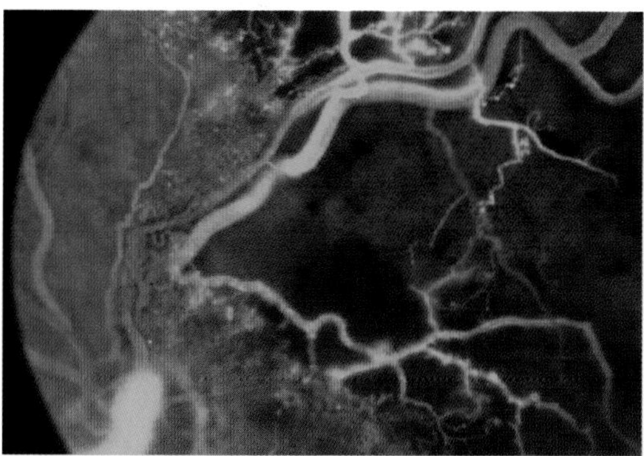

Fig. 2B: Superior temporal BRVO FFA vein occluded at A-V crossing Ischemic central retina and NV response at optic disc

- Capillary endothelial damage with increased permeability and non-perfusion
- Natural history depends on severity of the occlusion and the development of collateral channels.

ASSOCIATIONS

- Hypertension (75%)
- Diabetes mellitus
- Atherosclerosis
- Hypercoaguable states
- Ocular disease associations
  - Open angle glaucoma (10%)
  - Ocular inflammation such as Eales' disease and Behcet's disease.

INVESTIGATIONS

- Erythrocyte sedimentation rate
- Glucose tolerance test in non-diabetics
- Imaging by color and fundus fluorescein angiography
  - Venous filling delayed in obstructed vein
  - Capillary non-perfusion, areas of capillary non-perfusion variable
  - Retinal hemorrhage
  - Blocking background fluorescence
  - Staining of the venous wall especially close to the site of occlusion
  - Retinal leakage of dye with or without macular edema
  - Leakage of dye from neovascularization when present.

DIAGNOSIS

- Clinical diagnosis is obvious and supported by fundus fluorescein angiography.

TREATMENT AND PROGNOSIS

- Underlying medical condition to be treated
  - Branch vein occlusion study confirmed that eyes with macular edema and a visual acuity of less than 6/12 and duration of occlusion between 3 and 18 months who received argon laser grid photocoagulation did significantly better than controls at 3 years. On the other hand eyes with foveal ischaemia and hemorrhage were not included
- Where angiography confirms ischemia of the segment, quadrantic retinal photocoagulation should prevent neovascularization.
- If macular edema exists intraocular injection of Avastin worth the attempt to obtain some resolution of macular edema.
- Follow up required for at least 6 months to confirm absence of posterior or anterior segment neovascularization.

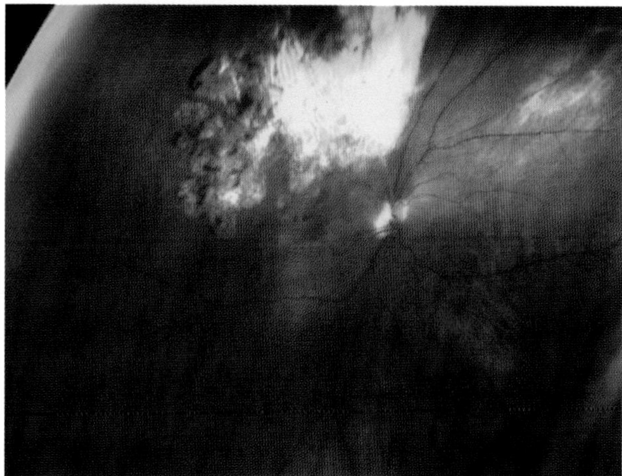

Fig. 3A: Superior temporal BRVO ischemic retinal with quadrantic PRP UCVA 6/12 20 years post-treatment

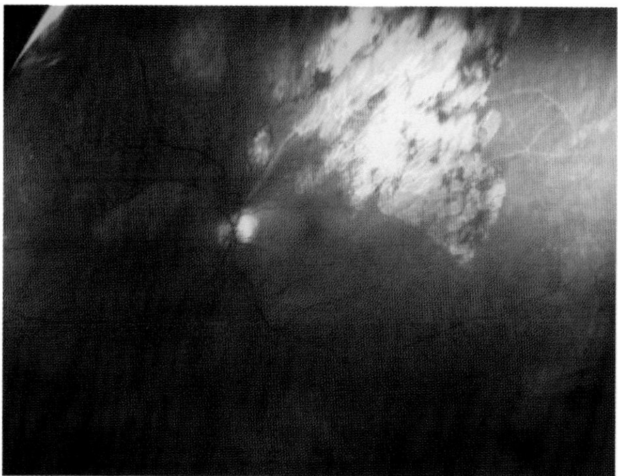

Fig. 3B: Fellow eye superior temporal BRVO ischemic retina with quadrantic PRP UCVA 6/6 20 years post-treatment

Malignant Hypertension Retinopathy

Emanuel Rosen (UK)

INTRODUCTION

Serious sight threatening retinopathy consequence of untreated hypertension with very high diastolic pressure.

CLINICAL SIGNS AND SYMPTOMS

- Malignant hypertension diastolic pressure > 120 mmHg
- Visual acuity better than 6/60
- Dilatation and increased tortuosity of retinal veins
- Optic disc edema
- Variable degree of intraretinal hemorrhages
- Macular edema and/or hemorrhage
- Cotton wool infarcts (when fresh) granular infarcts with passage of time (weeks)
- Visual fluctuations through to sudden visual loss
- Symptoms and appearances similar to ischemic central retinal vein occlusion.

COMPLICATIONS

- Cystoid macular edema
- Macular hemorrhage
- Vitreous hemorrhage
- Rubeosis iridis
- Neovascular glaucoma
- Tractional and rhegmatogenous retinal detachment.

PATHOGENESIS

- 50% of non-ischemic occlusions become ischemic in time.

SYSTEMIC FACTORS

- Systemic severe hypertension
- Atherosclerosis
- Diabetes mellitus often in association
- Renal failure.

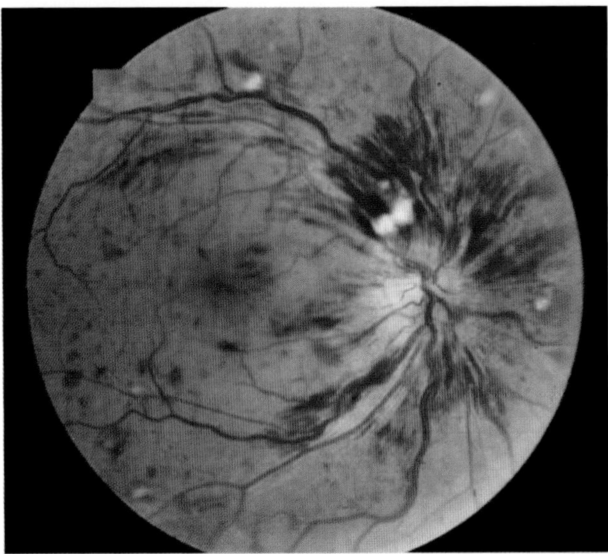

Fig. 1: Malignant hypertension (OD) typical round the clock hemorrhagic pattern congested veins and CWS indicating retinal ischemia

DIAGNOSIS

- Clinical appearances
- Fundus fluorescein angiography
  - Capillary non-perfusion

DIFFERENTIAL DIAGNOSIS

Shares many retinopathic features with other retinal vasculopathies such as diabetic retinopathy, vascular insufficiency retinopathy, central retinal vein occlusion.

PROGNOSIS

- Approximately 75% of visual acuity less than 6/12
- Better visual acuities associated with mild retinal ischemia
- Good initial visual acuity.

MANAGEMENT TREATMENT

- Hypertension treatment.

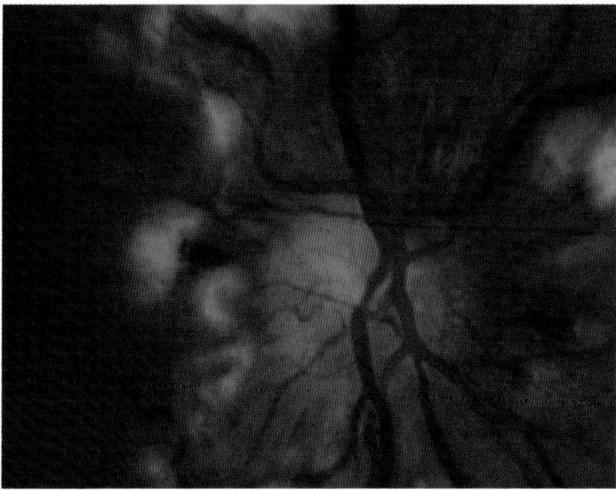

Fig. 2: Malignant hypertension—congested veins, papilledema and multiple CWS

Subhyaloid Hemorrhage

Shaifali Singla, Lalit Verma, Avnindra Gupta, Madhu Karna, Dinesh Talwar, HK Tewari (India)

INTRODUCTION

A hemorrhage at the macula causes sudden deterioration of the vision. The hemorrhage can be either subhyaloidal or subinternal limiting membrane subhyaloidal hemorrhage occurs at the interface between the posterior hyaloid and inner limiting membrane (ILM). Previously it was thought that subhyaloid and subinternal limiting membrane hemorrhage was same. But sub-ILM hemorrhage is located between the ILM and the retinal nerve fiber layer. It is now felt that true subhyaloid hemorrhages are probably quite rare. Sub-ILM hemorrhages have been described in a variety of clinical settings and often lead to severe visual impairment because of their predilection for the macular region. Subhyaloid hemorrhage can be caused by a variety of retinal disorders, the most common being valsalva retinopathy and Terson's syndrome. In addition, such hemorrhages may occur secondary to vascular diseases such as arteriosclerosis, hypertension, retinal artery or vein occlusion, diabetic retinopathy, retinal macroaneurysm, chorioretinitis, blood disorders as well as shaken baby syndrome, age related macular degeneration and can also occur spontaneously or as result of trauma.

SYMPTOMS AND SIGNS

1. Deterioration of visual acuity within seconds or minutes.
2. Slit lamp biomicroscopy reveales a dome shaped hemorrhage in the macular area.
3. OCT scan may be helpful in differentiating between subhyaloid and sub-ILM hemorrhages. In sub-ILM hemohage OCT scan just above the level of sedimented blood shows two distinct membranes; a single highly reflective band corresponding to the ILM and an overlapping patchy membrane with low optical reflectivity consistent with the posterior hyaloid.

COMPLICATIONS

Premacular subhyaloid hemorrhage is usually a benign condition that generally improves spontaneously in one to two months and rarely causes visual loss. However, the hemorrhage may cause permanent macular changes, formation of preretinal traction membrane and proliferative vitreoretinopathy.

26 years young computer professional male presented with sudden decrease in vision for the last two days. Visual acuity recorded was finger counting close to face in the right eye and 6/6 in the left eye. Anterior segment was normal in both the eyes and so was fundus examination in the left eye. Right eye fundus showed a large subhyaloid hemorrhage covering the whole of the macula.

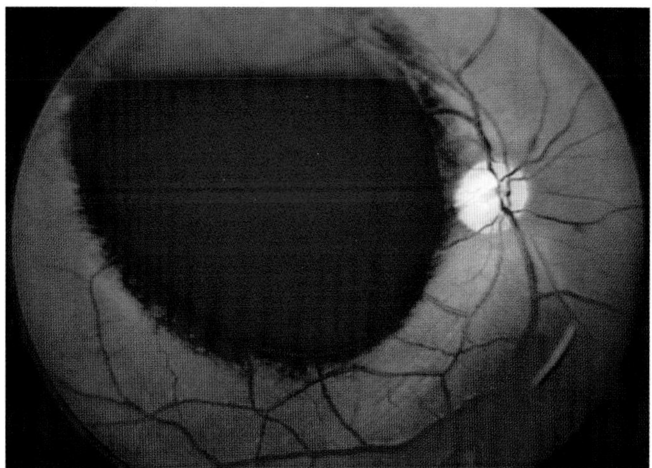

Fig. 1: Large subhyaloid hemorrhage

TREATMENT

Although treatment choices must consider the underlying disease, in clinical practice the primary aim of treatment is removal of the hemorrhage. In addition to the underlying disease, patients age, occupation, duration since onset of hemorrhage and the size of the hemorrhage are highly relevanrt factors affecting decisions regarding awaiting spontaneous resorption or administering treatment as well as regarding the type of treatment.

Observation for upto three months for spontaneous clearing of hemorrhage is a clinically accepted practice.

Laser drainage (hyaloidotomy) gives the entrapped blood a focal opening into the vitreous cavity and accelerates clearing and visual improvement.

In this patient conservative treatment option was discussed, but patient's occupation necessitated early visual rehabilitation. Hyaloidotomy option was then discussed with the patient and he opted for it. Hyaloidotomy was done in the most dependent part of the hemorrhage using double frequency YAG (532 nm). One minute after hyaloidotomy he felt better and his vision improved to 5/60 and after 10 minutes his vision was 6/36.

After 2 hours he regained vision of 6/9 in his right eye.

DIFFERENTIAL DIAGNOSIS

Subhyaloid Hemorrhage

Also known as premacular hemorrhage, preretinal hemorrhage.

Sub-ILM hemorrhage

Also known as macular hemorrhage.

PROGNOSIS

Although subhyaloid hemorrhage carries a good prognosis with conservative treatment but at times hyaloidotomy can be considered for faster visual rehabilitation. The only problem which hyaloidotomy can sometimes lead to is conversion of subhyaloid hemorrhage to intragel hemorrhage which may cause troublesome floaters.

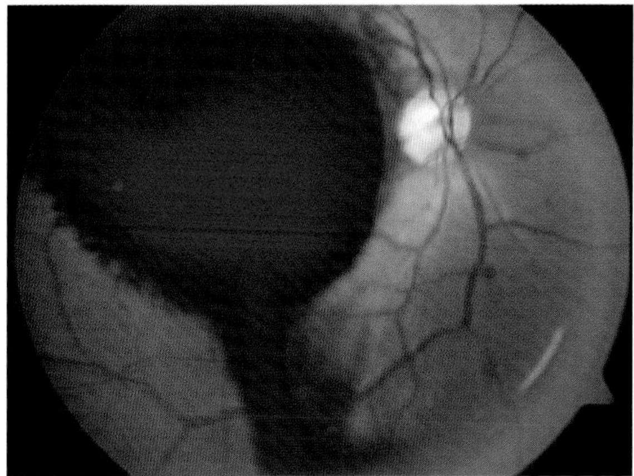

Fig. 2: One minute post-hyaloidotomy

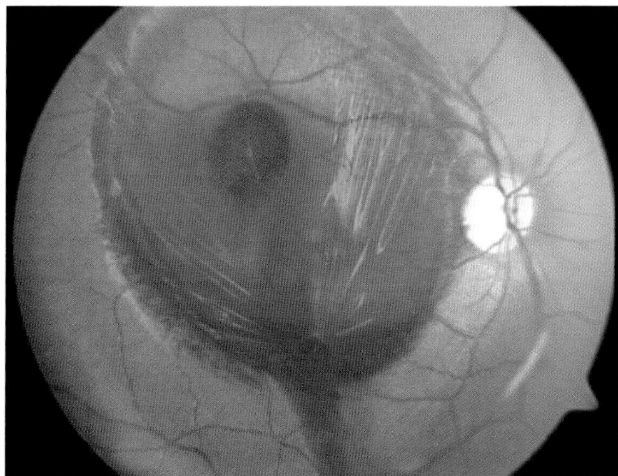

Fig. 3: Ten minutes post-hyaloidotomy

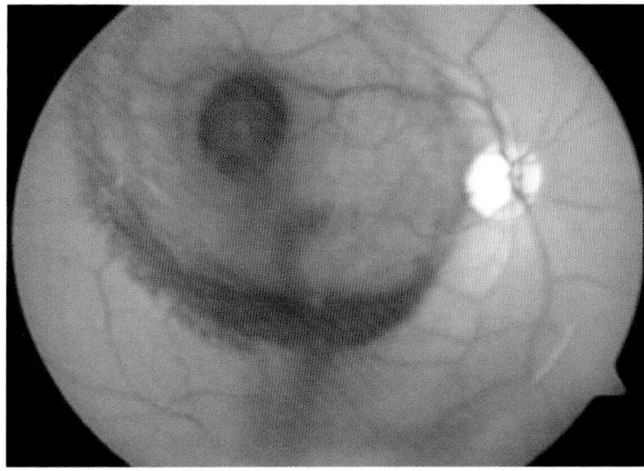

Fig. 4: Two hours post hyaloidotomy

CHAPTER FIVE

DIABETIC RETINOPATHY

- **DIABETIC RETINOPATHY – I**
  Javier Montero, Jose Ruiz Moreno, Amat-Peral P (Spain)
  - Nonproliferative Diabetic Retinopathy
  - Proliferative Diabetic Retinopathy
  - Diabetic Macular Edema
- **DIABETIC RETINOPATHY – II**
  T Mark Johnson (USA)
  - Nonproliferative Diabetic Retinopathy
  - Proliferative Diabetic Retinopathy
- **PROLIFERATIVE DIABETIC RETINOPATHY**
  Emanuel Rosen (UK)

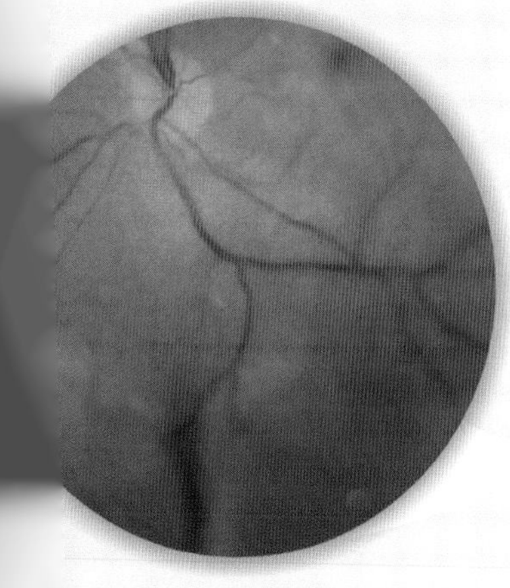

Diabetic Retinopathy–I

Javier Montero,Jose Ruiz Moreno, Amat-Peral P (Spain)

INTRODUCTION

A strict control of glycemia (fasting glycemia level under 110 mg/dL, HbA1c under 7%, diastolic arterial pressure under 80 mmHg, and systolic pressure under 140 mmHg, cholesterol levels under 200 mg/dL triglycerides under 150 mg/dL) is the best way to limit the progression of DR.

CLINICAL SIGNS AND SYMPTOMS (TABLE 1)

Nonproliferative DR

Microaneurysms/hemorrhages/lipidic or hard exudates/cotton wool spots/ vascular anomalies (veins: dilation, beading, duplication, loops, sheathing and perivascular exudates; arteries: local narrowing, occlusions and sheathing); intraretinal microvascular anomalies (IRMA).

Proliferative Diabetic Retinopathy (PDR)

First cause of severe vision loss in diabetics. New vessels on the optic disk and/ or the retina and into the hyaloid and vitreous cavity. Neovascularization is more frequent in the central 45° of the retina.

TABLE 1

Proposed disease severity level	*Findings on dilated ophthalmoscopy*
No apparent retinopathy	No abnormalities
Mild nonproliferative diabetic retinopathy	Microaneurysms only
Moderate nonproliferative diabetic retinopathy	More than just microaneurysms but less than severe nonproliferative diabetic retinopathy
Severe nonproliferative diabetic retinopathy	Any of the following: more than 2 intraretinal hemorrhages in each of 4 quadrants; definite venous beading in 2 quadrants; Prominent intraretinal microvascular abnormalities in 1 quadrant *And no* signs of proliferative retinopathy
Proliferative diabetic retinopathy	One or more of the following: neovascularization, vitreous/preretinal hemorrhage

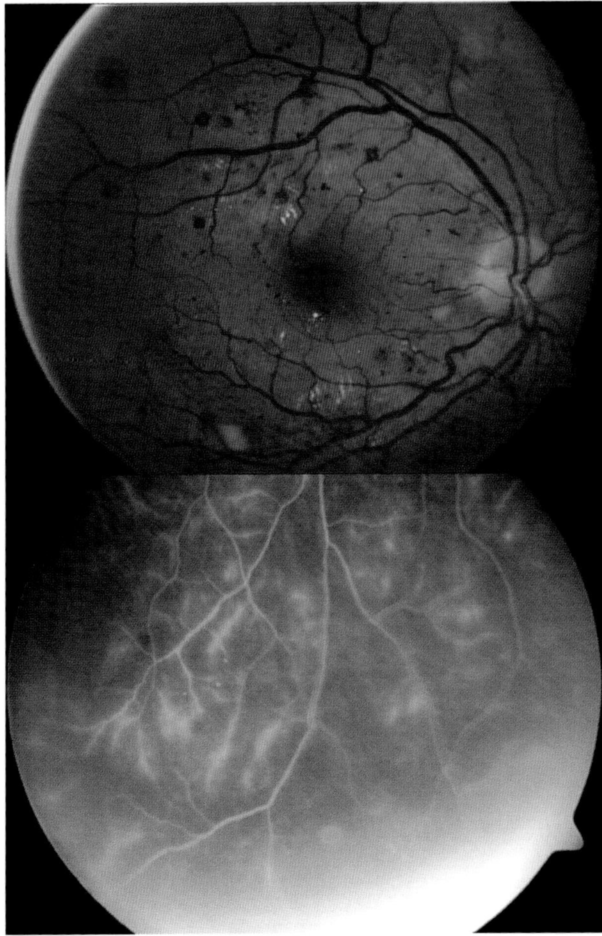

Fig. 1: Retinography and fluorescein angiography (FA) from one patient presenting peripheral ischemia. Notice the presence of hard exudates and vascular tortuosity

Diabetic Macular Edema (DME)

First cause of vision loss in diabetic patients. Fluid in the macula leaking from hyperpermeable capillaries, microaneurysms, IRMA or from the breakdown of the external blood-retinal barrier. DME is related with the levels of glycosilated hemoglobin, cardiovascular disease, diastolic hypertension, severe anemia, dyslipaemia, renal insufficiency, pregnancy, smoking habit and DR.

Usually as decreased visual acuity, color sensitivity, contrast sensitivity and dark adaptation.

Clinically significant DME (CSME): Retinal thickening within the central 500 microns from the fovea and/or hard exudates within the central 500 microns from the fovea with adjacent retinal thickening and/or areas of retinal thickening one disk area or bigger in size, at least in part within on disk diameter from the fovea.

Ophthalmic Examination

Biomicroscopy with dilated pupil and determination of best corrected visual acuity.

Fluorescein Angiography

Determination of ischemic areas, guidance of laser treatment in cases of clinically significant macular edema, ascertain the cause of unexplained visual acuity loss, identification of ischemic and neovascularized areas (occasionally).

B Scan

Vitreous hemorrhages, cataracts or any other media opacity, preparation for vitreoretinal surgery.

Optical Coherence Tomography (OCT)

Decision making of therapy, follow up of the treatment, clarification of fibroglial preretinal tissue and vitreoretinal traction.

Edema Staging

- E1: Diffuse macular thickening.
- E2: Cystoid macular edema.
  - — E2a: 2-4 central cysts with mild retinal thickening.
  - — E2b: Petaloidal cystic configuration or one large central cyst.
  - — E2c: Multiple coalescent cysts
- E3: Serous detachment.

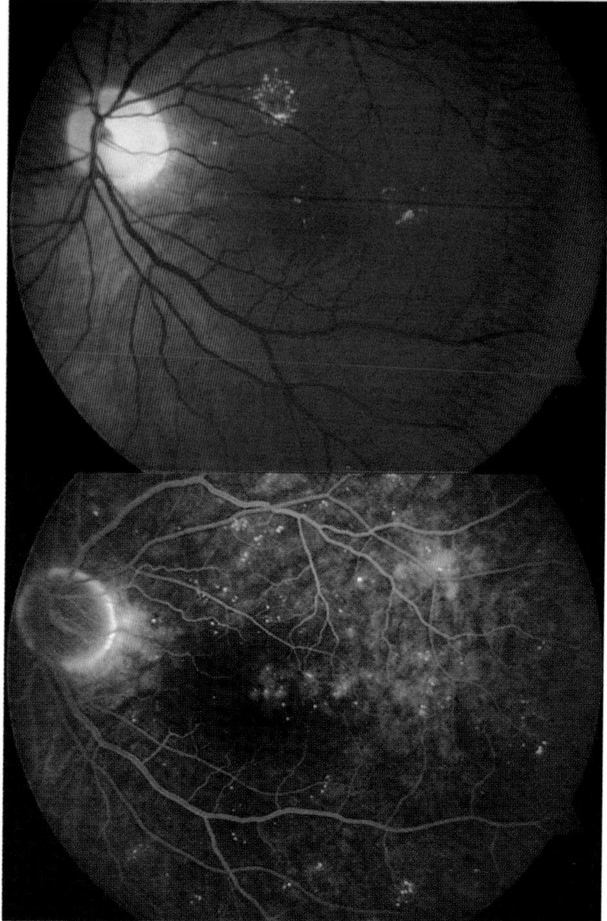

Fig. 2: Macular edema identification based on retinal thickening and presence of hard exudates in retinography. FA shows fluorescein leakage pinting out at the area to be treated

INVESTIGATION

Intravitreal Triamcinolone Acetate (TA)

As a unique therapy or in association with laser photocoagulation in doses 4 to 20 mg inducing reduction in macular edema (OCT and FA) and moderate improvement in visual acuity. Repeated injections every three to six months are frequently needed. Persistence of macular edema and ischemia may worsen visual prognosis.

In association with cataract surgery in patients with macular edema, or when media opacity hinders photocoagulation or the desired effect of the laser has not been achieved.

In association with vitrectomy in patients with diabetic retinopathy and tracional retinal detachment reducing the frequency of recurrent detachment and vitreoretinal proliferation.

Intravitreal Pegaptanib (0.3 mg every six weeks)

To treat CSME improving visual acuity reducing macular edema and need for focal photocoagulation. May also induce regression of retinal new vessels.

Intravitreal Bevacizumab (1.25 or 2.5 mg repeated on demand)

Induces cessation of fluorescein leakage from new vessels and reduction in the retinal area affected by neovascularization. The duration of the effect is limited and may be variable. May be associated with improvement in visual acuity. Injected 2 to 11 days before surgery may reduce vitreoretinal neovascular activity and is useful as adjuvant to vitreoretinal surgery, reducing the risk of bleeding during and after surgery. To reduce the duration of vitreous hemorrhages after vitrectomy. To treat anterior segment neovascularization by the injection of 1 mg in the anterior chamber or 1.25 mg. Intravitreal bevacizumab in non vitrectomized eyes may increase the risk of vitreoretinal traction from new vessels and subsequent tractional retinal detachments.

Intravitreal Ranibizumab

- To reduce macular edema and improve visual acuity.
- Protein kinase C inhibitors.

DIFFERENTIAL DIAGNOSIS

None of the lesions is pathognomonic of DR. Other vascular retinopathies (arterial hypertension, retinal vein occlusion), blood dyscrasias (anemia, policitemia, leukemia), increased plasmatic viscosity and other endocrine disorders should be considered.

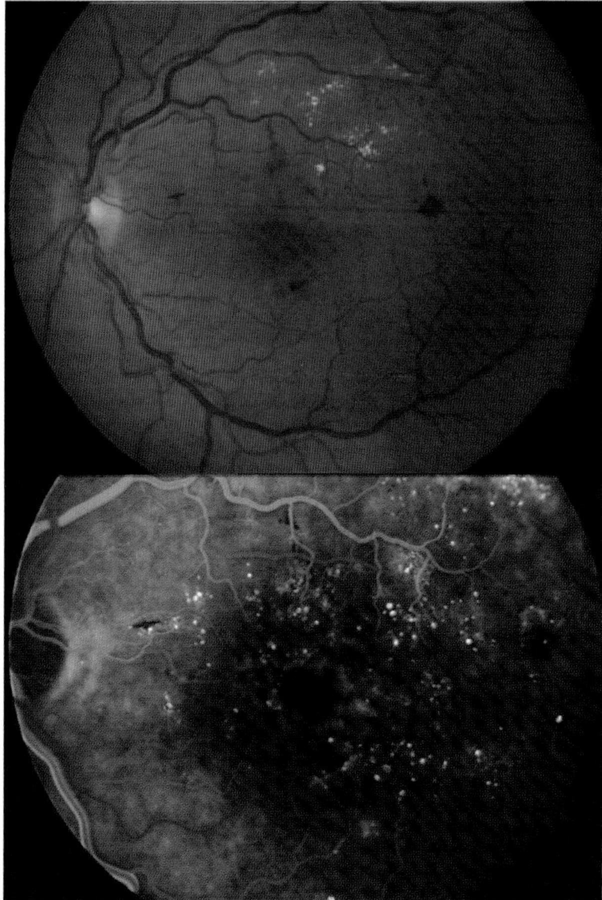

Fig. 3: Macular ischemia with increased foveal avascular zone with irregular borders, widened intercapillary areas in the perifoveal anastomotic circle, dilated and hyperfluorescent capillaries and appearance of microaneurysms near the fovea

TREATMENT

Laser Photocoagulation

Patients should be warned about the risks of laser photocoagulation. They should also be aware that the aim of laser treatment is not visual acuity gain but avoiding severe loss of vision.

Indications

DME: Always supported by a correct metabolic control of glycemia, blood pressure and hiperlipemia. Laser treatment is more useful in cases with focal than in diffuse DME. Laser treatment usually does not improve visual acuity and only reduces vision loss. Exposure time < 0.1 s, 75 to 100 microns. Treatment is performed on the aneurysms causing CSME located within 500 and 3000 microns from the fovea. Consider new treatment within 300 microns from the fovea in cases of persistent macular edema with visual acuity < 0.5 and preserved perifoveal capillary net. Microaneurysm > 4 microns may be treated by confluent laser treatment or grid laser.

Focal photocoagulation should be performed in cases of localized retinal thickening on the leaking areas causing CSME located within 500 and 3000 microns from the center of the fovea.

Grid laser (0.1 s exposure, 100 to 200 microns spots, distance between two contiguous impacts should be the diameter of one impact) should be performed on areas with diffuse retinal thickening causing CSME within 500 and 3000 microns from the center of the fovea; and/or on avascular zones associated with CSME located within 500 and 3000 microns from the center of the fovea.

There is a significant risk of vision loss associated with CSME within the central 500 microns urging laser treatment. Treatment is not so urgent in cases with normal visual acuity and hard exudates within 500 microns from the center of the fovea; in these cases laser is recommended whenever the risk for decreased visual acuity associated with laser treatment is small or the patient cannot be properly followed.

In cases with retinal thickening smaller than one disk area located within one disk diameter from the center of the fovea the risk of vision loss is low, so these patients may be followed and the treatment deferred. Non clinically significant macular edema does not require laser treatment, progression is slow and there is no evidence of benefit with laser treatment.

Patients should be examined 3 to 4 months after laser treatment and a new laser treatment should be considered in cases of persistence of the edema.

Proliferant DR is treated by panretinal laser in cases with transparent media in cases with neovascular glaucoma, rubeosis iridis and high risk PDR (optic disk neovascularization greater than ¼ of the disk area and/or optic disk neovascularization associated with vitreous hemorrhage, and/or retinal

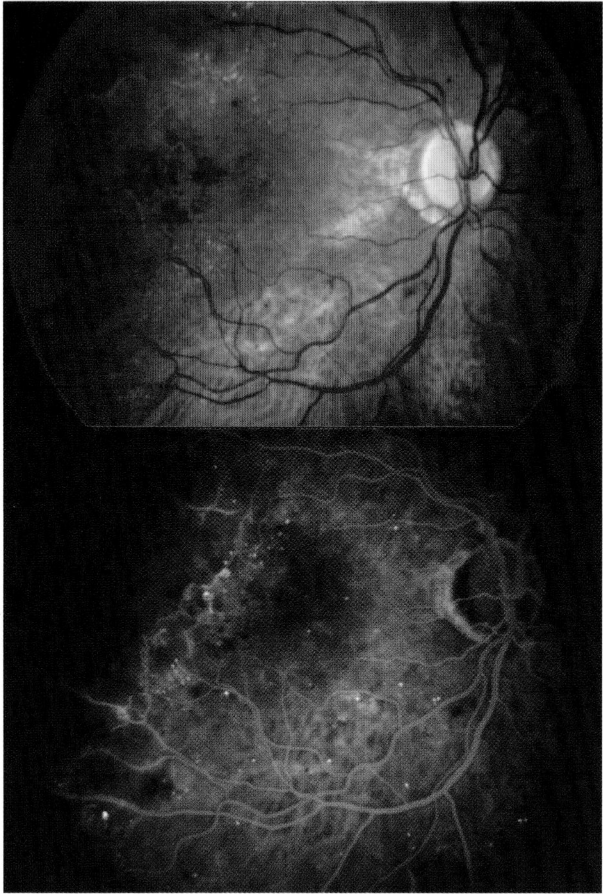

Fig. 4: Macular ischemia with increased foveal avascular zone. IRMA can be seen temporal to the fovea as anastomosis linking venous territories

neovascularization greater than ¼ of the disk area associated with vitreous hemorrhage).

The aim of panretinal laser is to achieve the destruction of ischemic retina reducing the production of proangiogenic factors stabilizing DR and reducing the risk of severe vision loss. 0.1 to 0.5 s exposure, 500 micron diameter, performed regularly, not affecting retinal vessels, and in the area between the equator of the eye and 3000 microns away from the fovea (1800 to 2000 impacts 500 microns wide; 2 to 4 sessions in 3 to 6 weeks). Control in 4 months time.

Complications: Pain, preretinal membranes. intraretinal, choroidal or intravítreal hemorrhages, subretinal fibrosis, choroidal neovascularization, choroidal effusion; macular photocoagulation may affect the fovea causing central scotoma.

Anterior segment complications: Corneal erosions, loss of endothelial cells, direct burns on the cornea, iris and crystalline lens.

Cryotherapy

Cryotherapy induces retinal ablation, reducing the production of proangiogenic factors. Cryotherapy is performed through the sclera, not requiring transparent media and reaching peripheral retina.

Indications

Persistence of neovascularization after panretinal laser, non transparent media, narrow pupils, persistent vitreous hemorrhages, neovascularization of the sclerotomies.

Side Effects

Vitreous contraction, intraocular inflammation.
Peribulbar or retrobulbar anesthesia. –70° C allowing the probe to freeze during 10 to 14 seconds, 10 to 12 applications per row in 3 to 4 rows.

Surgery

Indications of vitrectomy in patients with DR are:

- Vitreous hemorrhages, anterior segment neovascularization, fibrinoid syndrome
- Macular edema, macular pucker
- Rhegmatogenous/tractional retinal detachment, progressive fibrovascular proliferation
- Anterior hyaloidal fibrovascular proliferation, posterior hyaloidal opacification

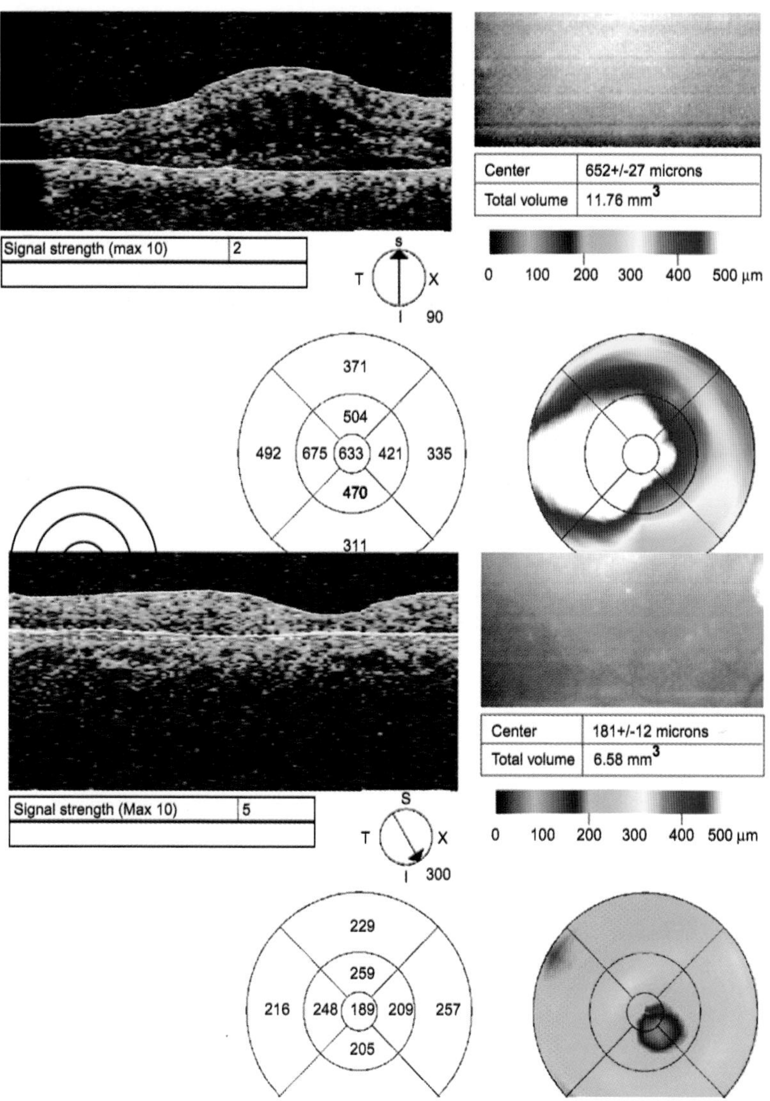

Fig. 5: Quantitative determinations of macular edema with OCT. Notice the reduction of macular edema (reduction in retinal thickness) after intravitreal injection of triamcinolone

PROGNOSIS

Visual prognosis may range from normal visual acuity to amaurosis. The appearance of DR and complications will be related to the control of the metabolic syndrome and arterial hypertension, the duration of the diabetic condition and early diagnosis and treatment.

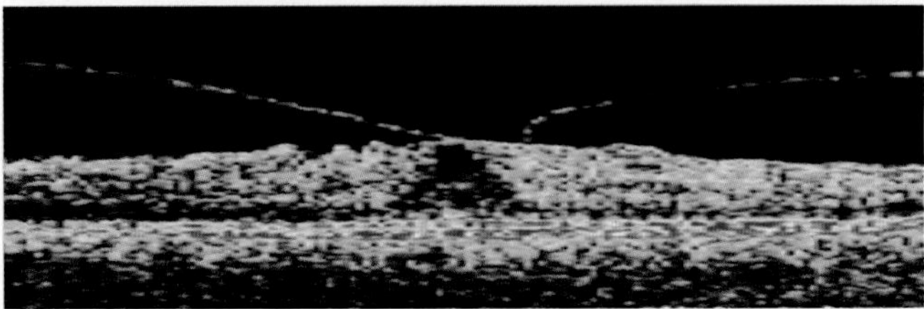

Fig. 6: Macular edema secondary to anterior traction from the posterior hyaloid in a diabetic patient

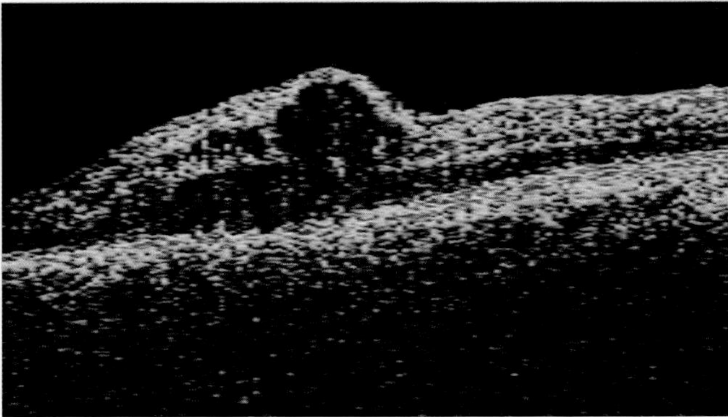

Fig. 7: Eversion of foveal depression as early stage macular edema in a diabetic patient

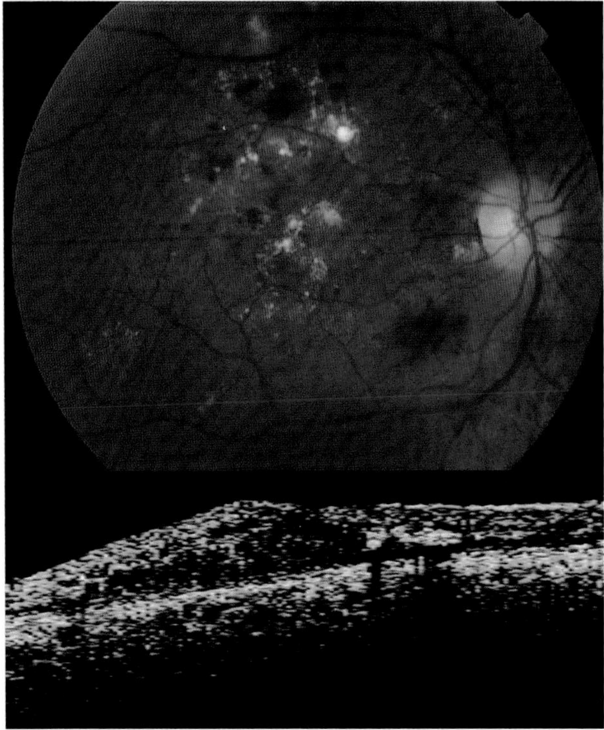

Fig. 8: Diffuse macular edema with hyporreflective retina. Notice the presence of a hyperreflective area corresponding to hard exudates

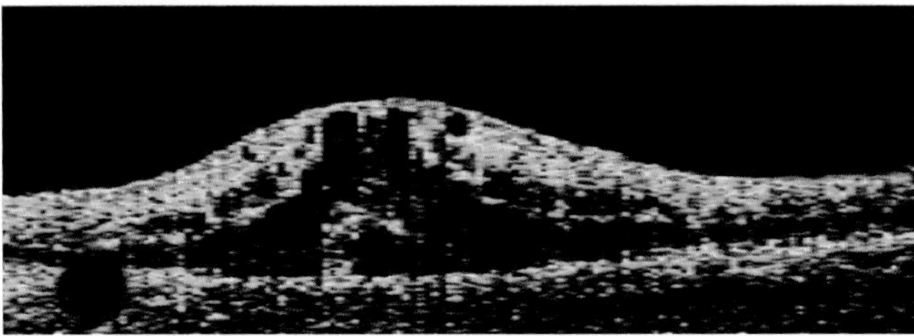

Fig. 9: Cystoid macular edema shown as hyporeflective rounded areas separated by thin normoreflective walls

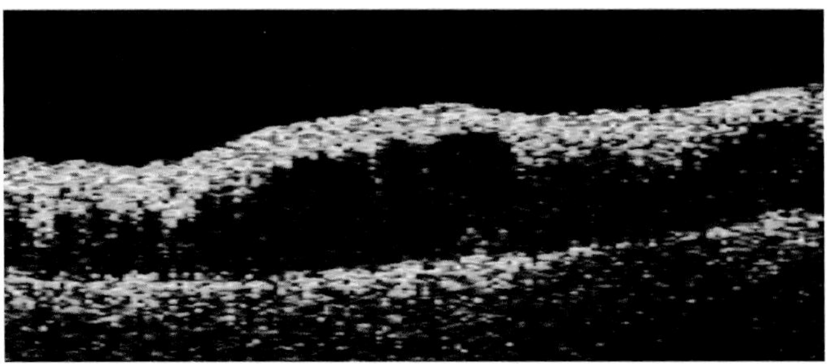

Fig. 10: Multiple cystic spaces and presence of subretinal fluid

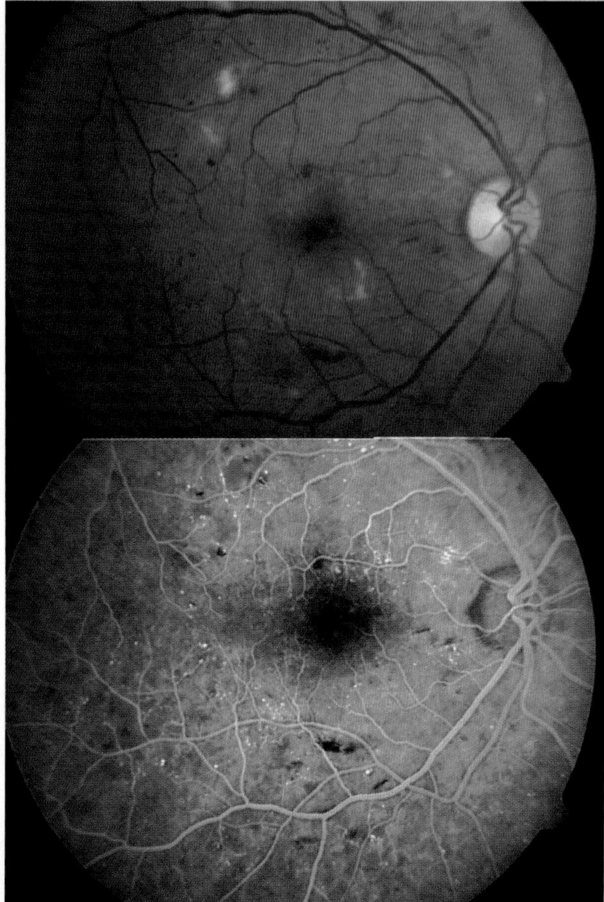

Fig. 11: Multiple microaneurysms can be seen as small red dots in the macula in retinography, and as hyperfluorescent dots in FA. Larger red lesions can be identified as hemorrhages by their angiographic behavior as hypofluorescent lesions

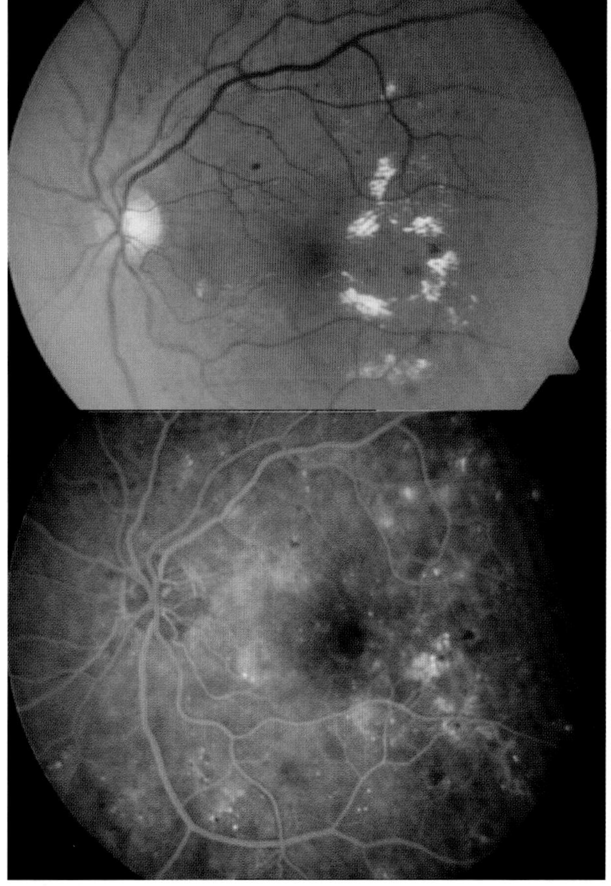

Fig. 12: Hard exudates located surrounding active microaneurysms

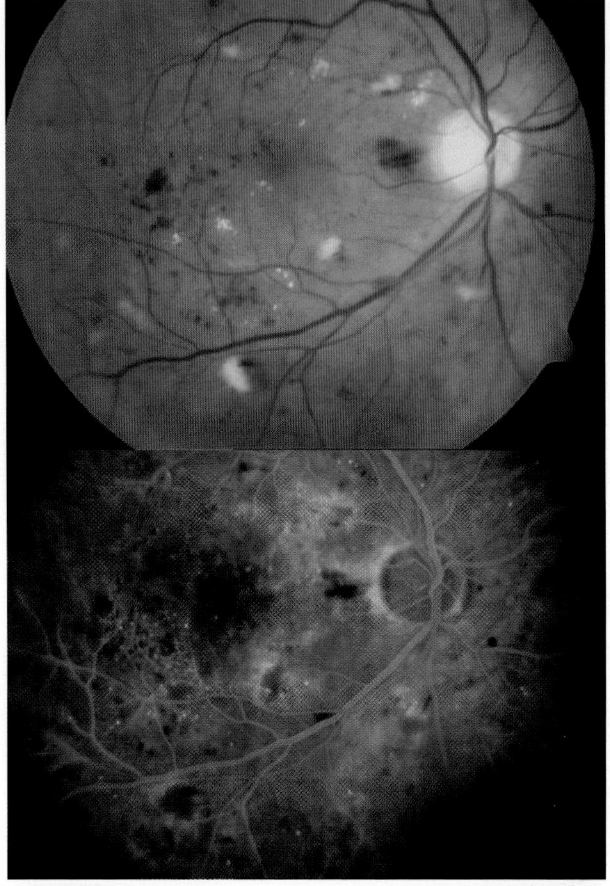

Fig. 13: Cotton wool spots appear as local hypofluorescent and low perfused areas, usually surrounded by dilated capillaries which leak and stain in FA

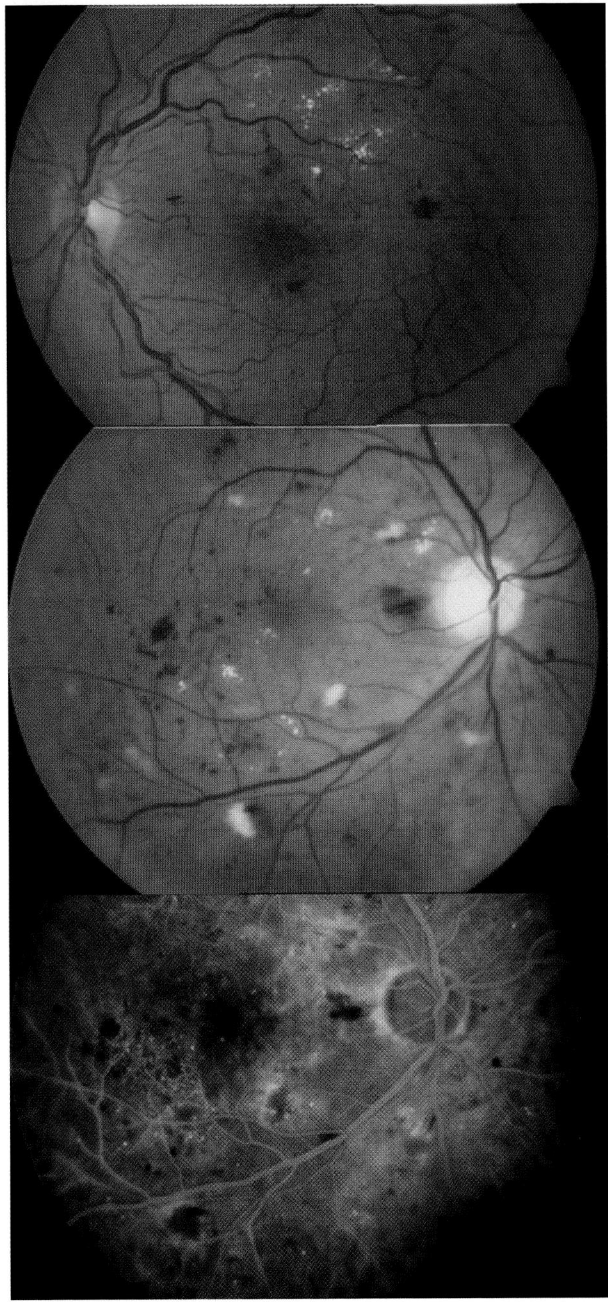

Fig. 14: Vascular anomalies may appear in veins as locally dilated areas, venous beading, duplication, loops, sheathing and perivascular exudates

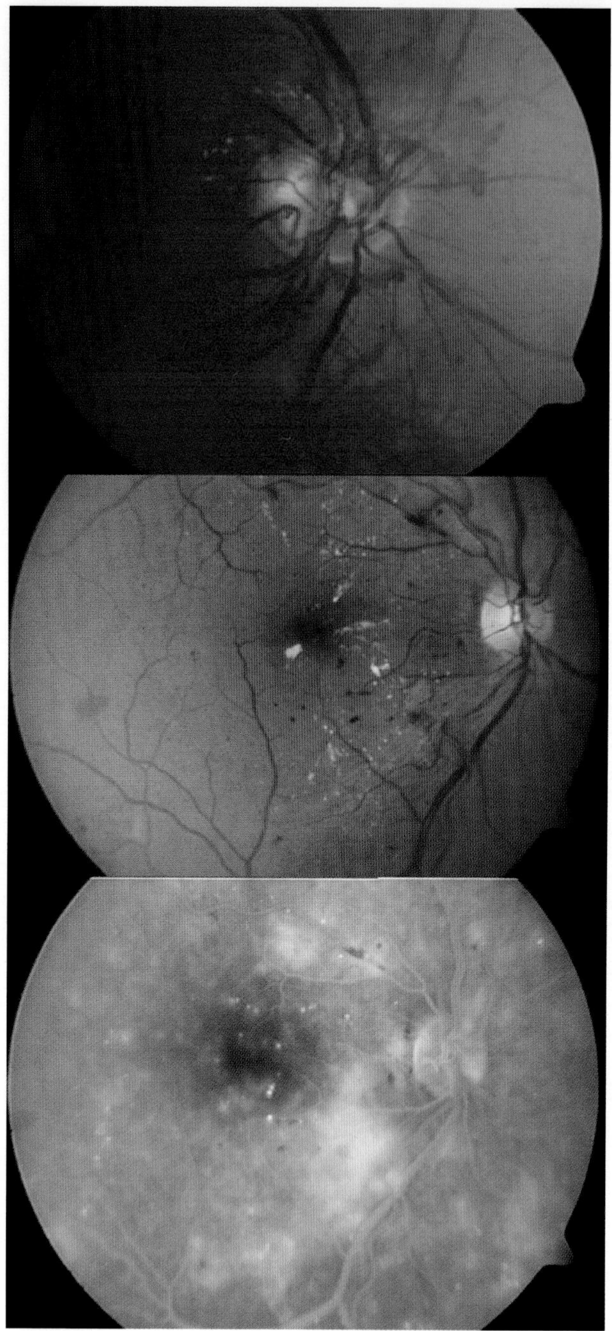

Fig. 15

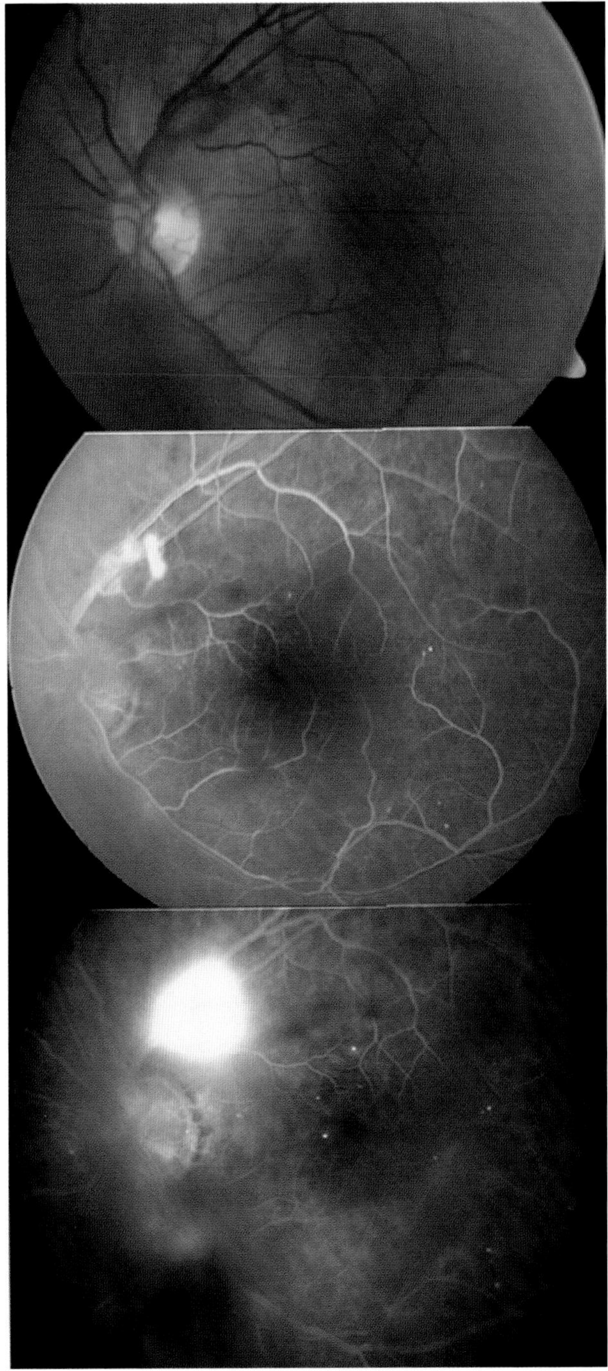

Fig. 16

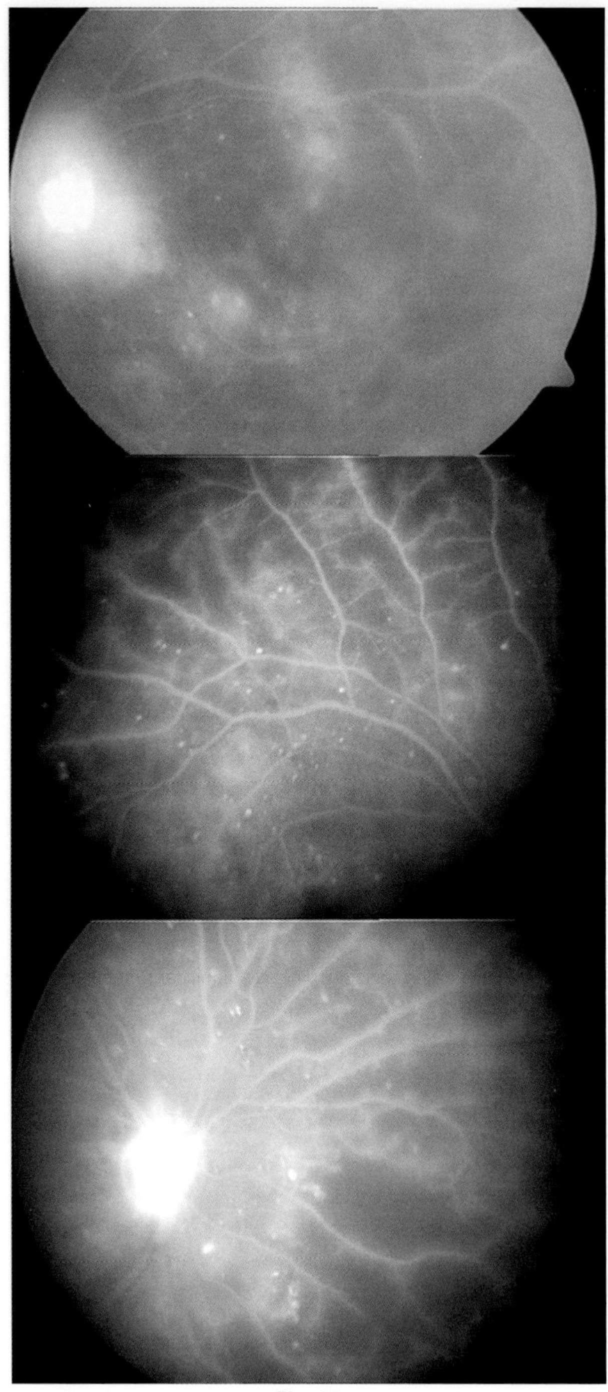

Fig. 17

Figs 15 to 17: FA shows ischemic arear limited by retinal neovascularization. Notice the intense leakage from retinal new vessels

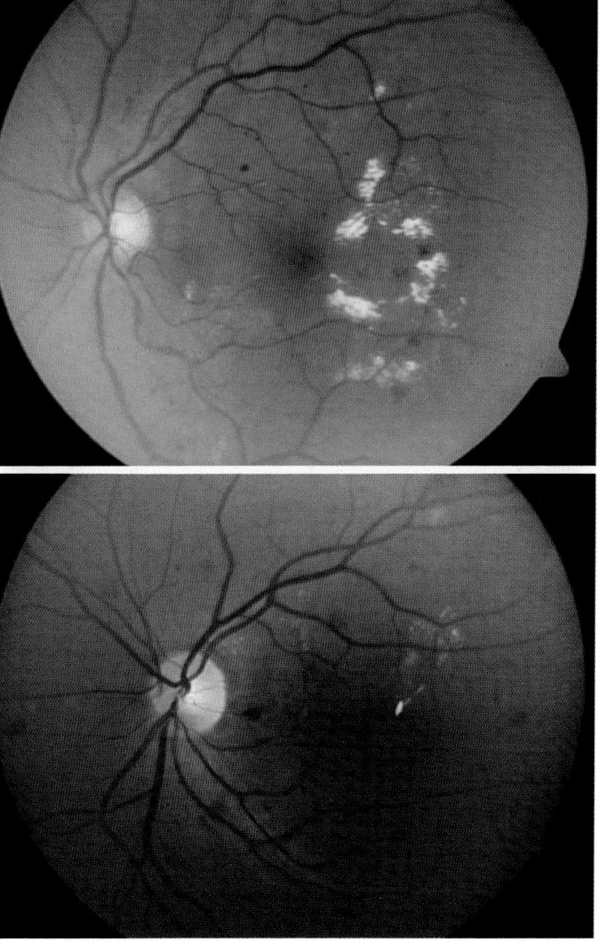

Fig. 18: Hard exudates causing clinically significant macular edema

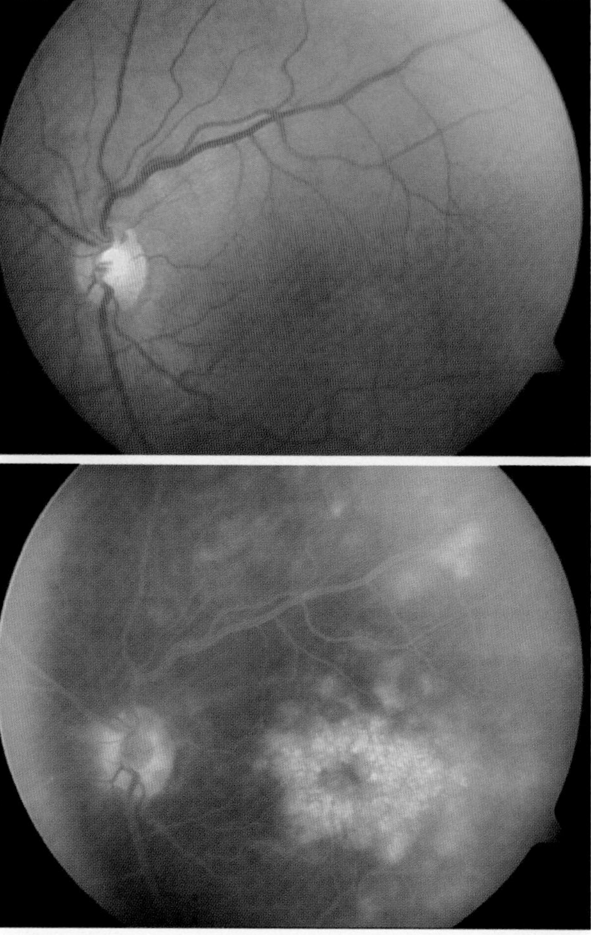

Fig. 19: Retinal thickening with marked diffuse macular edema

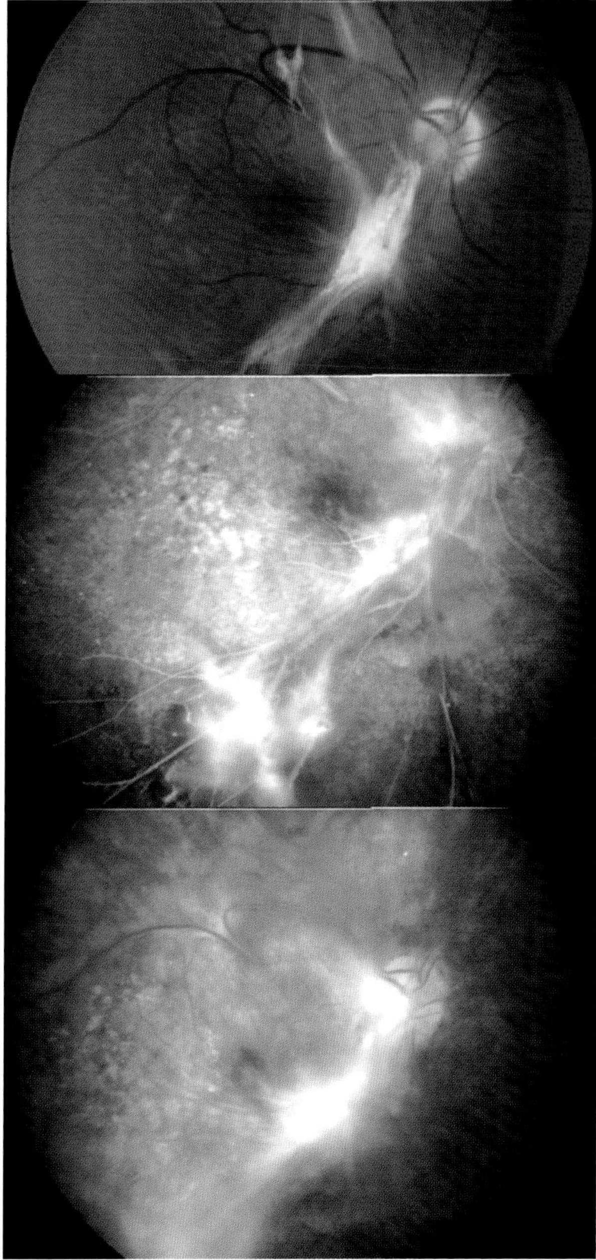

Fig. 20: Fibrovascular proliferation in PDR

Diabetic Retinopathy–II

T Mark Johnson (USA)

INTRODUCTION

Prevalence

- Prevalence of diabetes is increasing
- Estimated prevalence of diabetes in the United States is approximately 8% of the total population
  - — 30% of patients are undiagnosed
- All diabetics will develop some retinopathy
- The prevalence of retinopathy varies with:
  - — Type of diabetes
  - — Duration of diabetes
    - – Type I diabetes
      - - > 10 years duration: 70% have retinopathy
      - - > 30 years : 95% have retinopathy
    - – Type II diabetes
      - - > 16 years : 60% have retinopathy

Incidence

- 10 year incidence of retinopathy
  - — Type I diabetes without retinopathy at baseline
    - – 89% will develop some retinopathy
  - — Type II diabetes without retinopathy at baseline
    - – 79% will develop some retinopathy

CLINICAL SIGNS AND SYMPTOMS

Symptoms

- Asymptomatic
- Decreased visual acuity
- Floaters.

Signs

Nonproliferative Diabetic Retinopathy (NPDR)

- Retinal microaneurysms: outpouchings of the capillary walls
- Dot and blot-shaped hemorrhages

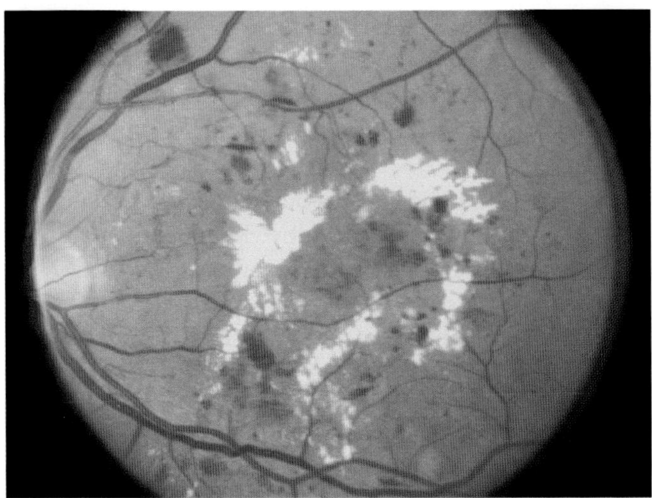

Fig. 1: Diabetic macular edema

- Venous caliber changes: venous "beading" and tortuosity
  — Indicative of increasing retinal edema
- Intraretinal microvascular abnormalities (IRMA): comprised of early neovascularization within the retina or shunting vessels in of poor capillary perfusion
- Cotton-wool spots: infarctions in the nerve fiber layer of the retina
- Higher risk of progression to Proliferative Retinopathy with:
  — Severe retinal hemorrhages in four quadrants
  — Venous beading in two quadrants
  — IRMA in two quadrants

Proliferative Diabetic Retinopathy (PDR)

- Neovascularization: on or near the optic disc (NVD) or elsewhere (NVE), often located at the watershed zone between perfused and non-perfused retina
- High Risk Proliferative Retinopathy
  — Any neovascularization with vitreous hemorrhage
  — Neovacsularization greater than ½ disk area
- Fibrovascular proliferation: often beginning at the optic disk and vascular arcades
- Pre-retinal hemorrhage: adjacent to or within areas of neovascularization
- Vitreous hemorrhage
- Tractional retinal detachment
- Rhegmatogenous retinal detachment: from retinal tears and holes secondary to traction

Diabetic Macular Edema

- Cystoid macular edema: leakage of capillaries into cystoid spaces within the outer plexiform layer of the retina
- Retinal thickening: within or adjacent to the center of the macula
- Hard exudates: lipid which precipitated as intraretinal fluid was absorbed
- Clinically Significant Macular Edema
  — Retinal thickening within 500 microns of center of FAZ
  — Hard exudates within 500 microns from center of FAZ associated with retinal thickening
  — Retinal thickening > 1 disk diameter within 1 disk diameter of the center of the FAZ

INVESTIGATIONS

Fluorescein Angiography

- Diabetic macular edema

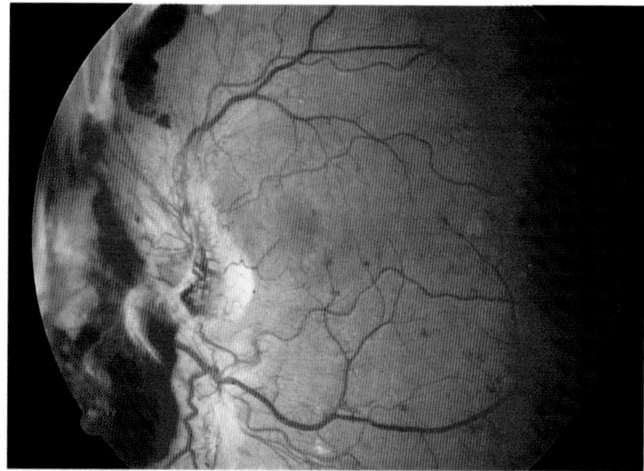

Fig. 2: Proliferative diabetic retinopathy

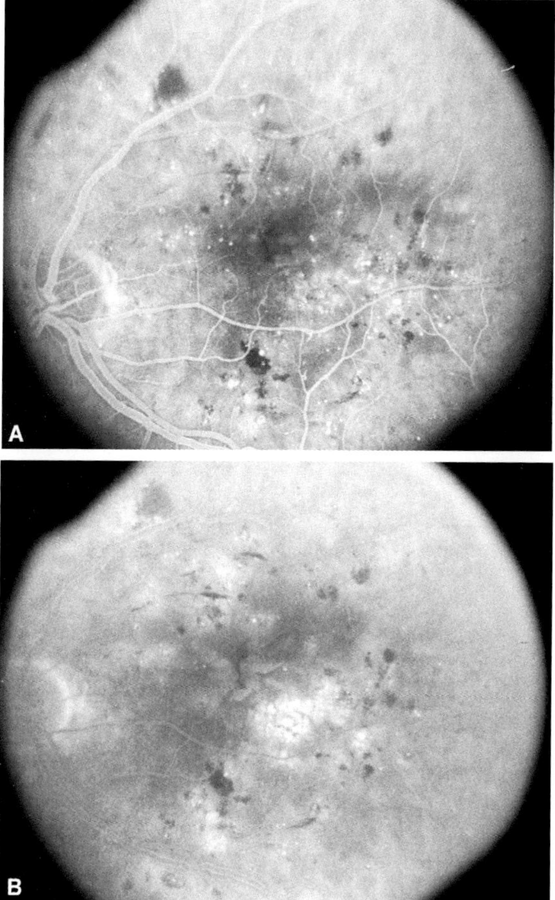

Figs 3A and B: Fluorescein angiography

- — Hyperfluorescent microaneuryms with late leakage
- — Diffuse late leakage
  - – Generalized vascular leakage
  - – Associated with midperipheral capillary nonperfusion
- — Capillary nonperfusion
- Proliferative retinopathy
  - — Early, preretinal vascular complexes that leak diffusely late
  - — Occur at margin of perfused and nonperfused retina

Optical Coherence Tomography

- Can localize and determine the extent of macular edema
  - — Volumetric maps may be useful in monitoring therapy
- Can determine the extent of tractional forces on the retina from fibrovascular proliferation.

Ultrasonography

Indicated if posterior segment cannot be visualized due to vitreous hemorrhage or other media opacification.

Differential Diagnosis

- Branch retinal vein occlusion
- Central retinal vein occlusion
- Anemia
- Hypertensive retinopathy
- Radiation retinopathy
- Blood dyscrasia
- Parafoveal telangiectasis.

TREATMENT

Prevention

Indications

Primary and secondary prevention of retinopathy.

Methods

- Intensive therapy to maintain glucose control
- Hemoglobin A1C should be maintained < 7%.

Results

Large trials demonstrate beneficial effects of excellent glycemic control in type I and type II diabetes.

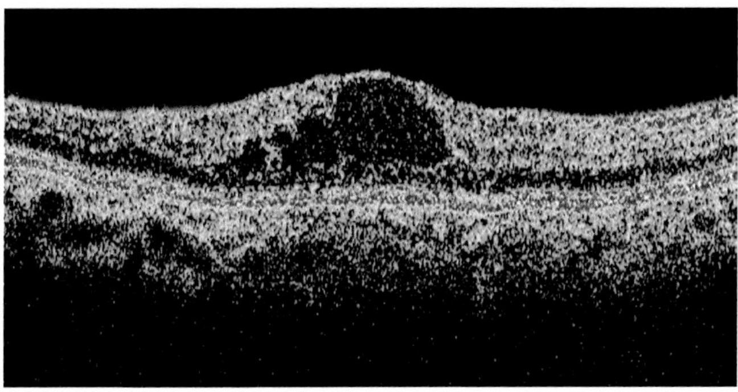

Fig. 4: Optical coherence tomography

Ophthalmic Screening Eye examination

- Baseline exam
  - — Type I: 5 years after onset or in puberty
  - — Type II: At time of diagnosis
- Follow up is determined by the severity of retinopathy
  - — 1 year incidence of progression to PDR
    - Mild NPDR : 0.8%
    - Moderate NPDR : 3%
    - Severe NPDR : 40%

Laser Photocoagulation

- Focal laser treatment indications:
  - — Indications
    - Clinically significant macular edema
  - — Methods
    - Focal application of laser to microaneurysms to achieve light blanching
      - Grid laser may be applied to areas of diffuse retinal thickening
  - — Results
    - Randomized trial of laser has demonstrated a significantly reduced risk of visual loss with laser therapy
      - Fewer patients regained significant amounts of vision
    - Focal laser may be less effective in cases of extensive diffuse macular edema
- Panretinal photocoagulation
  - — Indications
    - High-risk PDR
    - Nonhigh-risk in PDR in patients with poor compliance
    - Severe NPDR in select patients

- — Methods
    - 1600 – 2000 200 micron burns in retinal periphery
    - Multiple sessions reduces risk of choroidal effusion
- — Results
    - PRP reduces the risk of severe visual loss in patients with high risk PDR
    - PRP reduces risk of severe visual loss in non high risk PDR and severe NPDR, however, the risk of severe visual loss is lower in these patient groups

Corticosteroids

Indications

Non-responsive macular edema.

Methods

Intravitreal or sub Tenon triamcinolone.

Results

- Numerous case series demonstrate clear reduction in retinal edema
    - — No large randomized trials published to date
- May be associated with significant visual improvement in some cases
- Effects of treatment may be transient with edema recurring in 4 to 6 months.

Anti VEGF Therapy

Indications

- Non-responsive macular edema
- Proliferative diabetic retinopathy.

Methods

- Serial intravitreal injections
- Ongoing studies examining the role of pegaptanib sodium, bevacizumab and ranibizumab.

Results

- Proliferative diabetic retinopathy
    - — post injection rapid regression of neovascularization
    - — unclear what the long term durability of treatment will be
    - — likely will have a role in combination with laser
- Diabetic macular edema

— post-injection improvement of macular edema noted
— unclear what long term durability of treatment will be
— ongoing clinical trials in progress.

Surgical

Indications

- Non clearing vitreous hemorrhage
- Vitreo-macular traction with visual loss
- Tractional retinal detachment.

Methods

- Pars plana vitrectomy
- Complete removal of posterior hyaloid and associated epiretinal membranes
- Complete photocoagulation.

BIBLIOGRAPHY

1. Adamis AP, Altaweel M, Bressler NM, et al. Changes in retinal neovascularization after pegaptanib (Macugen) therapy in diabetic individuals. Ophthalmol. 2006;113:23-8.
2. DCCT Group. The effect of intensive treatment of diabetes on the development and progression of long term complications in insulin dependent diabetes mellitus. New Engl J Med 1993;329:977-86.
3. Diabetic Retinopathy Study Group. Indications for photocoagulation. Report #14. Int Ophth Clin 1987;27(4);239-253, Winter.
4. Diabetic Retinopathy Study Group. Photocoagulation treatment of proliferative diabetic retinopathy. Report #8. Ophth 1981;88;583-600.
5. ETDRS Group. Photocoagulation for diabetic macular edema:report number 4. Int Ophth Clin. 1987;27;265-72.
6. ETDRS Group. Treatment techniques and clinical guidelines for photocoagulation of diabetic macular edema. Ophth 1987;94;761-74.
7. ETDRS Study Group. Early photocoagulation for diabetic retinopathy. Ophth. 1991;98 (suppl):766-85.
8. Klein R, et al. The Wisconsin study of diabetic retinopathy II. Prevalence and risk of diabetic retinopathy when age at diagnosis is less than 30 years. Arch Ophth 1984;102:520-26.
9. Klein R, et al. The Wisconsin study of diabetic retinopathy III. Prevalence and risk of diabetic retinopathy when age at diagnosis is greater than 30 years. Arch Ophth 1984;102:527-32.
10. Klein R, Klein B, Moss SE, et al. The Wisconsin Epidemiologic Study of Diabetic Retinopathy XIV : 10 year incidence and progression of diabetic retinopathy. Arch Ophth 1994;112;1217-28.

Proliferative Diabetic Retinopathy

Emanuel Rosen (UK)

INTRODUCTION

Advanced form of diabetic retinopathy in response to retinal ischaemia. Will lead to blindness unless treated by retinal photocoagulation. Pan retinal photocoagulation usually required.

CLINICAL SIGNS AND SYMPTOMS

New vessel formation at optic nerve head (NVD) and elsewhere in retina (NVE).

COMPLICATIONS

- Retinal bleeding at all levels
- Intravitreal hemorrhage
- Retinal traction detachment
- Retinal rheumatogenous detachment
- Maular traction
- Macular oedema.

PATHOGENESIS

Angionenic factors (vascular growth factors) respond to retinal ishemia.

INVESTIGATIONS

- Retinal fluorescein angiography
- OCT retina.

DIAGNOSIS

Ophthalmoscopy

DIFFERENTIAL DIAGNOSIS

Hypertensive retinopathy, retinal vascular occlusive disease, retinopathies of anemia and leucemia.

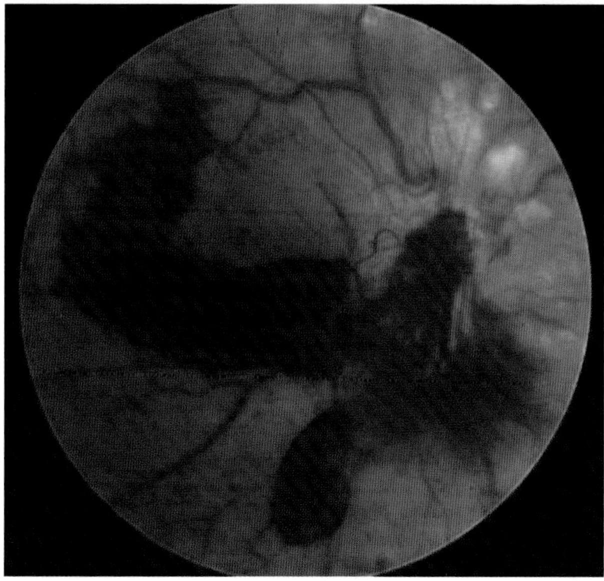

Fig. 1: Proliferative diabetic retinopathy with NVD and intravitreal hemorrhage

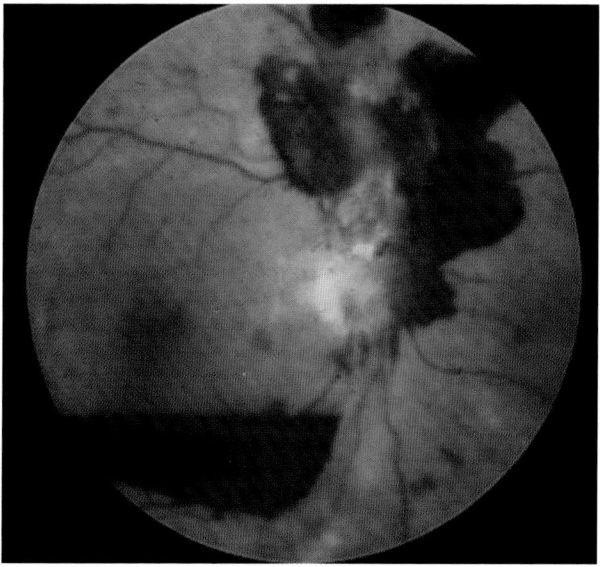

Fig. 2: Proliferative diabetic retinopathy with NVD and Sub-hyaloid pooled hemorrhage

TREATMENT AND PROGNOSIS

- Pan-retinal photocoagulation
- Vitrectomy
- Retinal surgery

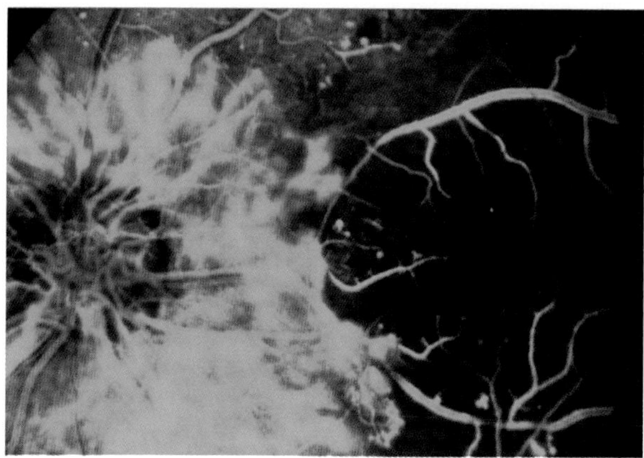

Fig. 3: FFA ischemic diabetic retinopathy with gross NVD showing. Typical NV incontinence to fluorescein molecules

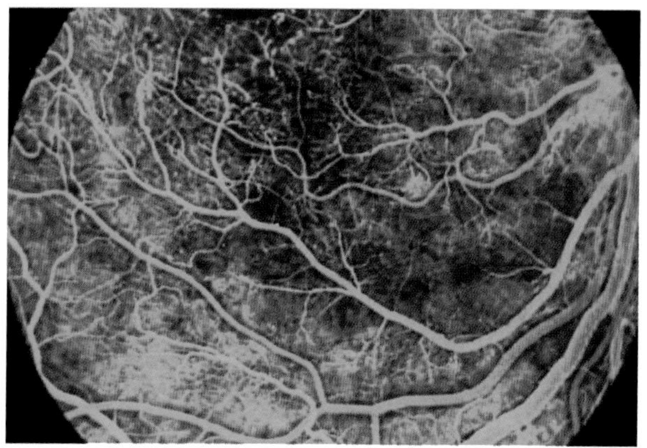

Fig. 4: FFA Diabetic retinopathy showing general retinal capillary permeability enabling microcirculation visualisation

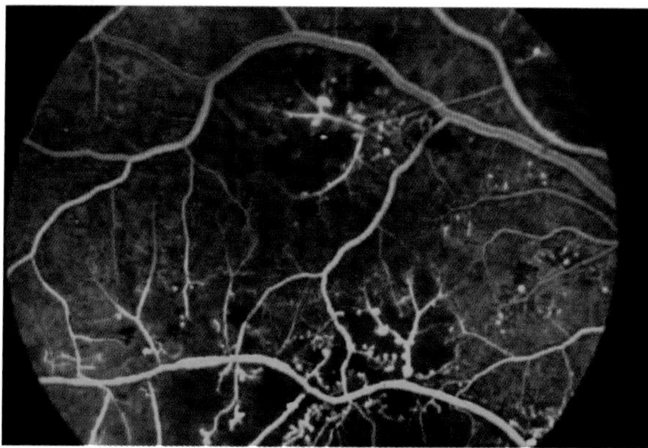

Fig. 5: FFA diabetic retinopathy showing ischemic areas (capillary non-perfusion), arteriolar calibre variations and attenuation with multiple micro-aneurysms and hemorrhages (black)

CHAPTER
SIX

PEDIATRIC DISEASES

- **RETINOPATHY OF PREMATURITY**
  Anjli Hussain, Nazimul Hussain, Sundaram Natarajan (India)
- **BEST'S DISEASE OR BEST'S VITELLIFORM MACULAR DYSTROPHY**
  Nazimul Hussain, Anjli Hussain (India)
- **GYRATE ATROPHY**
  Nazimul Hussain, Anjli Hussain (India)

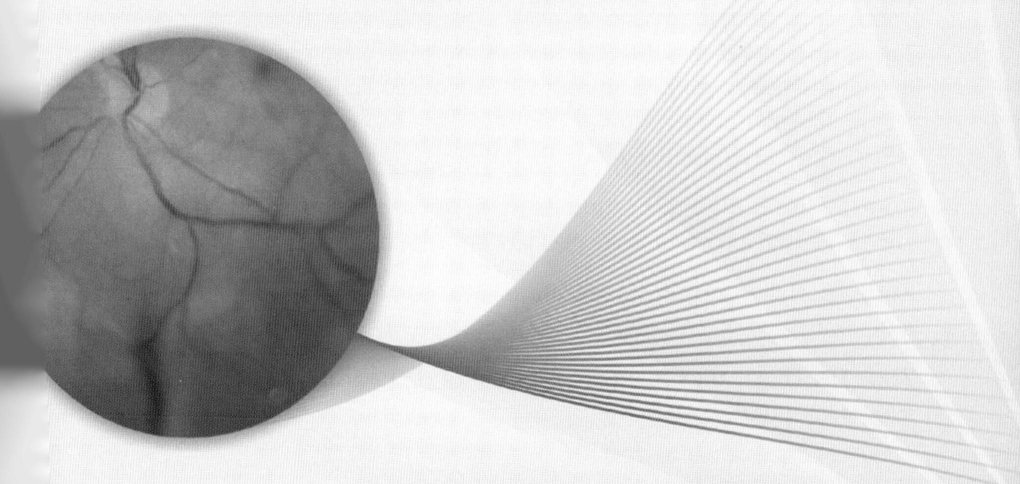

Retinopathy of Prematurity

Anjli Hussain, Nazimul Hussain, Sundaram Natarajan (India)

INTRODUCTION

Retinopathy of prematurity (ROP) is a potentially blinding eye disorder that primarily affects premature infants weighing 1250 grams or less, that are born before 31 weeks of gestation (A full-term pregnancy has a gestation of 38–42 weeks). The smaller an infant is at birth, the more likely that infant will develop ROP. The incidence of ROP worldwide ranges from 21.3% to 64.5%, and the estimated incidence in India is 38- 42.3%. The disease improves and leaves no permanent damage in milder cases of ROP. About 90 percent of all infants with ROP are in the milder category and do not need treatment. However, infants with more severe disease can develop impaired vision or even blindness. ROP is a multifactorial disease. Low birth weight, low gestational age and supplemental oxygen therapy following delivery have been consistently associated with ROP.

CLASSIFICATION AND CLINICAL SIGNS

An International classification of Retinopathy of Prematurity (ICROP) is followed world wide for documentation of ROP findings. The antero-posterior extent or the location was divided into 3 zones (zones1-3), the circumferential extent into clock hours (1-12) and severity of the disease in 5 stages (stage1-5). The presence of dilated and tortuous vessels denotes an aggressive, potentially sight threatening component and is called the **PLUS** disease.

LOCATION OF THE DISEASE (ZONES)

The normal blood vessels of the retina progress from optic nerve posteriorly to the edge of the ora serrata anteriorly. The location of ROP is a measure of how far this normal progression of blood vessels has reached before the disease takes over. Three circular zones are defined with the optic disc at the center.

Zone I: This is the area around the optic nerve and the macula. The radius of zone I is equal to two times the distance between the disc and the fovea.

Zone II: This is up to ora serrata on the nasal side and up to the equator temporally.

Zone III: This is the remaining crescent of retina from the equator to the ora serrata temporally.

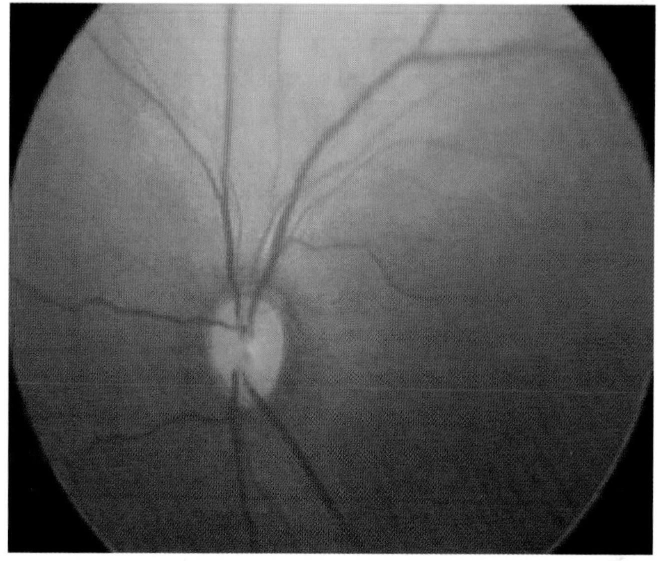

Fig. 1: A mature retina in a neonate
(Courtesy: Anjli Hussain, Ex. Consultant, L.V. Prasad Eye Institute, Hyderabad)

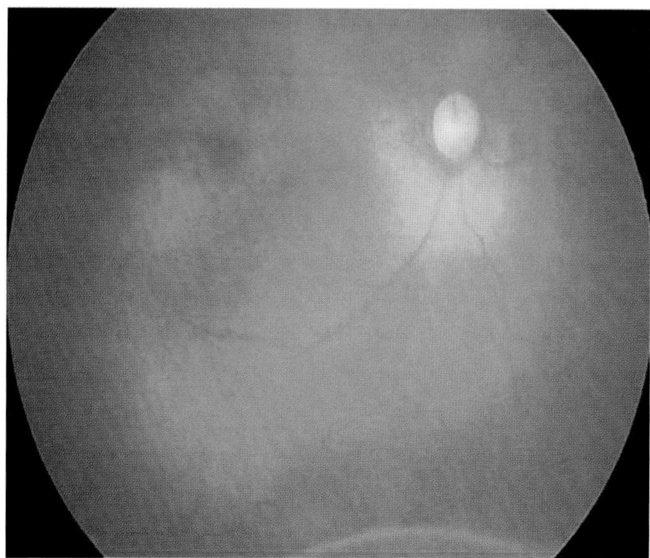

Fig. 2: Zone 1 immature retina
(Courtesy: Anjli Hussain, Ex. Consultant, L.V. Prasad Eye Institute, Hyderabad)

EXTENT OF THE DISEASE (CLOCK HOURS)

The extent of ROP is defined by how many clock hours of the eye circumference is diseased.

PLUS DISEASE

Plus disease is characterised by abnormal dilated vessels on the iris and or engorgement and tortuosity of the blood vessels in the retina. Additional findings include retinal haemorrhages, poorly dilating pupil and hazy media.

Stages of the disease (severity): A white line separating the clear normal red retina from the sharply contrasting underdeveloped gray retina characterizes *stage 1* ROP.

Stage 2 ROP shows a rolled ridge of scar tissue, which may be limited to a small area or encircle the entire inside of the eye, around the middle of the eye.

Stage 3 ROP is characterized by the development of abnormal new blood vessels and fibrous scar tissue on the edge of the ridge seen in stage 2. These vessels are lifted off from the surface and project into the vitreous cavity.

Stage 4 ROP occurs due to pulling of the retina by the scar tissue. As a result retina separates from the wall of the eyeball. Depending on the extent of RD stage 4 is further subdivided into Stage 4A (sparing macula) and 4B (involving macula).

Stage 5 ROP involves complete RD with the retina assuming a partial or closed funnel configuration. The infants usually develop a white reflex in the eye (leukocoria)

RUSH DISEASE

This is zone I ROP with plus disease. In this the progression is rapid and fulminant. In this new vessels are initially flat and in groups and later tend to get elevated into the vitreous cavity and may rapidly progress in nasal retina. This is also termed ***Fulminant ROP/Type II ROP or Posterior Zone I ROP***.

Threshold ROP is defined as zone I or II ROP stage 3 more than 5 contiguous or 8 cumulative clock hours with plus disease present. **Pre-threshold ROP** is defined as any stage of ROP in zone I with plus disease or ROP stage 3 with plus disease with 3 contiguous or 5 interrupted clock hours of retinal involvement in zone II but less than threshold.

A. **Aggressive posterior ROP:** This is most virulent form of ROP observed in the tiniest of babies. This is new terminology for Rush disease or type 2 fulminant ROP where posterior pole vessels show increased dilatation and tortousity in all 4 quadrants out of proportion to peripheral retinopathy. It progresses rapidly and does not progress through classic stages 1-3 and may appear only as a flat network of neovascularisation at the deceptively featureless junction of vascularised and non-vascularized retina.

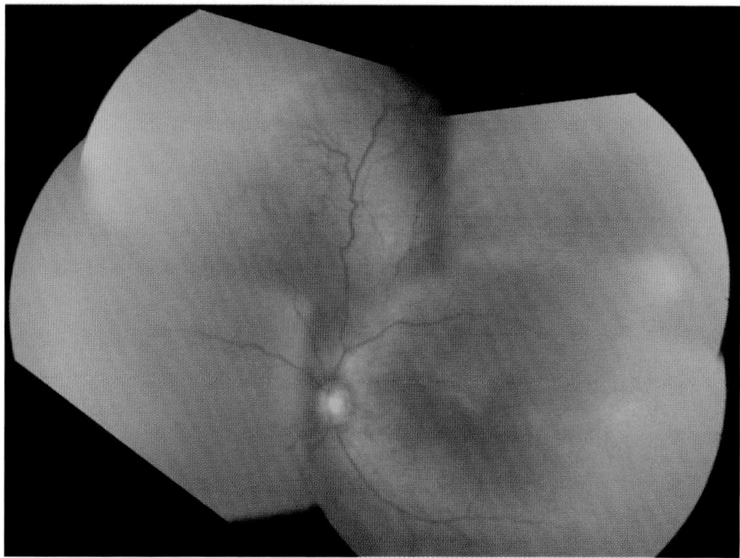

Fig. 3: Zone II stage 1 disease
(Courtesy: Anjli Hussain, Ex. Consultant, L.V. Prasad Eye Institute, Hyderabad)

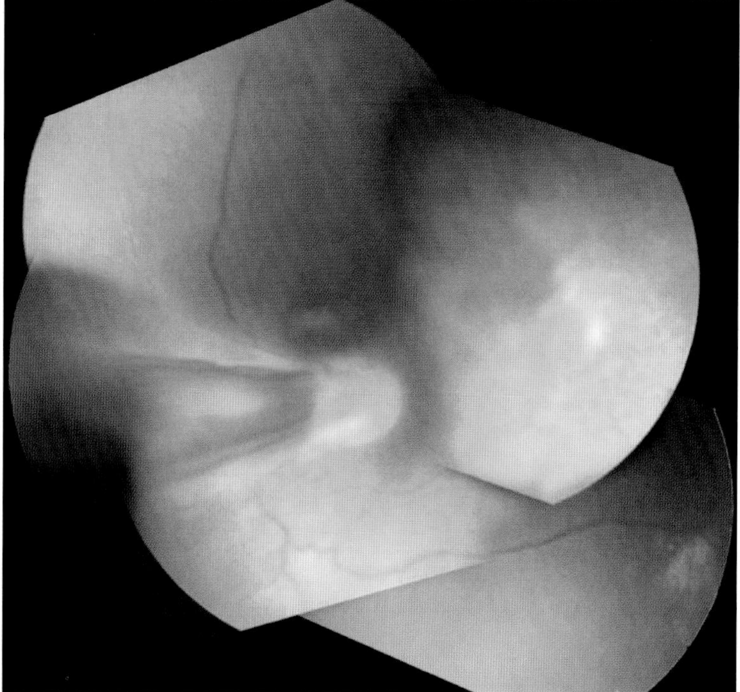

Fig. 4: Stage 4b ROP. Note the macular detachment and the falciform fold
(Courtesy: Anjli Hussain, Ex. Consultant, L.V. Prasad Eye Institute, Hyderabad)

B. **Preplus disease:** This is in between normal posterior pole vessels and frank plus disease. This is defined as vascular abnormalities of the posterior pole that are insufficient for the diagnosis of plus disease but that shows more arterial tortuosity and venous dilatation than normal and may later progress to plus disease.

SCREENING FOR ROP (INVESTIGATIONS)

Proper planning is a key component of efficient screening in a neonatal intensive care unit (NICU). The screening protocol at each NICU should be based on published recommendation and preferences of screening ophthalmologists and neonatologist.

In Indian population, significant number of infants fall outside the screening criteria than the high income group countries, so screening criteria suiting Indian population were proposed as follows:

1. Birth weight of less than or equal to 1700 grams.
2. Gestational age at birth of less than or equal to 34-35 weeks.
3. Exposed to oxygen for more than 30 days.
4. infants weighing less than 1200 grams at birth and those born at 24-30 weeks gestational age are at particular high risk of not only developing ROP but also developing it earlier, in more aggressive form. Hence definite need to screen these babies at the earliest
5. Other factors that can increase the risk of ROP and where the screening should be considered are other premature babies (<37 weeks and/or <2000 grams) with
   - Respiratory distress syndrome
   - Sepsis
   - Multiple blood transfusions
   - Multiple birth (twins/triplets)
   - Apnoeic episodes
   - Intraventricular hemorrhage
   - Pediatricians has index of concerns for ROP

TIME FOR SCREENING THE INFANTS AT RISK

Screen all eligible babies at

- 31 weeks PCA or 3-4 weeks after birth, whichever is earlier.
- Infants weighing less than 1200 grams at birth and those born at 24-30 weeks gestational age are screened early, usually not later than 2-3 weeks after birth.
- No examination needed in first 2 weeks of birth.
- Next date of examination to be decided by the ophthalmologist based on initial findings.
- Complete one screening session definitely before **Day 30** of life.

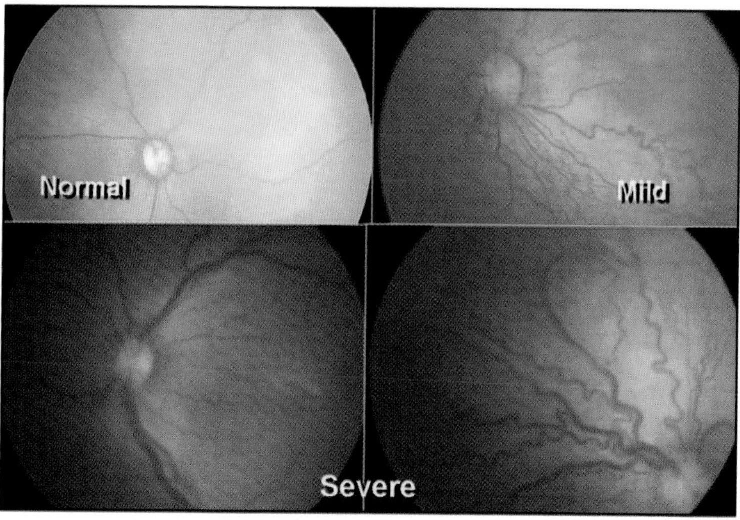

Fig. 5: Various grades of Plus disease
(Courtesy: Anjli Hussain, Ex. Consultant, L.V. Prasad Eye Institute, Hyderabad)

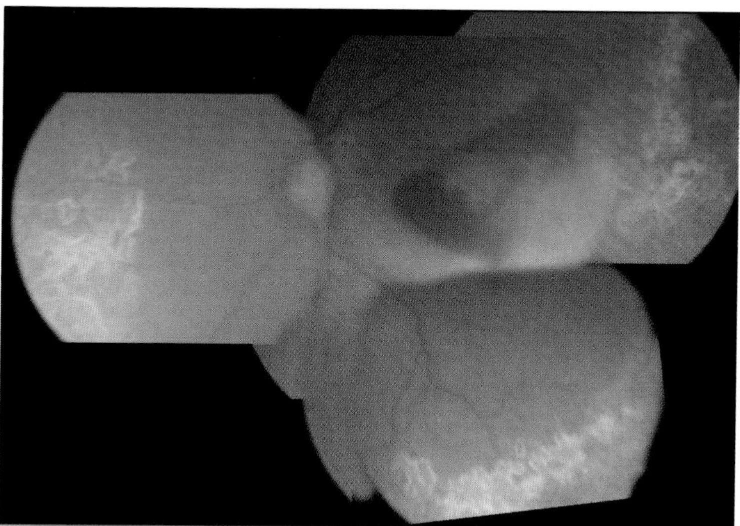

Fig. 6: Regress ROP following laser. Note: the preretinal hemorrhage
(Courtesy: Anjli Hussain, Ex. Consultant, L.V. Prasad Eye Institute, Hyderabad)

Ideally, a fixed time should be arranged for screening. Dilatation can be started by the NICU staff, 15-20 minutes before arrival of the Ophthalmologist. Babies, should be evaluated in an appropriate temperature controlled, clean environment where risk of hypothermia, infections and apnea are minimum. For in-patients in NICU, the screening can be done in temperature-controlled environment of the incubator. The room illumination should be low to avoid glare and annoying reflexes during examination with the indirect ophthalmoscope and viewing lens.

The child should be fed and burped preferably an hour before examination so as to minimize the risk of vomiting after instillation of drops. The pupils are dilated using 0.5-1% tropicamide and 2.5% phenylepherine instilled twice 10 minutes apart, about 15-20 minutes before the due time of evaluation. Due to small size of the palpebral fissure, detailed examination may require use of a self-retaining pediatric size wire speculum. A wire vectis or a pediatric depressor is useful to stabilize the globe and visualize the periphery.

DIFFERENTIAL DIAGNOSIS

1. Familial Exudative Vitreoretinopathy (FEVR)
   - Mostly autosomal dominant and observed in full term infant
   - Avascular peripheral retina with associated changes with progression of the disease. They are vascular buds at the junction of the vascular and avascular retina, dragging of vessels in the posterior pole and retina folds
   - Often associated with subretinal exudates and advanced disease can lead to total retina detachment.
2. Congenital Falciform fold
3. Incontinentia pigmenti
   - 33% have ocular defects
   - Associated with retinal hypopigmentation, peripheral nonperfusion with intravitreal neovascularisation (important finding), retinal detachment, microphthalmia, cataracts and strabismus
   - Systemic affections: Cutaneous (100%), CNS and structural.
4. Toxocara canis infection
   - Parasitic infection of the eye and are mostly unilateral
   - Posterior segment findings: Peripheral granuloma, posterior pole granuloma, chronic endophthalmitis.
   - Peripheral retinal locations is most common
5. Causes of leukocoria: this represents Stage 5 ROP

TREATMENT

The indications for treatment of threshold ROP (5 or more contiguous or 8 cumulative clock hours of stage 3+ ROP either in Zone I or Zone II) were initially proposed by the CRYO-ROP study for those stages of the disease that are likely to result in adverse visual outcomes. The ETROP Study proposes newer criteria for early treatment of eyes that have more than 15% risk of adverse outcomes. Retinal ablation should be considered for any eye with type 1 ROP that includes the following;

1. Zone I, any stage ROP with plus disease.
2. Zone I, stage 3 ROP with or without plus disease
3. Zone II, stage 2 or 3 ROP with plus disease.

Plus disease is defined in this case as at least 2 quadrants of dilation and tortuosity of the posterior retinal blood vessels. The treatment should be done at the earliest, preferably within 24 hours and not later than 72 hours. The aim of treatment is to ablate the whole of the avascular retina as rapidly and completely as possible with minimum side effects. Treatment for acute ROP can be done either by laser photoablation or cryotherapy. Laser effect is usually apparent within one week of adequate laser therapy. An alternate to cryotherapy and LIO ablation is to use a transconjunctivo-scleral laser diopexy. The main indication for the use of TCSDL is for initial management of severe cases of threshold ROP in situations where LIO is difficult or unavailable. Disadvantages of cryotherapy can be circumvented.

Signs that indicate disease has reached a quiescent phase of acute ROP after retinal ablation include:

- Pupil dilates well
- There is no rubeosis
- Media is clear
- Vascular dilatation and tortuosity are absent
- Feeder vessels to proliferation/ hemorrhages are 'silent 'and not dilated or tortuos
- No increase in traction
- All elevated focal areas have an avascular base with no feeder vessels.

Lens sparing vitrectomy and scleral buckle have been used to manage stage 4A ROP. Lens sparing vitreous surgery can interrupt progression of ROP from Stage 4A to stages 4B or 5 by directly addressing transvitreous traction resulting from fibrous proliferation. The surgical goal for stage 5 ROP is to reattach as much as retina as possible. Form vision can be preserved following vitrectomy for stage 5 ROP.

INFERENCES

Start screening for ROP between 20 to 30 days of life, earlier (20 days) for smaller babies (less than 30 weeks gestational age and 1500 grams birth weight). One screening session should be completed before day 30 of life. The critical factor to ensure better outcomes are to screen early, follow-up weekly or more closely, watch out for Plus and/or new vessels and treat such eyes vigorously for full retinal ablation of avascular retina . ROP is a continuous race against time with a very small window of opportunity of 7-10 days where optimum treatment outcomes with least complications can be achieved. Surgical interventions offer the potential for preservation of vision for eyes with ROP related retinal detachment; especially if it is directed prior to macular distortion.

Best's Disease or Best's Vitelliform Macular Dystrophy

Nazimul Hussain, Anjli Hussain (India)

INTRODUCTION

Best's disease is inherited as an autosomal dominant disease. The true prevalence of Best's disease is unknown. It is a bilateral macular dystrophy characterized by subretinal accumulation of yellowish material in the macular area. It is slowly progressive and eventually results in retinal pigment epithelial (RPE) and photoreceptors atrophy. At the end stage, impairs severely the central vision.

CLASSIFICATION AND CLINICAL FEATURES

Stage 1

This is characterized by normal fundus finding but associated by abnormal electro-oculogram.

Stage 2 or Pre-vitelliform Stage

The lesions appear as yellow subfoveal pigment disturbance associated with RPE mottling with small yellow spot.

Stage 3 or Vitelliform Stage

This is characterized by a yellow orange slightly elevated lesion. Visual acuity is maintained at this stage. This appears like a "egg yolk".

Stage 4 or Scrambled Egg Stage

Here, the vitelliform appearance gets ruptured and appears granular. This gives a scrambled egg appearance. Visual acuity starts reducing at this stage.

Stage 5 or Pseudohypopyon Stage

Here the yellowish subretinal material collects in the inferior part of the cyst giving a pseudohypopyon appearance.

Stage 6 or Atrophic Stage

Eventually the subretinal material gets absorbed and RPE atrophy occurs with minimal scarring. Visual acuity (VA) is impaired significantly at this stage.

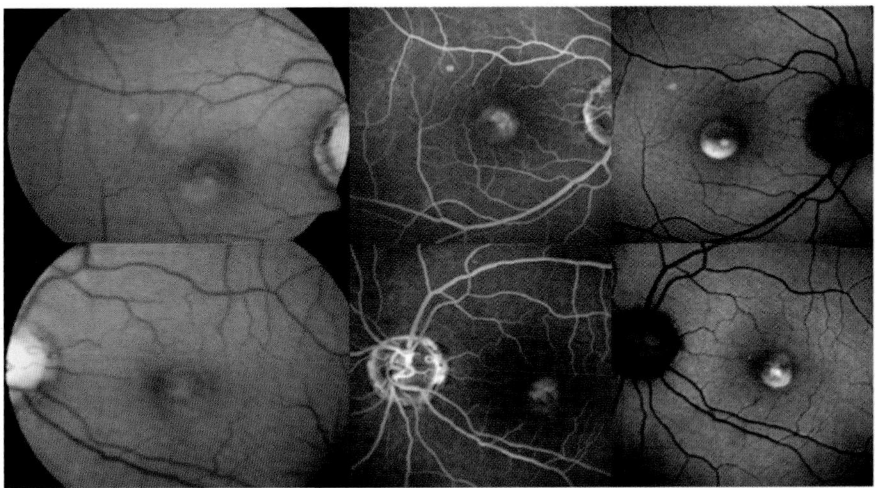

Fig. 1: Pseudohypopyon stage in the right eye and later stage in the left eye

Each patient may not follow each stage and may skip one or the other stage. Mutation in VMD 2 gene is associated with Best's disease. Most patients have VA of 20/40 or better. Despite better VA, patients complain of metamorphopsia and lacunar scotoma causing difficult reading ability. Choroidal neovascularization (CNV) may occur as a complication.

INVESTIGATIONS

Best's disease is characterized by normal electroretinogram (ERG) and abnormal electro-oculogram (EOG). The Arden ratio is usually greater than 1.7 on exposure to light. However, this response is blunted by changes in illumination where the ratio falls below 1.5. Dark adaptation is normal in Best's disease. In general, EOG is distinctly abnormal with complete absence of light induced rise.

Fundus fluorescein angiographic (FFA) finding depends on the stage of the disease. FFA is useful in detecting the extent RPE abnormality and presence of CNV.

DIFFERENTIAL DIAGNOSIS

1. Pattern dystrophy: They appear almost similar to best's disease as there is a phenotypic overlap. Molecular diagnostic testing may help to differentiate between the two.
2. Stargardt's disease: They can have poor VA at early stage and usually worse in comparison to the fundus lesion. Has dark choroid or masked appearance in FFA.
3. Age related macular degeneration (AMD): In the late stage with atrophic scar, CNV or RPE abnormality, best's disease may simulate AMD.
4. Traumatic maculopathy.

MANAGEMENT

There is no definite treatment for this disorder. The management mainly includes genetic counseling and support services to improve the quality of life. When VA is impaired, low vision services is a definite advantage.

INFERENCE

Best's disease is a abnormality of the RPE associated with accumulation of yellowish lipofuschin like material in the macula. Known genetic mutation occurs at VMD2 gene. Genetic counseling and low vision services are essential when needed.

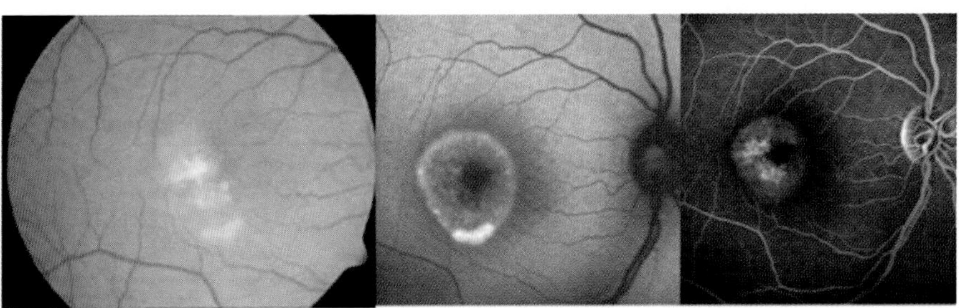

Fig. 2: Late showing RPE atrophy and minimal scarring

Gyrate Atrophy

Nazimul Hussain, Anjli Hussain (India)

INTRODUCTION

Gyrate atrophy of the choroid and retina is a rare autosomal recessive disorder associated with hyperornithinemia. Hyperornithinemia is due to the deficiency of ornithine aminotransferase. The precise pathomechanism is unknown.

CLINICAL FEATURES

It usually presents in the first decade with night blindness and high myopia, subsequent development of posterior subcapsular cataracts by second decade, progressive constriction of visual fields, and eventual loss of central acuity in the fourth to fifth decades. Clinical features also follow a slowly progressive time course. One usually observes circular, well circumscribed regions of chorioretinal atrophy with hyperpigmented margins in the midperiphery. These regions enlarge and coalesce in a scalloped pattern, spread anteriorly and posteriorly and eventually encroach on the macula, threatening central vision.

Natural history study of gyrate atrophy has shown that central visual loss can begin at any age. Visual acuity decreased rapidly in phakic eyes within less than ten years. Even after cataract extraction, there was transient improvement of vision especially in young patients; subsequently visual loss was slow until macula was involved. The study also quotes that macular involvement is often difficult to perceive ophthalmoscopically except in adult eyes where obvious chorioretinal atrophy could be seen. The macular changes noted were primarily pigmentary dystrophy or atrophic patches. Macular changes were seen in 30% at 20 years and 60% at the age of 30 years.

INVESTIGATIONS

On fundus fluorescein angiography, one may observe leakage at the margins of healthy and affected tissue, with hyperfluorescence within the gyrate lesions. Besides atrophic or pigmentary macular changes, fundus fluorescein angiography and optical coherence tomography study showed additional changes like epiretinal membranes, cystoid macular edema and macular hole. Sparsely available anecdotal reports suggest that cystoid macular edema may precede macular hole formation in eyes with gyrate atrophy. Since recent literature shows that such macular changes are seen in the younger age, it can be speculated that the atrophic changes in the macula may be a late sequelae of the same. A macular complication of foveal atrophy has also been reported. Natural history of gyrate atrophy suggests 43% macular involvement.

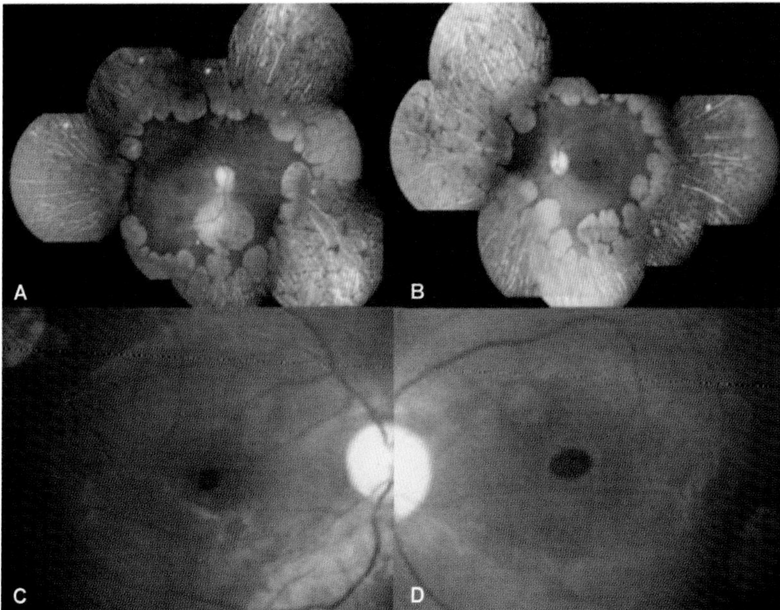

Figs 1A to D: Shows the montage color fundus photograph of both the eyes (A & B) multiple coalescent areas of choroidal atrophy with scalloped edges. Magnified photograph of the macula shows a thin foveal roof with pseudo appearance of macular hole (C) in the right eye. The left eye showed appearance of full thickness macular hole (D)

An electrophysiological test usually reveals early impaired scotopic and photopic responses, which becomes extinguished as the disease progresses.

Biochemical test for amino acid analysis will show increase plasma ornithine level.

TREATMENT

Therapeutic regimen is directed towards reducing the plasma ornithine level. In majority of the patients, a diet low in arginine results in lower plama ornithine level. In pyridoxine responsive individuals, vitamin B_6 may be tried.

DIFFERENTIAL DIAGNOSIS

1. Retinitis pigmentosa
2. Other causes of night blindness.

INFERENCE

Gyrate atrophy is a rare autosomal recessive disorder associated with hyperornithinemia. Amino acid analysis for plasma ornithine level is essential to restrict arginine free diet.

CHAPTER SEVEN

INFLAMMATORY AND INFECTIVE DISORDERS OF RETINA

Ajay Aurora, Alay Banker, Vikrant Sharma, Neeraj Sanduja (India)

- Toxoplasmosis
- Toxocariasis
- Vogt-Koyanagi-Harada Syndrome
- Sarcoidosis
- CMV Retinitis
- Acute Retinal Necrosis (ARN)
- Progressive Outer Retinal Necrosis (PORN)
- Frosted Branch Angiitis
- Treatment of Viral Retinitis
- Ocular Tuberculosis

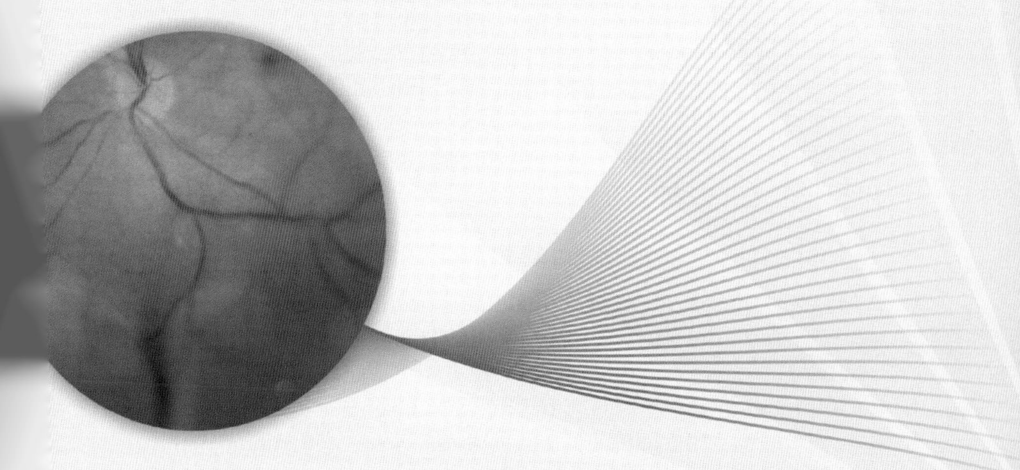

Inflammatory disorders of the retina could be primary where the inflammation starts in the retinal tissue and there is a spill over into the adjacent choroid and vitreous or it may start in the adjacent choroid or vitreous and involve the retinal tissue secondarily. The diseases that involve the retina secondarily from the adjacent choroid will be discussed in the chapters dealing with uvea.

The pathological changes in retinal inflammations can broadly have the following course: Initially in response to an insult there is a vascular response leading to accumulation of inflammatory cells and exudates extravascularly. Typically this accumulation occurs around the blood vessels and is clinically manifested as sheathing. Exudation in the retinal tissue leads to its opacification and separation. Edema in macular area could lead to minimal separation/crowding of photoreceptors. Crowding of photoreceptors in the macula leads to macropsia while their separation leads to micropsia. Further, straight lines could appear wavy and with further increase in exudation there develops a detachment of sensory retina leading to a decreased visual acuity which usually develops on a rapid course. Associated capillary damage may present as retinal hemorrhages which may be superficial or deep . Occasionally this bleeding may be significant and can present as blood underneath the internal limiting membrane or may breakthrough the ILM to present as subhyaloid or vitreous hemorrhage. Like with inflammatory response elsewhere in the body fibrous tissue can form on the retinal tissue, underneath it and within it as well. This may lead to retinal scarring, folding, traction causing it to detach and impairment/loss of its function.

Retinal inflammations affect retinal pigment epithelium (RPE) as well. Due to exudation, this is however obscured during the acute phase. The RPE cells may get disrupted leading to release of pigment that is picked up by the wandering macrophages. Some of these cells migrate along the blood vessels while others transform into fibroblasts and lay down fibrous tissue that binds the retinal tissue together and clinically may present as a retinal scar in the later stages. Clinically above changes may be seen as an area of depigmentation surrounded by pigment and is typically labeled as a chorioretinal scar. Occasionally with the disruption of the ILM, aberrant vessels may grow into the vitreous as a neovascular tuft. Similarly choroidal neovascular membrane can form rarely.

Following findings help one to differentiate between an acute and healed inflammatory retinal lesion:

Acute/Active Retinal Inflammatory Lesion

1. A "Fuzzy" opacification of retina that is normally transparent.
2. Vitreous haze detected as hazy media. This is because of exudation. 90D or a contact lens exam will reveal cells in the posterior vitreous.
3. Sheathing of blood vessels with "fuzzy" margins.
4. Retinal edema or detachment. It may be associated with retinal hemorrhages.

Healed Retinal Inflammatory Lesion

1. Above signs of activity are not visible.
2. Area of depigmentation surrounded by area of hyperpigmentation. This may be focal (chorioretinal scar) and of varying sizes or may be diffuse as salt and pepper fundus.
3. Blood vessels are reduced to "white cords".
4. Fibroglial scars with secondary affects on retina: traction, distortion and detachment.

Various inflammations and infections of the retina are listed below and will be discussed individually:

1. Toxoplasmosis
2. Toxocariasis
3. Vogt Koyonagi Harada syndrome
4. Sarcoidosis
5. Cytomegalovirus retinitis
6. Herpesvirus hominis infection
7. Ocular tuberculosis

TOXOPLASMOSIS

INTRODUCTION

- Its probably the commonest type of retinochoroiditis caused by an obligate intracellular protozoan *Toxoplasma gondii*
- 20-70% of normal adult US population has serologic evidence of previous toxoplasmosis.

CLINICAL FEATURES

- Most cases of adult toxoplasmosis are thought to be the reactivation of healed congenital lesions though a recent UK study estimated that 66% to 86% of ocular toxoplasmosis was due to posnatally acquired infection.
- The active lesion is a focal area of retinochoroiditis with mild to severe overlying vitritis (visible as vitreous haze and cells)
- It has predilection for the posterior pole
- The active lesion usually occurs adjacent to an edge of healed previous lesion — *Satellite lesion*
- Lesion associated with severe vitritis may give appearance of *'headlight in the fog'*
- Morphological variants:
  - Large destructive lesion
  - Punctate inner retinal lesion
  - Punctate outer (or deep) retinal lesion.

DIFFERENTIAL DIAGNOSIS

- Other causes of retinitis: Sarcoidosis, tuberculosis, syphilis, viral and fungal infections.

INVESTIGATION

- A characteristic clinical lesion with serologic evidence of toxoplasmosis (indirect fluorescent antibody and ELISA)
- Local production of *T. gondi* IgG in the aqueous humor: More frequently noted in recurrent rather than primary ocular toxoplasmosis
- PCR of ocular fluids for *Toxoplasma* DNA: More frequently found in primary ocular toxoplasmosis than recurrent disease.

TREATMENT

- In immunocompetent patients its generally self limiting and small peripheral lesions need not be treated.

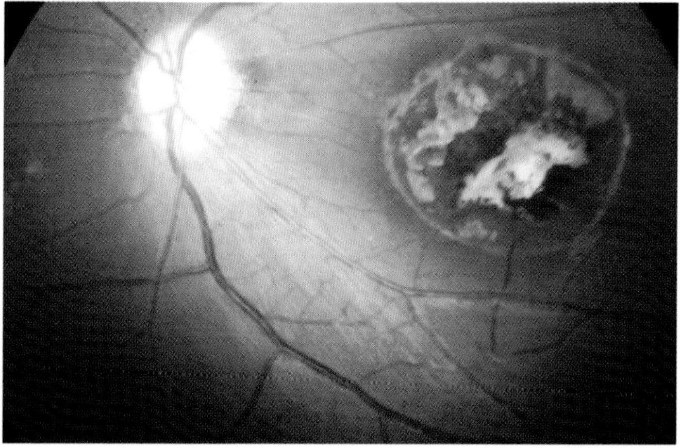

Fig. 1: Fundus photo of left eye showing *Toxoplasma* scar

- Indication for treatment:
  - Lesion within temporal arcade or,
  - In close proximity to disc or,
  - Associated with severe vitritis or,
  - In immunocompromised patients (all lesions in AIDS patients need treatment irrespective of size or location).
- Triple drug therapy
  - Pyrimethamine two 50 mg loading doses 12 hours apart, then 25 mg by mouth twice daily
  - Sulfadiazine 2 gm loading dose, then 1 gm by mouth four times daily
  - Prednisone 20 to 40 mg by mouth once daily
  - Folinic acid 3 to 5 mg by mouth twice weekly

  Antimicrobials to be continued for 3 to 4 weeks.

PROGNOSIS

- A lesion in the macular region is the cause of visual loss in 88% cases
- In other cases the vision is lost due to large destructive peripheral lesion
- Visual loss was independent of the number of previous episodes but correlated with the duration of active disease.

TOXOCARIASIS

INTRODUCTION

- Caused by infestation with nematode *Toxocara canis* (dog tapeworm)
- Systemic effect of *Toxocara* infestation is termed visceral larva migrans.
- Affected patients are usually young.

CLINICAL FEATURES

- *Toxocara* endophthalmitis is usually unilateral and may take one of the four forms
  - Posterior pole "granuloma":
    - Children, 6 -14 years
    - 0.75 to 6.0 mm, subretinal or intraretinal white or grey mass, frequently associated with membranes/traction bands running from the mass to adjacent retina
    - May present as squint.
  - Peripheral granuloma:
    - Usually presents later in the life as it is generally asymptomatic.
    - May be preceded by diffuse endophthalmitis that resolves over time and media clears
    - May be localized or have bands running from the granuloma to other parts of retina
  - Chronic endophthalmitis:
    - Younger age (2-9 years),
    - Presenting feature is leukocoria and decreased vision
    - History negative for trauma, intraocular surgery or metastasis; positive history of pica
    - External signs of ocular inflammation absent; AC may have hypopyon and evidence of granulomatous iridocyclitis
  - Atypical presentation
    - Inflammation and swelling of optic nerve head
    - Motile subretinal nematode
    - Diffuse chorioretinitis

DIFFERENTIAL DIAGNOSIS

- Retinoblastoma
- Other forms of endophthalmitis and uveitis
- ROP
- FEVR
- Coat's disease

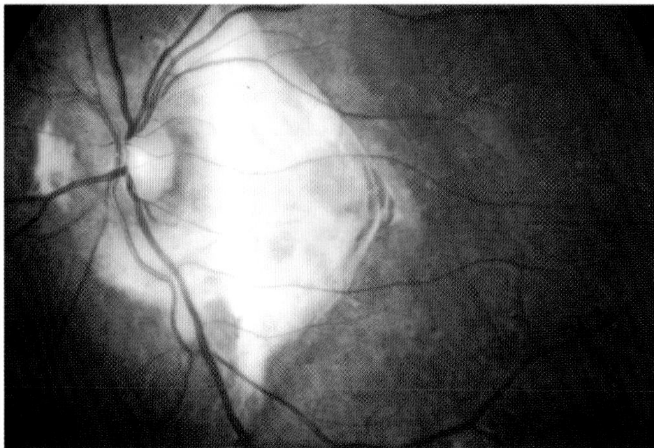

Fig. 2: Unilateral large subretinal healed posterior granuloma: presumed *Toxocara*

- PHPV
- Idiopathic optic neuritis.

INVESTIGATIONS

- ELISA for antibodies in the serum and intraocular fluid against second stage larval secretory antigen
- Cytology of aqueous humor and vitreous demonstrating eosinophils. Occasionally remnants of *Toxocara* may be seen in vitreous samples.

TREATMENT

- Depends on the stage of inflammation
- An asymptomatic peripheral lesion needs no treatment.
- Medical management: Periocular and/or systemic steroids.
- The role of antihelminthics is controversial
- Surgical intervention: Retinal detachment or macular traction. Scleral buckle may be used, vitrectomy is preferred
- Laser photocoagulation around the larva

PROGNOSIS

- Ocular *Toxocara* is a major cause of visual loss in young.

VOGT-KOYANAGI-HARADA SYNDROME

INTRODUCTION

- It's a systemic disorder involving eye, ear, skin and meninges characterized by bilateral non traumatic granulomatous, uveitis with extraocular manifestations like poliosis, vitiligo and dysacusis and may be associated with serous retinal detachment and CSF pleocytosis.
- Usually affects adults, has predilection for dark pigmented races, increased prevalence in patients having HLA DR4 and DW 15 haplotype.

CLINICAL FEATURES

- Clinical course typically follows a pattern of:
  - *Prodromal stage*: Viral like illness 3-5 days
  - *Uveitic stage*: Acute uveitis, several weeks
  - *Chronic stage (convalescent stage):* Integumentory and uveal depigmentation, lasts months to years depending in therapeutic intervention.
  - *Chronic recurrent stage:* Resolving chronic uveitis interrupted with recurrent anterior uveitis.

Ocular and Extraocular Features (Revised International Criteria)

Complete Vogt-Koyanagi-Harada disease (criteria 1 to 5 must be present)

1. No history of penetrating ocular trauma or surgery preceding the initial onset of uveitis.
2. No clinical or laboratory evidence suggestive of other ocular disease entities.
3. Bilateral ocular involvement (a or b must be met, depending on the stage of disease when the patient is examined).

a. *Early Manifestations of Disease*

1. There must be evidence of a diffuse choroiditis (with or without anterior uveitis, vitreous inflammatory reaction, or optic disk hyperemia), which may manifest as one of the following:
   a. Focal areas of subretinal fluid, or
   b. Bullous serous retinal detachments.
2. With equivocal fundus findings; both of the following must be present as well:
   a. Focal areas of delay in choroidal perfusion, multifocal areas of pinpoint leakage, large placoid areas of hyperfluorescence, pooling within

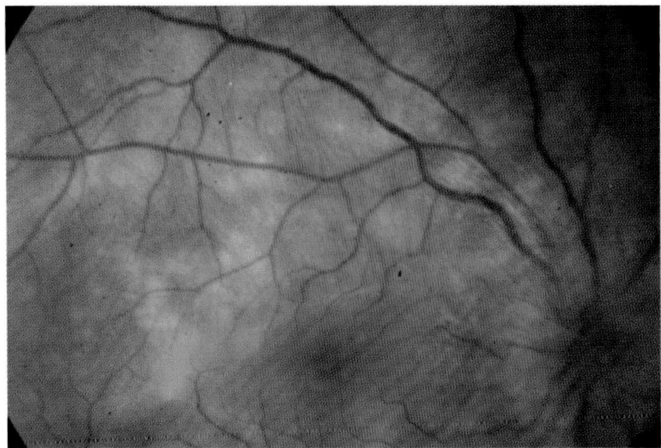

Fig. 3: Color photo of the right eye showing active stage of Vogt-Koyanagi-Harada syndrome

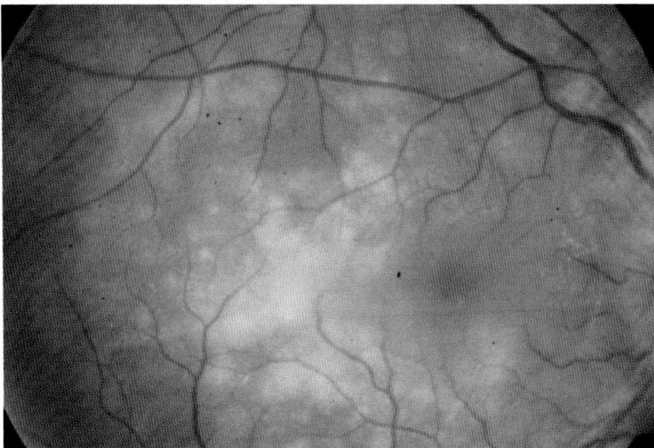

Fig. 4: Color photo of the right eye showing active stage of Vogt-Koyanagi-Harada syndrome

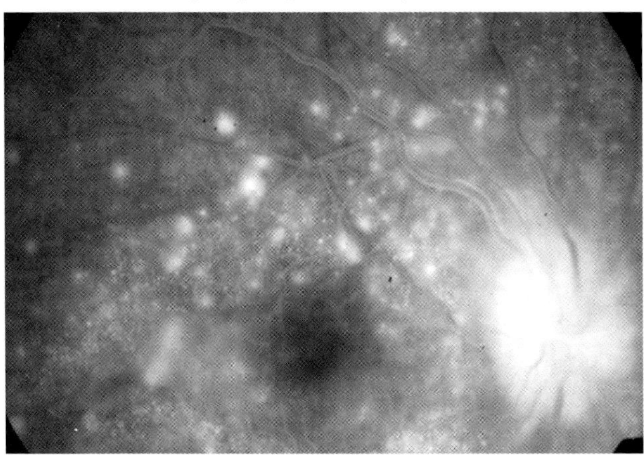

Fig. 5: Early phase of FFA in the active stage of Vogt-Koyanagi-Harada syndrome

subretinal fluid, and optic nerve staining (listed in order of sequential appearance) by fluorescein angiography, and

b. Diffuse choroidal thickening, without evidence of posterior scleritis by ultrasonography.

b. Late Manifestations of Disease

1. History suggestive of prior presence of findings from 3a, and either both (2) and (3) below, or multiple signs from (3):
2. Ocular depigmentation (either of the following manifestations is sufficient):
   a. Sunset glow fundus, or
   b. Sugiura sign.
3. Other ocular signs:
   a. Nummular chorioretinal depigmented scars, or
   b. Retinal pigment epithelium clumping and/or migration, or
   c. Recurrent or chronic anterior uveitis.
4. Neurological/auditory findings (may have resolved by time of examination).
   a. Meningismus (malaise, fever, headache, nausea, abdominal pain, stiffness of the neck and back, or a combination of these factors; headache alone is not sufficient to meet definition of meningismus, however), or
   b. Tinnitus, or
   c. Cerebrospinal fluid pleocytosis.
5. Integumentary finding (*not* preceding onset of central nervous system or ocular disease).
   a. Alopecia, or
   b. Poliosis, or
   c. Vitiligo.

Incomplete Vogt-Koyanagi-Harada disease (criteria 1 to 3 and either 4 or 5 must be present)

1. No history of penetrating ocular trauma or surgery preceding the initial onset of uveitis, and
2. No clinical or laboratory evidence suggestive of other ocular disease entities, and
3. Bilateral ocular involvement.
4. Neurologic/auditory findings; as defined for complete Vogt-Koyanagi-Harada disease above, or
5. Integumentary findings; as defined for complete Vogt-Koyanagi-Harada disease above.

Probable Vogt-Koyanagi-Harada disease (isolated ocular disease; criteria 1 to 3 must be present)

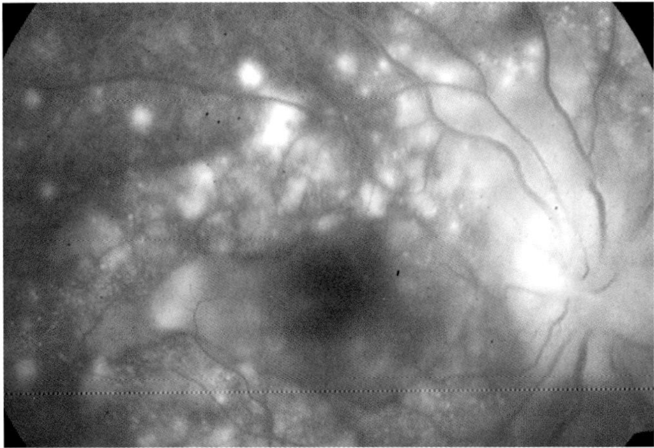

Fig. 6: Late phase of FFA in the active stage of Vogt-Koyanagi-Harada syndrome

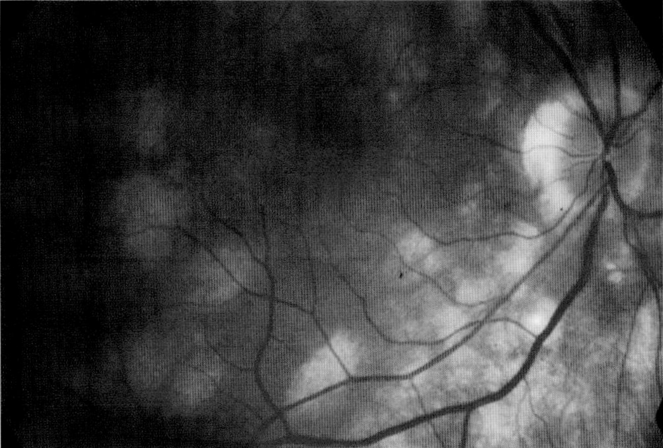

Fig. 7: Healed stage of Vogt-Koyanagi-Harada syndrome showing sunset fundus

1. No history of penetrating ocular trauma or surgery preceding the initial onset of uveitis.
2. No clinical or laboratory evidence suggestive of other ocular disease entities.
3. Bilateral ocular involvement as defined for complete Vogt-Koyanagi-Harada disease above.

DIFFERENTIAL DIAGNOSIS

- Sympathetic ophthalmia
- Uveal effusion syndrome
- Posterior scleritis
- Primary intraocular lymphoma
- Uveal lymphoid infiltration
- Acute posterior multifocal Placoid pigment epitheliopathy
- Sarcoidosis.

INVESTIGATIONS

- Diagnosis of VKH is predominantly clinical
- VKH without extraocular changes may benefit with following investigations:
  - Lumbar puncture: CSF pleocytosis, mainly lymphocytes
  - FFA: Punctuate hyperfluorescent dots that enlarge and stain the surrounding SRF; late phase multiple serous RD; in chronic stage "moth eaten appearance".
  - Ultrasound: Diffuse low to medium reflective thickening of posterior choroids, serous RD, vitreous opacities
  - OCT: Helps in monitoring resolution of serous RD, macular edema and CNVM.

TREATMENT

- Systemic steroids are the mainstay of the treatment; patients unresponsive to or who have intolerable side effects to steroids may need cytotoxic agents.
- Corticosteroids:
  - Oral prednisone 100-200 mg initially; then taper gradually over 3-6 months
  - Pulse IV methylprednisolone 1 g/day for 3 days followed by gradual tapering of oral prednisolone over 3-6 months
  - IV methylprednisolone 100-200 mg/day for 3 days followed by gradual tapering of oral prednisolone over 3-6 months
- Immunosuppressive agents

   - Cyclosporin 5 mg/per day
- Cytotoxic agents:
   - Azathioprine 1-2.5 mg/kg per day
   - Mycophenolate mofetil 1-3 g/day
   - Cyclophosphamide 1-2 mg /day
   - Chlorambucil 0.1 mg/kg per day, doses adjusted every three weeks to a maximum of 18 mg /day

PROGNOSIS

- VKH patients treated with initial high dose steroids followed by gradual tapering over 3-6 months fare better
- Eyes having better VA at presentation fare better
- If VKH develops at advanced stage, visual prognosis is worse
- Complications of chronic VKH include: Cataract, glaucoma, choroidal neovascularization, subretinal fibrosis and optic atrophy.

SARCOIDOSIS

INTRODUCTION

- It's a chronic granulomatous disease of unknown etiology affecting many organs of the body especially the lungs, skin, lymphoid system, bones and eyes. Posterior segment lesions occur in 14-28% cases of ocular sarcoid.

CLINICAL FEATURES

- Ocular features
  - It may present as acute or chronic granulomatous iridocyclitis.
  - Vitreal involvement (commonest posterior segment manifestation of ocular sarcoid) may present as diffuse vitritis or, less commonly, as cotton ball opacities called "snowballs" or "string of pearls".
  - Perivascular sheathing is the second commonest feature of posterior segment sarcoidosis, Severe periphlebitis gives a characteristic appearance of candle wax drippings. Occasional cases develop branch retinal vein occlusion.
  - Infrequently it may present as retina, choroidal or optic nerve granuloma.

DIFFERENTIAL DIAGNOSIS

- Pars planitis
- Eales disease
- Vogt-Koyanagi-Harada syndrome.

INVESTIGATIONS

- Chest X-ray abnormal in 90% patients with pulmonary sarcoid
- Histological biopsy: non-caseating granuloma from lymph nodes, lung, skin, liver, conjunctiva and salivary gland.
- ACE (Serum Angiotensin Converting Enzyme) level is abnormal in active sarcoidosis and reflects total body granuloma content
- Serum calcium, urinary calcium, serum lysozye and serum immunoglobulin: are all non-specific and nondiagnostic.

TREATMENT

- Systemic and periocular steroids are the mainstay of treatment

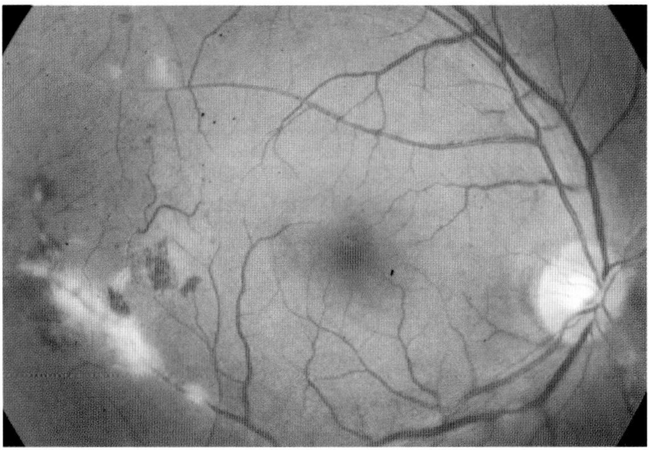

Fig. 8: A case of sarcoidosis with vasculitis

- Patients having side-effects of corticosteroids can be put on corticosteroid sparing agents like: hydroxychloroquine, methotrexate, azatioprine, mycophenol mofetil or cyclosporine.

PROGNOSIS

- Factors associated with lack of improvement of visual acuity of less than 20/40 are:
  - Delay in presentation to uveitis subspecialist of greater than 1 year
  - Development of glaucoma
  - Presence of intermediate or posterior uveitis.

CMV RETINITIS

INTRODUCTION

CMV retinitis is the most common infection, seen in 15-40% of patients with HIV disease, more so when CD4 cell count is less than 100 cells per cubic mm.

CLINICAL FEATURES

- The classic CMV retinitis: *(cottage cheese with catsup or pizza pie retinopathy)* scattered yellow-white areas of necrotizing retinitis with variable degree of hemorrhage without much vitreous involvement is the hallmark of CMV retinitis.
- The other descriptions are the "Granular" variety and "Frosted Branch Angiitis". Often, the retinitis follows a perivascular distribution.
- Usually starts in the periphery and so patients either have no subjective complaints, or may complain of floaters. If the retinitis begins in the posterior pole, the patient may notice a visual field deficit.
- Rhegmatogenous retinal detachment (13.5-29% of patients with CMV retinitis) may occur during the active or healed phase of the disease.
- Other findings associated with CMV retinitis include perivasculitis, vascular attenuation and vessel closure, venous occlusions, as well as vitritis, anterior uveitis, and papillitis.

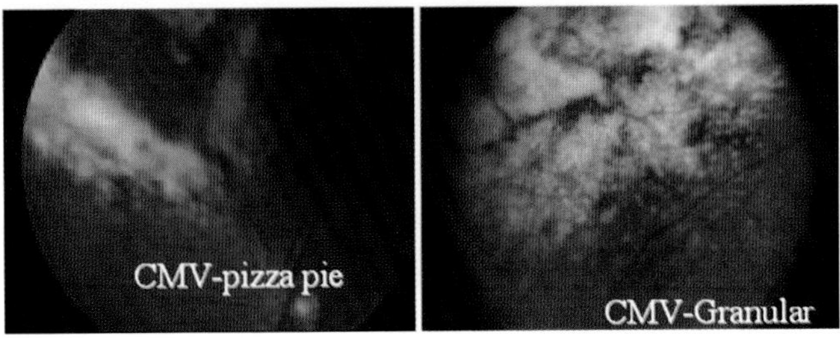

Fig. 9: Cytomegalovirus retinitis

VARICELLA ZOSTER VIRUS DISEASE: ACUTE RETINAL NECROSIS (ARN)

INTRODUCTION

- It's characterized by necrotizing retinitis mainly affecting otherwise healthy individuals of either sex and any age.

CLINICAL FEATURES

- The classic triad described for ARN is as follows:
  - Arteritis and periphlebitis of retinal and choroidal vasculature
  - Confluent necrotizing retinitis with a predilection for peripheral retina. The posterior pole remains largely unaffected and patient may retain reasonably good vision.
  - Moderate to severe vitritis
  - The usual cause of visual loss is development of rhegmatogenous Retina detachment which occurs as a result of hole formation at the junction of involved and uninvolved retina.
- Rarely may develop *ischemic optic neuropathy* caused by thrombotic arteriolar occlusion and infiltration of nerve by inflammatory cells.

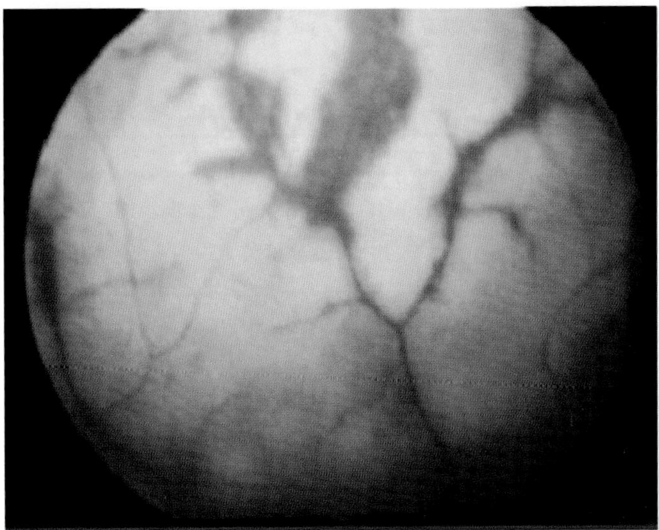

Fig. 10: Acute retinal necrosis

PROGRESSIVE OUTER RETINAL NECROSIS (PORN)

INTRODUCTION

- It's a variant of necrotizing herpetic retinopathy representing a distinct form of ARN, which usually affects immunocompromised patients.

CLINICAL FEATURES

- It's a rapidly progressive necrotizing retinitis, characterized by deep retinal opacification without granular borders.
- With progression there is clearing of areas around retinal vessels, giving a *"cracked mud"* appearance.
- There is no or little intraocular inflammation and an early involvement of posterior pole – features which differentiates it from ARN.

TABLE 1: Differentiating features of three types of viral retinitis in AIDS

	ARN	*PORN*	*CMV retinitis*
Immune status	Healthy	Immunosuppressed	Immunosuppressed
Laterality	Bilateral 30-80%	Bilateral 71%	Bilateral 30-50%
Visual loss	Severe	Early loss of vision	Only if involves macula
Anterior uveitis	Mild to moderate	Mild	Mild
Vitreous reaction	Significant vitritis	Minimum/No vitritis	Minimum/no vitritis
Retinal involvement	Full thickness	Deep outer retinal involvement	Full thickness involvement with granular border
Classic appearance	Late swiss-cheese	Cracked mud	Pizza -pie
Vasculitis	Common	Uncommon	Seen but not common
Retinal hemorrhages lesion	Common	Uncommon	Common in active
Retinal detachment	Common	Common	Less common
Progression	Rapid	Rapid	Slow

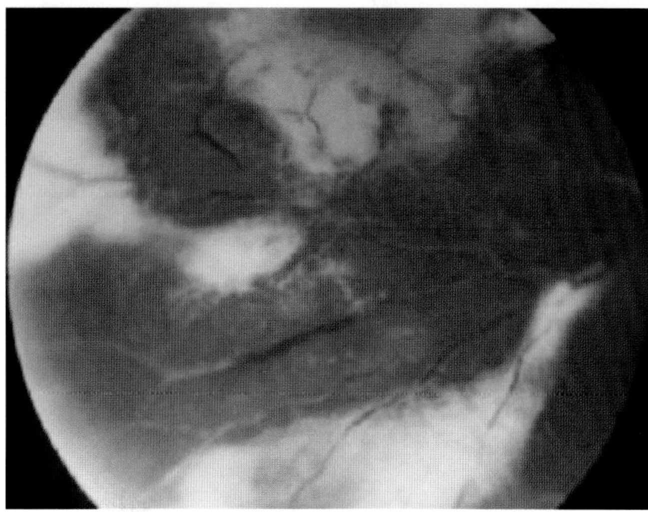

Fig. 11: Progressive outer retinal necrosis

FROSTED BRANCH ANGIITIS

Is essentially a severe form of idiopathic vasculitis which effects the entire retina. Although both arteries and veins are affected venules tend to be more affected. Cytomegalovirus retinitis (CMV), Toxoplasmic chorioretinitis, systemic lupus erythematosus, Crohn's disease, large cell lymphoma and acute lymphoblastic leukemia have been described as disorders associated with frosted branch angiitis.

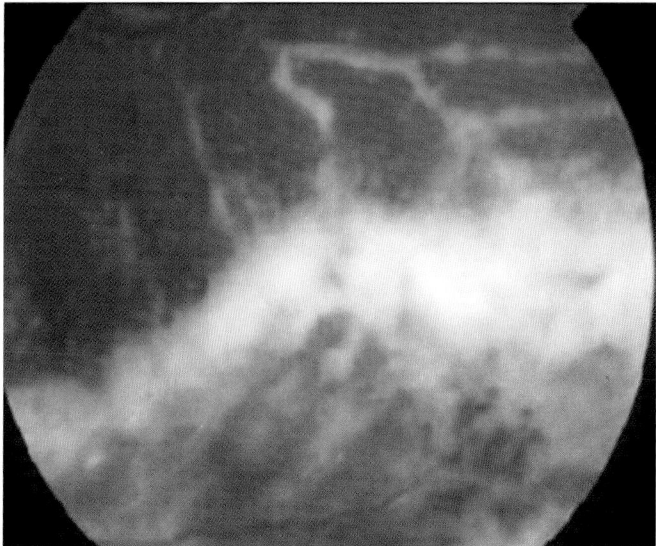

Fig. 12: Frosted branch vein angiitis

TREATMENT OF VIRAL RETINITIS

The treatment of viral retinitis may be systemic, local, or a combination of the two. The following are the various treatment modalities that are available for use.

GANCICLOVIR

- Ganciclovir is a nucleoside analogue that acts as a competitive inhibitor and faulty substrate for CMV DNA polymerase.
- Induction dose of 5 mg/kg every 12 hours for 14 to 21 days; followed by maintenance doses of 5 mg/kg/day,
- Major side effect:
  - Neutropenia (15-40% cases).
  - Other adverse effects include thrombocytopenia, anemia, nausea, vomiting, and elevated liver enzymes.
- Resistance to the drug is known.

FOSCARNET

- Foscarnet is a pyrophosphate analogue that inhibits DNA polymerase of CMV and other herpesviruses and reverse transcriptase
- Induction dose of 90 mg/kg twice a day for 14-21 days; followed by a maintenance dose of 90-120 mg/kg/day
- Major side effects are nephrotoxicity and hypocalcemia causing arrhythmias and seizures.

Combinations of foscarnet and ganciclovir are more effective in the treatment of recurrent or resistant retinitis than is continued monotherapy.

ACYCLOVIR

- Acyclovir (9-2[2-hydroxyethoxymethyl] guanine; acycloguanosine) is a nucleoside analogue that selectively targets infected cells only by a virally encoded enzyme, thymidine kinase, to phosphorylate it into an active form.
- The recommended intravenous dose is 1500 mg/m^2/day divided into three daily doses for 7 to 10 days. This should be followed by an oral therapy of 800 mg fives times daily for 14 weeks.

CATHETER-LESS THERAPY

The use of intravenous ganciclovir or foscarnet requires long-term indwelling catheter. As the risk of catheter-related sepsis is high and these lines are expensive to maintain and are associated with a substantial negative impact on quality of life, recently, there has been great interest in developing therapies that do not require an indwelling catheter. The following are the catheterless treatment options:

1. Oral ganciclovir
2. Intravenous cidofovir
3. Ganciclovir intraocular implant

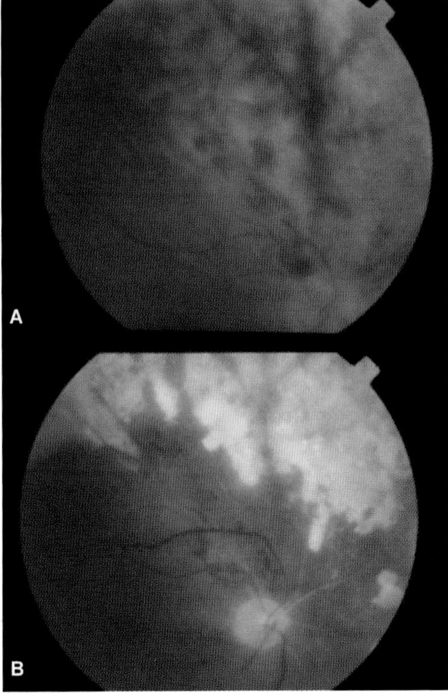

Figs 13A and B: Pretreatment (A) and post-treatment (B) CMV retinitis

4. Intravitreal injections (ganciclovir, foscarnet, cidofovir, fomivirsen).
5. Oral valganciclovir.

Ganciclovir Intraocular Implant

- Is a sustained-release drug delivery device that contains about 4.5-6 mg of ganciclovir. It is placed into the vitreous cavity through a 5-6 mm incision in the pars plana and sutured to the sclera . The drug diffuses into the vitreous cavity by passive diffusion at the rate of 1 mg/hour over a 6-8 month period. After that, the device is usually surgically removed and/or replaced with a new device.
- Adverse events include retinal detachments (12% cases), endophthalmitis (1.7%), and transient vitreous hemorrhage (7.8%). However, as with all local treatments, there is a risk of CMV disease in the fellow eye (up to 40% cases) and extraocular CMV disease (10.3%).

Retinal Detachment Secondary to CMV Retinitis

This is the most common situation one comes across in AIDS patients. There are multiple areas of necrotic retina, which can harbor fine holes that may not be visible. Pars plana vitrectomy with belt buckle with a high viscosity silicone oil (5000 CS) tamponade may be needed in most cases. The oil needs to be kept for a long-time while the CMV status needs to be managed. No extra precautions except wearing double gloves and avoiding direct contact with blood/vitreous fluid are necessary during the surgery.

OCULAR TUBERCULOSIS

- Ocular tuberculosis may present as:
  - Chronic granulomatous iridocyclitis
  - Periphlebitis (Eale's disease)
    - Second most commonest manifestations of ocular tuberculosis after iridocyclitis
    - Perivenous accumulation of whitish material (presumably edema and inflammatory cells)
    - These cases are generally treated with steroids but some benefit with antituberculous treatment
  - Choroiditis:
    - Can occur focally or diffusely with either indolent or military tuberculosis
    - Choroiditis is deep, usually subvenous and heals with deep scars. Rarely can break through into vitreous
    - HIV positive patients may present with multifocal lesions of military tuberculosis
  - Serpiginous choroiditis
  - Ethambutol optic neuropathy.

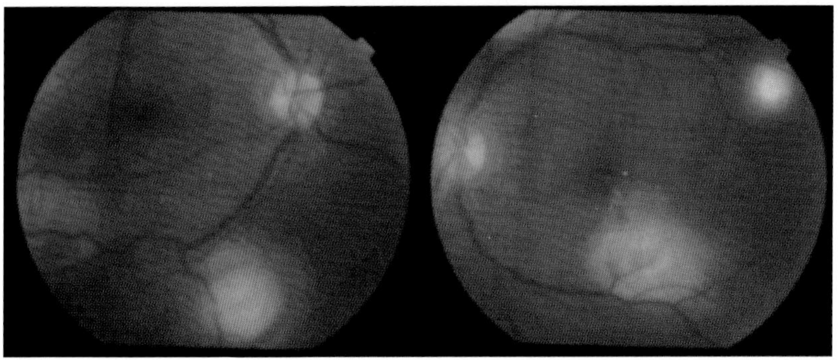

Fig. 14: Fundus photograph showing multiple choroidal tubercles

CHAPTER EIGHT

VITREOUS DISEASES

- **ASTEROID HYALOSIS**
  Soumen Mondal, S Natarajan (India)
- **HEREDITARY VITREORETINOPATHIES**
  Soumen Mondal, Supriya Dabir, S Natarajan (India)
  - Stickler's Syndrome
  - Wagner's Disease
  - Familial Exudative Vitreoretinopathy
  - Fabre-Goldmann Disease
  - Hereditary Retinoschisis
- **VITREOUS OPACITIES**
  Ashok Garg (India)

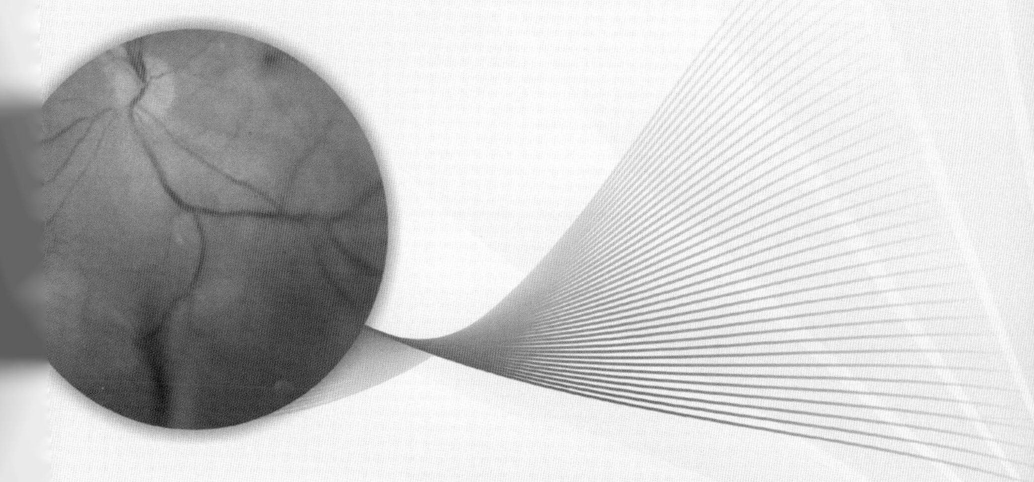

Asteroid Hyalosis

Soumen Mondal, S Natarajan (India)

INTRODUCTION

First described by Benson in 1894[1] as small spheres scattered in the vitreous, asteroid hyalosis is seen in about 2% of patients.

CLINICAL SIGNS AND SYMPTOMS

Usually present unilaterally, asteroid hyalosis does not cause any symptom, but rarely patient may complain of floaters.

Clinically, it manifests as small, round to oval refractile opacities suspended into the vitreous which are often associated with vitreous collagen.[2] The asteroid bodies move with the vitreous (along with eye movement) and their location is not affected by gravity as shown in Figure 1. Interestingly, eyes with asteroid hyalosis do not have posterior vitreous detachment.

DIFFERENTIAL DIAGNOSIS

Synchisis scintillans or cholesterolosis bulbi is characterized by glistening, angular crystalline bodies that float freely in the vitreous cavity and tend to settle inferiorly due to gravity. It is mostly seen after vitreous hemorrhage.

Vitreous amyloidosis has a bilateral presentation in which "glasswool" like deposits are seen in the vitreous. They may be preferentially located perivascularly with progression over the years leading to visual compromise.

MANAGEMENT

Being an innocuous condition, it does not require any treatment at all. In rare situations like poor visualization of the fundus, inability to perform laser photocoagulation, inability to find retinal breaks in retinal detachment. Vitrectomy can be contemplated.[2]

REFERENCES

1. Benson AH. Diseases of the vitreous. A case of 'monocular asteroid hyalites'. Trans Ophthalmol Soc UK 1894;14:101.
2. Rutar T, Reinke MH, D'amico DJ, Bhisitkul RB. Disease of the vitreous. In: Albert DM, Miller JW Albert (Eds): Jacobiec's Principles and practice of ophthalmology, 3rd (edn). Saunders Elsevier, Philadelphia 2008;2387:2401.

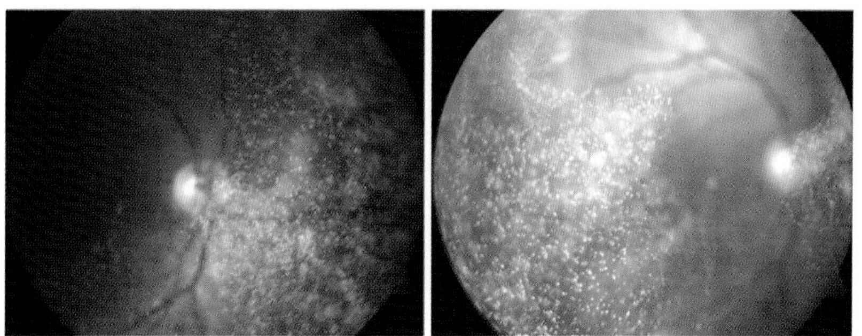

Fig. 1: Asteroid hyalosis

Hereditary Vitreoretinopathies

Soumen Mondal, Supriya Dabir, S Natarajan (India)

STICKLER'S SYNDROME

INTRODUCTION

First reported in 1965,[1] Stickler's syndrome or hereditary progressive arthroophthalmopathy is a progressive, debilitating connective tissue disorder with systemic and ocular manifestations and is of varying severity. It is inherited in an autosomal dominant fashion with variable penetrance.

CLINICAL SYMPTOMS AND SIGNS

Ocular: Progressive axial myopia with vitreous syneresis is seen. A characteristic finding in the posterior segment is the presence of an optically empty vitreous cavity. Vitreous membranes can be seen which are relatively dense, avascular and freely mobile. In the retina, peripheral radial lattice - like degeneration are seen which are often associated with RPE hyperplasia, vascular sheathing and sclerosis. Single large or multiple retinal breaks can be seen.[2] Retinal detachment occurs in 30% patients in the first decade of life. Other ocular associations are presenile cataract, ectopia lentis and glaucoma.

Systemic: Maxillary hypoplasia, bifid uvula, high arched palate, Pierre Robin sequence (micrognathia, cleft palate, glossoptosis) abnormal teeth and malocclusion are some of the orofacial abnormalities seen. Musculoskeletal abnormalities like osteoarthritis, spondyloepiphyseal dysplasia, muscular hypoplasia and hypotony, marfanoid habitus are commonly manifested. Conductive and sensorineural hearing loss are other common systemic findings.

INVESTIGATION

ERG: ERG is reduced.

FFA: Areas of paravascular pigmentary degeneration manifests zone of window defect with blockage of choroidal fluorescence at the areas of pigment deposits.

TREATMENT

Barrage laser or cryopexy should be done irrespective of presence or absence of symptoms. In case of retinal detachment, repair by buckling or vitreous surgery is done (as appropriate) though results are not very encouraging (inadequate drainage of subretinal fluid due to liquefied vitreous).

INFERENCE

A hereditary arthroophthalmopathy, Stickler's syndrome manifests with liquefied, optically empty vitreous cavity, peripheral radial or paravascular lattice-like retinal degenerations and retinal breaks. They frequently lead to rhegmatogenous retinal detachment. All peripheral degeneration seen in Stickler's syndrome is to be aggressively treated.

REFERENCES

1. Stickler GB, Belau PG, Farell FJ, et al. Hereditary progressive arthroophthalmopathy. Mayo Clin Proc 1965;40:433-55.
2. Van Balen ATM, Falger ELF. Hereditary hyaloideoretinal degeneration and palatoschisis. Arch Ophthalmol 1970;83:152-85.

WAGNER'S DISEASE

Wagner's hyaloideoretinal dystrophy or Wagner's disease is a rare vitreoretinopathy with autosomal dominance inheritance pattern.

CLINICAL SIGNS AND SYMPTOMS

Liquefaction of vitreous with absence of scaffolding is seen most commonly, which presents as an optically empty vitreous. Also seen are equatorial, preretinal grayish white membranes. With time, progressive chorioretinal atrophy is seen. Patients with Wagner's disease have an increased risk of having rhegmatogenous retinal detachment. Other associated ocular findings are low myopia and cortical cataract. Unlike Stickler's syndrome, there is no systemic association.

TREATMENT

Prophylactic treatment to all breaks should be done. Contrary to Stickler's syndrome, rhegmatogenous retinal detachment in Wagner's disease has a better outcome following scleral buckling surgery.

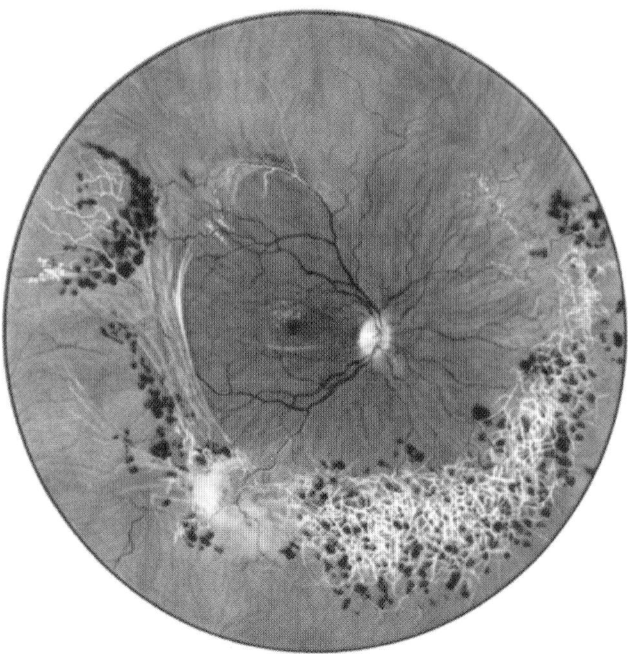

Fig. 1: Peripheral retinal degeneration in Wagner's disease

FAMILIAL EXUDATIVE VITREORETINOPATHY

Inherited in an autosomal dominant pattern, Familial Exudative Vitreoretinopathy is characterized by failure of the temporal retinal periphery to vascularize.

CLINICAL SIGNS AND SYMPTOMS

Presenting in late childhood, initially, areas of white without pressure are seen which are associated with peripheral attachments and vitreous degeneration. Later on, telangiectasis is seen in retinal periphery which may further progress to fibrovascular proliferation and ridge formation due to vitreous traction. These in turn, may lead to tractional retinal detachment and subretinal exudation.

INVESTIGATION

FFA: Peripheral nonperfusion with vascular straightening and abrupt termination.

TREATMENT

Prognosis of this condition is generally poor. Vitrectomy for tractional retinal detachment has been successful in selected cases.

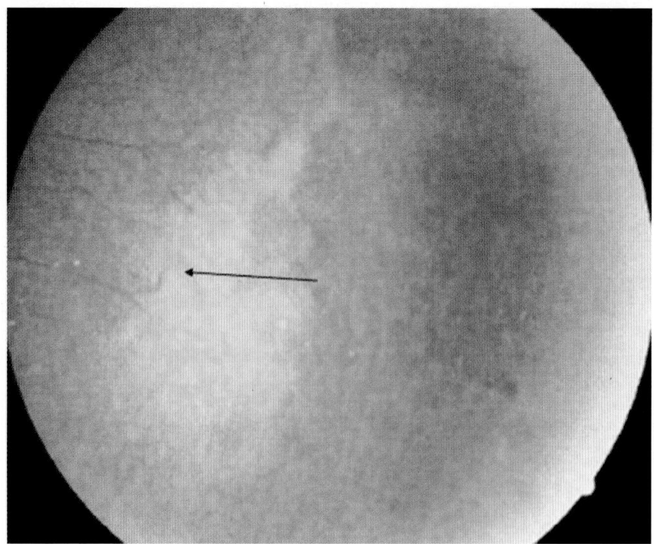

Fig. 2: FEVR - Typical abrupt cessation of vessels at mid-periphery with fimbriated edge of vessels

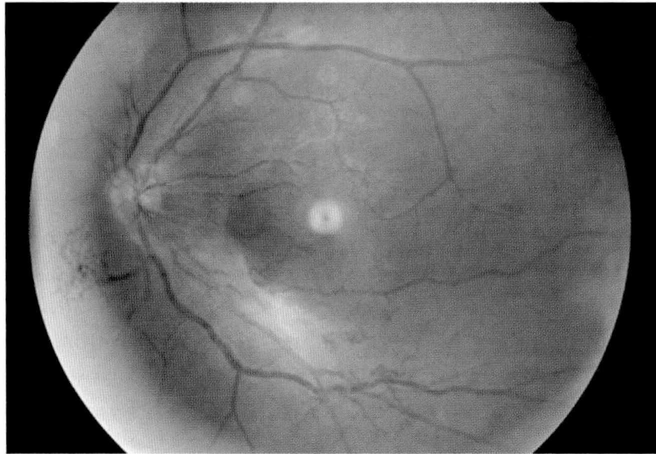

Fig. 3: FEVR — Thick preretinal vitreous causing minimal TRD

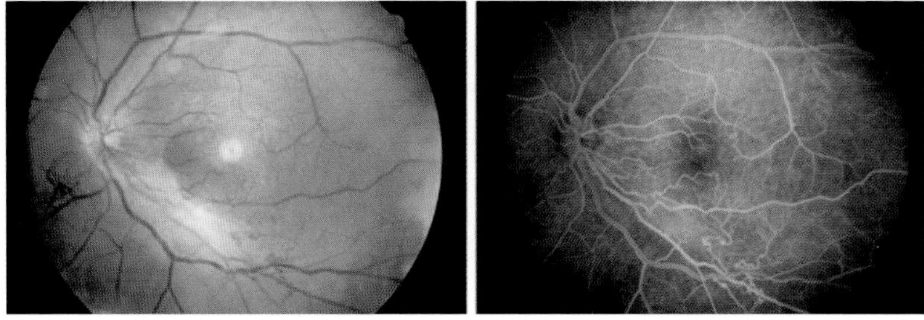

Fig. 4: FEVR — Thick preretinal vitreous causing minimal TRD, vascular distortion also seen

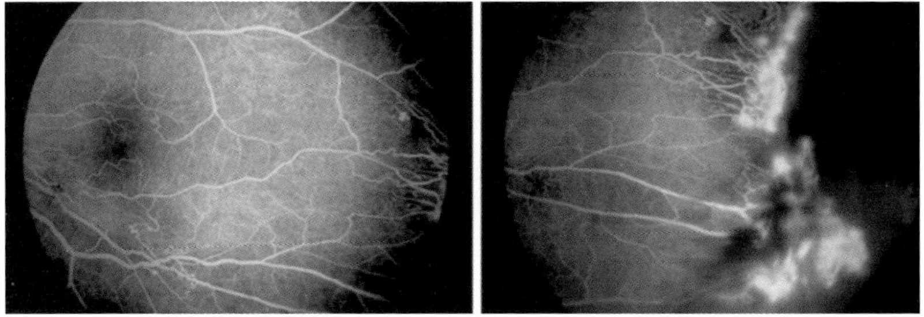

Fig. 5: FFA of the same patient showing avascular retina at mid-periphery with diffuse leakage from abnormal vessels

FABRE-GOLDMANN DISEASE

Fabre-Goldmann Tapetoretinal dystrophy or Fabre-Goldmann disease is a bilateral, progressive disease inherited in an autosomal recessive pattern.

CLINICAL SIGNS AND SYMPTOMS

Usually the child presents with defective vision and nyctalopia. Clinical examination reveals features of peripheral congenital retinoschisis as well as pigmentary retinopathy.

Peripheral retinal degenerative changes like chorioretinal atrophy and pigment clumping are seen in areas of schisis, along with arteriolar attenuation and occasionally waxy disk pallor. There may be associated vitreous syneresis. Retinal detachment may occur at any time.

INVESTIGATION

ERG: Markedly reduced or absent a-wave and b-wave amplitudes.

TREATMENT

Early diagnosis, genetic counseling and vigilance for retinal detachment is warranted.

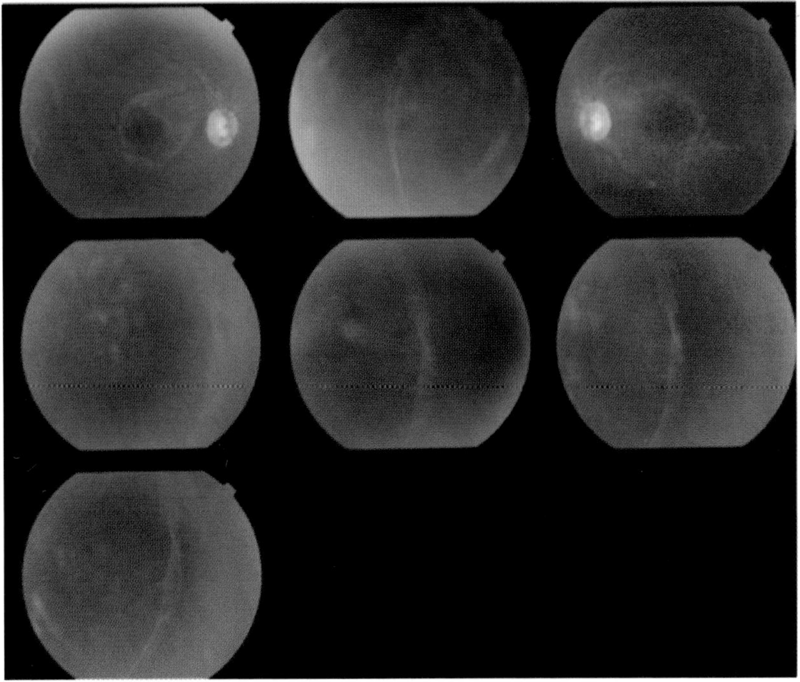

Fig. 6: Fabre-Goldmann Disease

HEREDITARY RETINOSCHISIS

A rare vitreoretinal dystrophy with an X-linked transmission pattern, hereditary retinoschisis presents in the first or early second decade.

Foveal retinoschisis is seen in almost 100% cases.[1] Initially the foveal lesion may have a stellate appearance formed by intraretinal microcystoid spaces which enlarges over time tocoalsce and rupture. Peripheral schisis predominantly involves the inferotemporal quadrant. The inner layer contains the internal limiting membrane and the nerve fiber layer whereas the outer layer contains the rest of the outer retina. Avascular or vascular vitreous veils may appear in extreme cases which probably represents various combinations of retinoschisis and inner layer holes.[2] There may also be peripheral perivascular sheathing, dendritiform lesions and neovascularization of the retina.

Complications of the dystrophy include vitreous and intraschisis hemorrhage and retinal detachment.

INVESTIGATION

ERG: In eyes with peripheral schisis, there is decrease in b-wave amplitude in photopic and scotopic testing.

OCT: Cystoid changes characterizing the foveal retinoschisis can be documented by OCT.

Management: Prophylactic laser to peripheral retinoschisis has been found to be of no benefit.[3] Scleral buckling surgery for retinal detachment has a variable success rate. Vitreous hemorrhage and posterior break might require a vitrectomy procedure. Genetic counseling is a must for patients and family members.

REFERENCES

1. Ide CH, Wilson RJ. Juvenile retinoschisis. Br J Ophthalmol 1973;57:560-63.
2. Sarin LK, Green WR, Dailey EG. Juvenile retinoschisis: congenital vascular veils and hereditary retinoschisis. Am J Ophthalmol 1964;57:793-96.
3. Turut P, et al. Analysis of results in the treatment of retinoschisis in X-linked congenital retinoschisis. Graefes Arch Clin Exp Ophthalmol 1989;227:328-31.

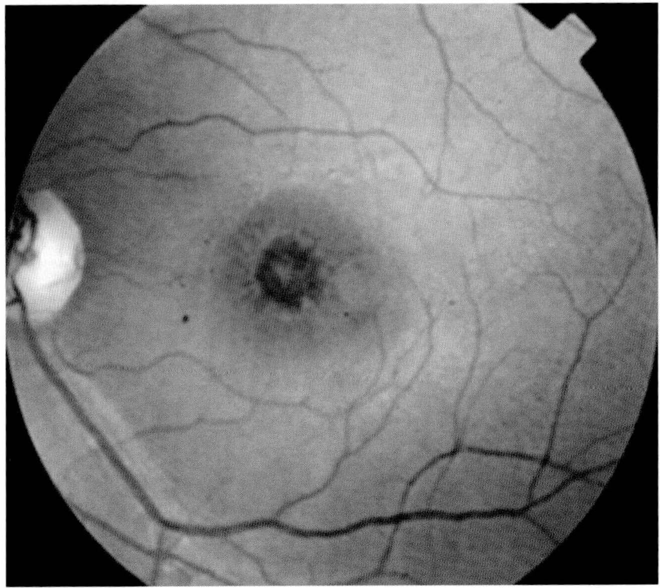

Fig. 7: X-linked retinoschisis — cystoid changes at macula

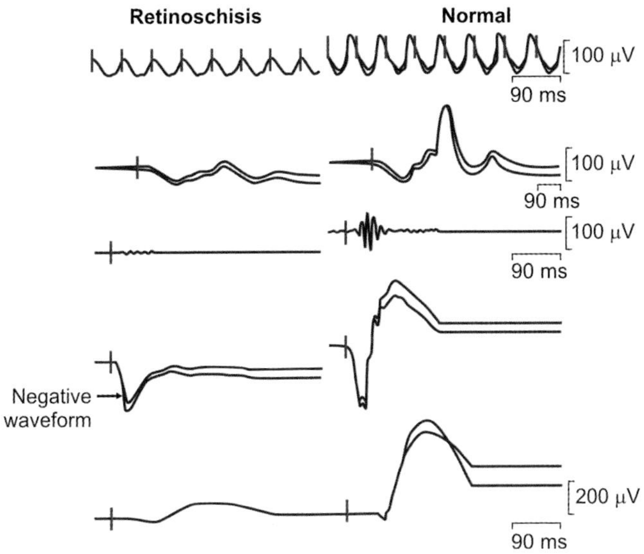

Fig. 8: ERG — B wave amplitude reduced

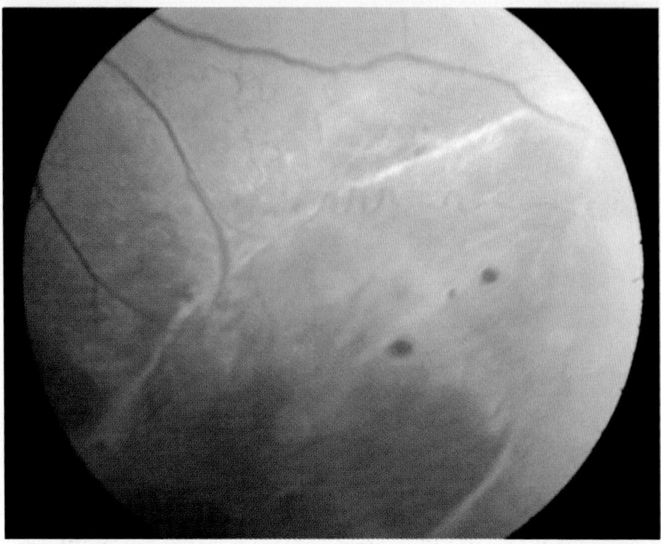

Fig. 9: Inner layer holes in retinoschisis

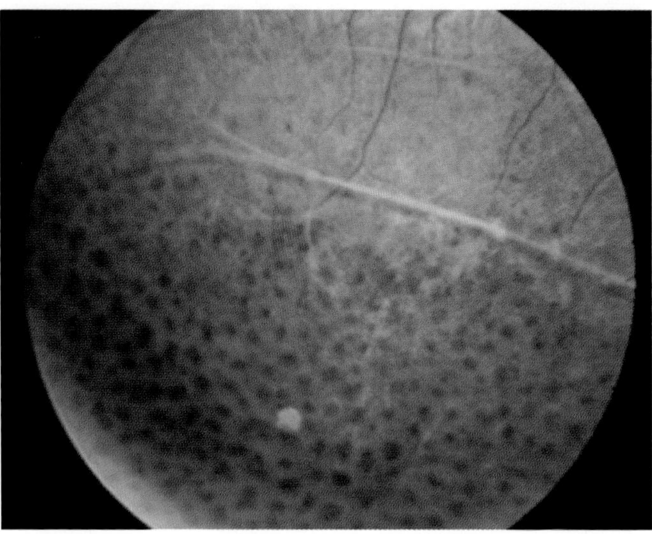

Fig. 10: X-linked retinoschisis — mottled appearance of retinal pigment epithelium

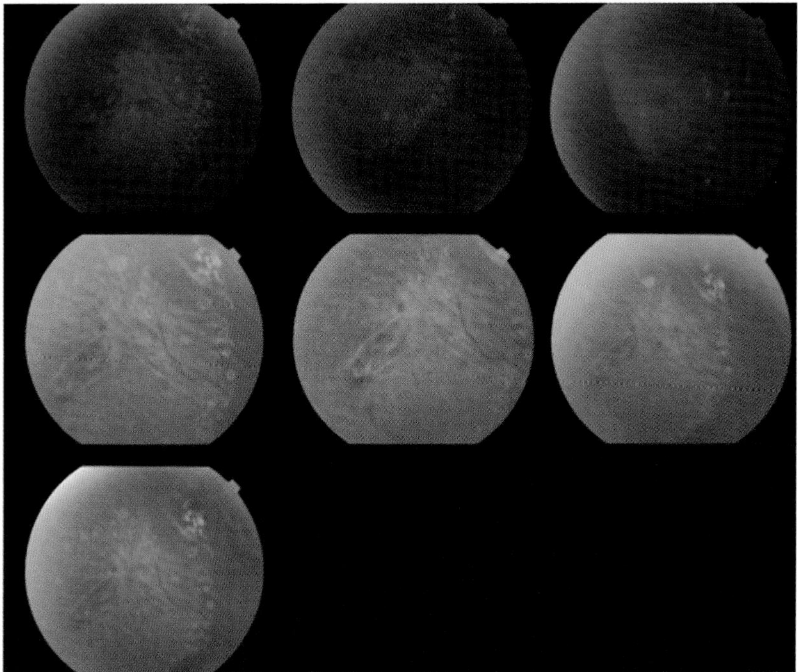

Fig. 11: Peripheral retinoschisis

Vitreous Opacities

Ashok Garg (India)

INTRODUCTION

- Vitreous is an inert, jelly like transparent structure which subserves optical functions.
- Any relatively non-transparent structure present in it shall form an opacity.
- Vitreous opacity may be single or multiple depending upon the causative factor or may be developmental or degenerative.

Pathophysiology

A. For single vitreous opacities
   - Developmental vitreous opacities
   - Anterior hyaloid remanant (Mittendorf's dot)
   - Foreign body
   - Dislocated lens
   - Parasitic cysts
   - Vitreous detachment
   - Vitreous cylinders

B. For multiple scattered vitreous opacities
   - Vitreous degeneration as seen in older and Myopic persons
   - Inflammatory vitreous opacities
   - Amyloid degeneration
   - Myelomatosis
   - Hemorrhagic opacities
   - Tumor cell opacities
   - Plasmoid vitreous
   - Synchysis scintillans
   - Asteroid hyalosis

CLINICAL SIGNS AND SYMPTOMS

Symptoms

- Vitreous opacities appear as black spots floating in front of the eye.
- Dense opacities may cause marked fall in vision.

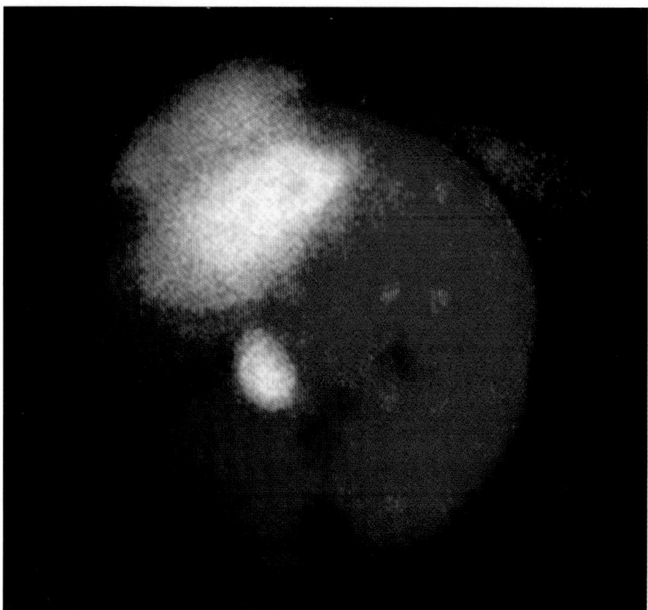

Fig. 1: Inflammatory vitreous opacities

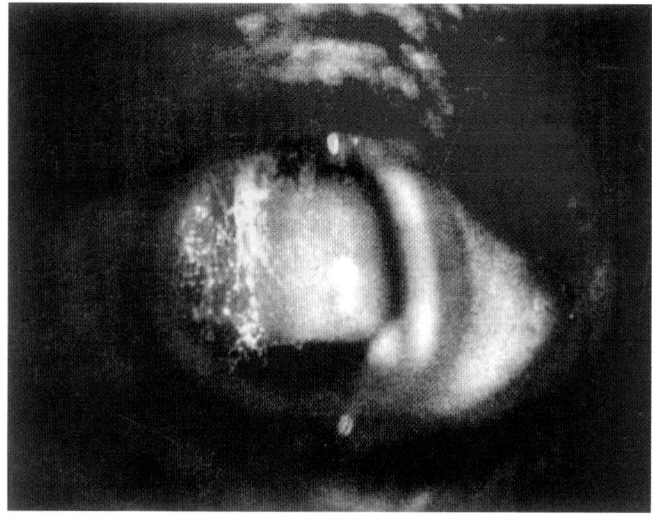

Fig. 2: Asteroid hyalosis

Signs

- Vitreous opacities are best seen on slit-lamp examination.
- These are also visible by the ophthalmoscope with a + 8D lens.
- These are seen as mobile opaque matter in the vitreous.

INVESTIGATIONS

- On echography, minimal heterogeneity within the normal homogenous vitreous called vitreous opacities are among the most common findings
- This pathological change in vitreous is seen as point like lesions.
- Vitreous opacities in senile vitreous degeneration appear as point like echo source with a spike height usually less than 5 percent at tissue sensitivity.
- Echogram of Asteroid Hyalosis shows a medium to high (40-100%) reflectivity with central vitreous distribution as typical finding.
- Calcium soaps that accumulate in the vitreous can be easily identified and echoes demonstrated in this condition are very intense and may persist at sensitivity settings as low as 50 dB.

DIFFERENTIAL DIAGNOSIS

(a) Opaque sheets anterior to the vitreous as.
   - Elschnig pearls after ECCE.
   - Normal posterior capsule following ECCE.
   - Soemmerring ring.
   - Vitreous adhesions to iris, capsule or IOL.

(b) Pseudoglioma leukokoria
   Scattered opacities as seen in:
   - Amyloid disease
   - Ankylosing spondylitis
   - Crystalline deposits
   - Heterochromic uveitis
   - Multiple myeloma
   - Pigment cells
   - Snowball opacities
   - Toxoplasmosis
   - Retinoblastoma
   - Whipples disease
   - Vitreous degeneration – Wagner's disease
   - Dislocated lens
   - Foreign body
   - Vitreous detachment

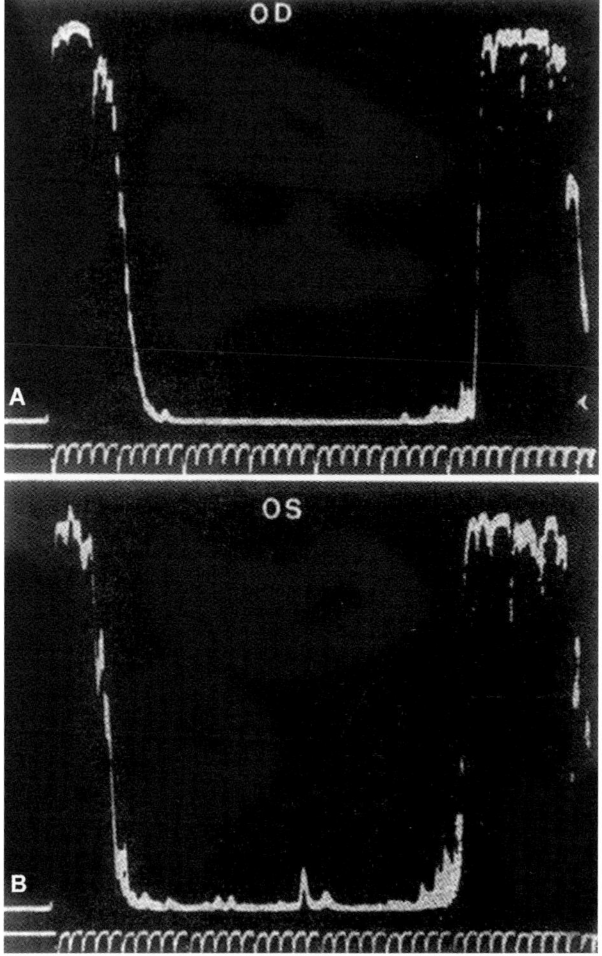

Figs 3A and B: Echogram showing bilateral low reflective spikes of vitreous opacities in senile vitreous degeneration

TREATMENT

- Muscae, volitantes need no treatment.
- For inflammatory vitreous opacities treatment of underlying cause like uveitis or retinochoroiditis is required.
- The earlier treatment of vitreous opacities advocated was aspiration alone without replacement which has been out of favour now.
- For vitreous replacement with automated vitrectomy instruments, physiological saline with other additives like glutathione and adenosine have been recommended.
- Pars plana vitrectomy and 25 G TCV vitrectomy have been advocated for vitreous opacities as a result of vitreous hemorrhage, trauma, vitreous traction bands or membranes.

PROGNOSIS

- Small and few scattered vitreous opacities are not harmful and do not obscure the vision and fundus details.
- Vitreous opacities of Grade 2+ or more require immediate medical and surgical intervention to maintain visual acuity.

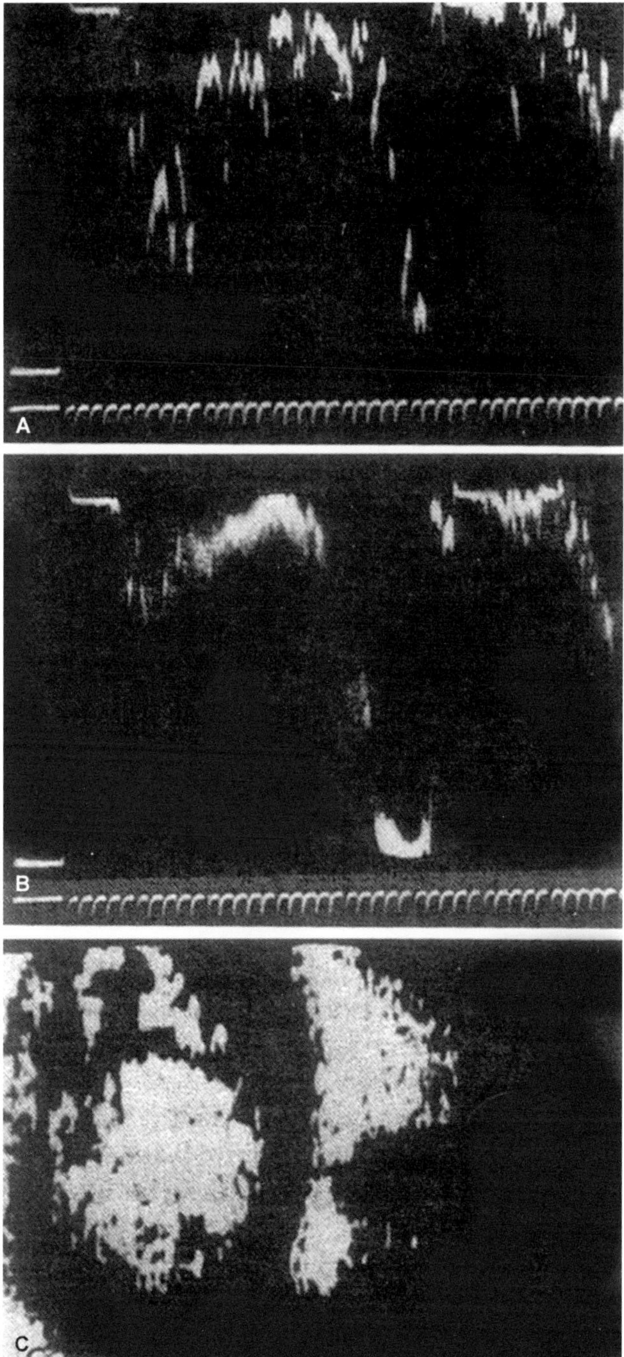

Figs 4A to C: Typical Echogram of Asteroid Hyalosis (A) High reflectivity, (B) Non-specific spike of marked after movement, (C) Central distribution

CHAPTER NINE

RETINAL DETACHMENT

- **RETINAL DETACHMENT**
  Neeraj Sanduja, Ajay Aurora (India)
  - Rhegmatogenous RD
  - Tractional RD
  - Exudative RD

- **EXUDATIVE RETINAL DETACHMENT**
  Hsi Kung Kuo (Taiwan)
  - Vogt-Koyanagi-Harada Syndrome
  - Sympathetic Ophthalmia
  - Toxemia of Pregnancy
  - Choroidal Metastasis
  - Choroidal Hemangioma
  - Coat's Disease

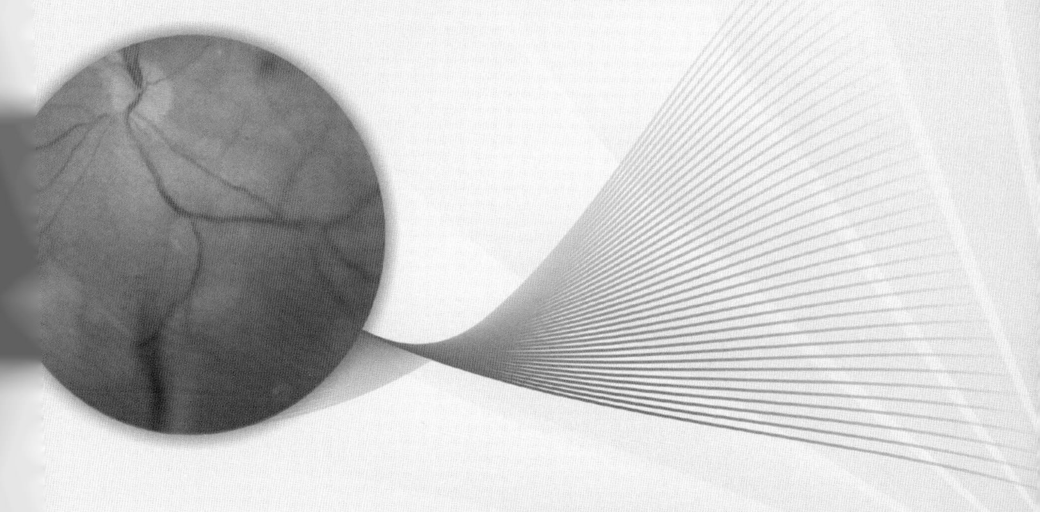

Retinal Detachment

Neeraj Sanduja, Ajay Aurora (India)

INTRODUCTION

Retinal detachments (RD) are the results of separation of the sensory retina from the retinal pigment epithelium (RPE).
Phakic non traumatic retinal detachment occurs in approximately 5-12 persons per 100,000 per year.

Types of RDs

Rhegmatogenous RD

Results from a hole, tear, or break in the neuronal layer allowing fluid from the vitreous cavity to seep in between and separate sensory and RPE layers.

Tractional RD

Results from traction from inflammatory or vascular fibrous membranes on the surface of the retina, which tether to the vitreous.

Exudative RD

Results from extravasation of fluid into the subretinal space from choroid or retinal blood vessels in absence of retinal hole.

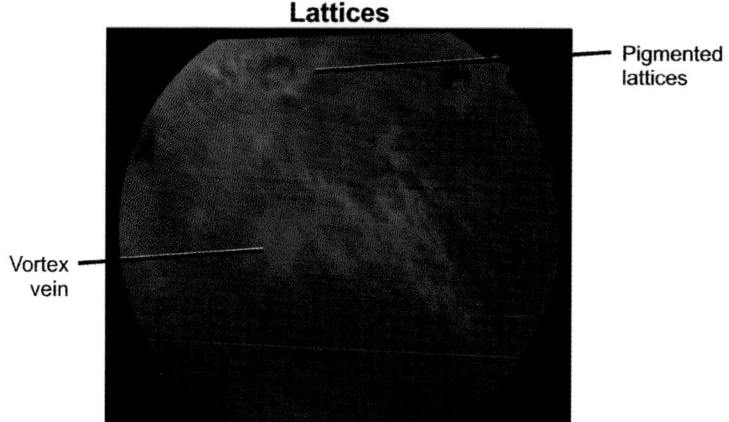

Fig. 1: Circumferential pigmented lattices located anterior to equator

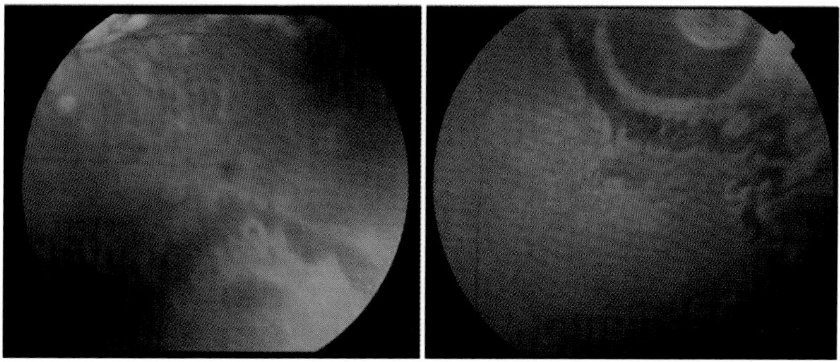
Fig. 2: Old pigmented laser marks around horse shoe tear

RHEGMATOGENOUS RETINAL DETACHMENTS

PATHOGENESIS

- Development of posterior vitreous detachment (PVD) which may cause retinal break by traction on the retina.
- Ocular trauma.

Vitreous cavity fluid then passes through the tear causing detachment of the sensory retina from the RPE.

CONDITIONS PREDISPOSING TO RD

Peripheral Retinal Tufts

Small, peripheral reinal elevations caused by focal areas of vitreous traction.

Degenerative Retinoschisis

- Results from the progression of peripheral cystoid degeneration
- Usually bilateral
- Separation of retinal layers can take place at level of outer plexiform layer or at nerve fiber layer
- Outer layer breaks may lead to retinal detachment.

Lattice Degeneration

- Lattice degeneration is seen in the form of elongated well demarcated white or pigmented patches lying circumferentially or radially around the retinal periphery, being characterized in well established cases by a network of branching white lines.
- There is discontinuity of the internal limiting membrane of the retina, an overlying pocked of liquefied vitreous, adherence of vitreous at the margin of lesion and varying degree of atrophy of inner retinal layer.
- Causes 20-30 % of all retinal detachments.
- Detachment is caused by a tear beginning posterior to or at the end of the lattice degeneration or by means of atrophic retinal holes in lattice itself.

Myopia

Myopia with refractive error greater than 8 diopters accounts for 10% of all retinal detachments.

Rhegmatogenous RD

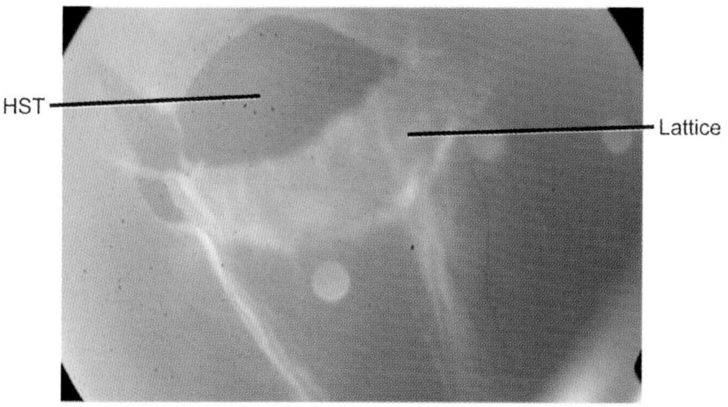

Fig. 3: Horse shoe tear (HST) at edge of lattice with retinal detachment

Rhegmatogenous RD

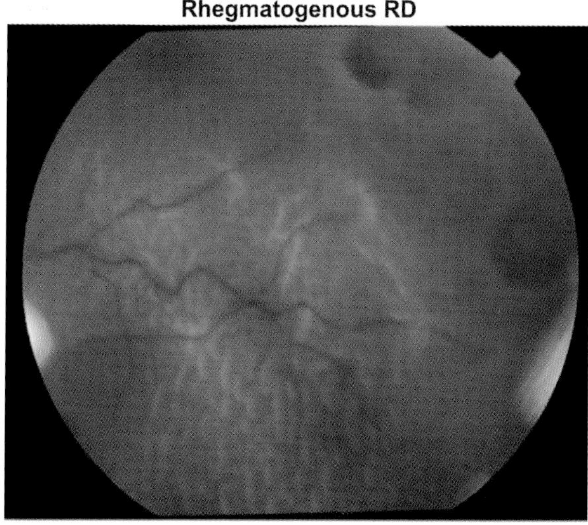

Fig. 4: Fundus photograph left eye—detached retina with whitish retinal folds with 2 horse shoe shape tears superiorly and temporally

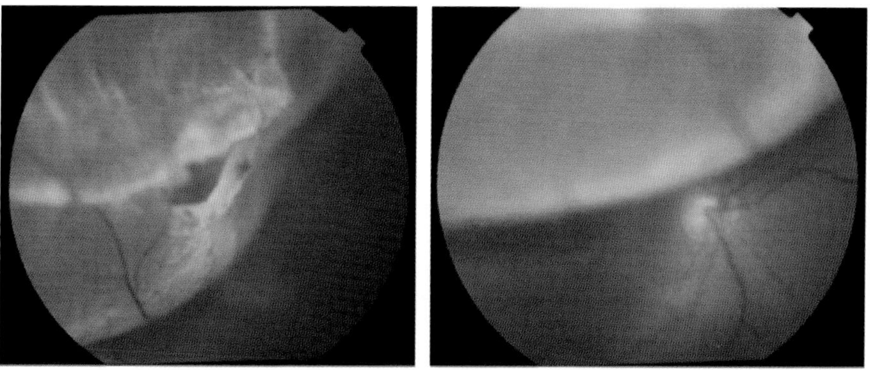

Fig. 5: Bullous RD with bulla overhanging macula with posterior retinal break

Cataract Surgery

- Incidence of retinal detachment after
- Intra-capsular cataract extraction (ICCE)- 2-5%
- Extra-capsular cataract extraction (ECCE) with or without IOL - 1.4%
- YAG capsulotomy- 3.2%.

Trauma

- Blunt trauma can lead to retinal dialysis in inferotemporal or superonasal region
- May result in giant retinal tear especially in myopic eyes
- Penetrating injury is often followed by vitreous band formation, and this band contraction may lead to retinal detachment.

DIFFERENTIAL DIAGNOSIS

- Posterior vitreous detachment
- Peripheral retinal lesions (e.g. enclosed oral bays, meridional folds, cystic retinal tufts, lattice degeneration)
- Myopia
- Senile retinoschisis
- Cataract extraction
- Trauma
- Intraocular inflammation/infection
  - Acute retinal necrosis syndrome
  - Cytomegalovirus retinitis
  - Ocular toxocariasis
  - Ocular toxoplasmosis
  - Pars planitis
- Colobomas of the choroid and retina
- Coloboma of the lens (giant retinal tear)
- Stickler syndrome
- Goldmann-Fabre syndrome
- Marfan syndrome
- Homocystinuria
- Ehlers-Danlos syndrome.

SYMPTOMS

a Floaters:
  - Ring like shadow (Weiss ring).
  - Shower of dot like black spots (Vitreous hemorrhage caused by retinal break or avulsed blood vessel)
  - Cobweb like

Rhegmatogenous RD

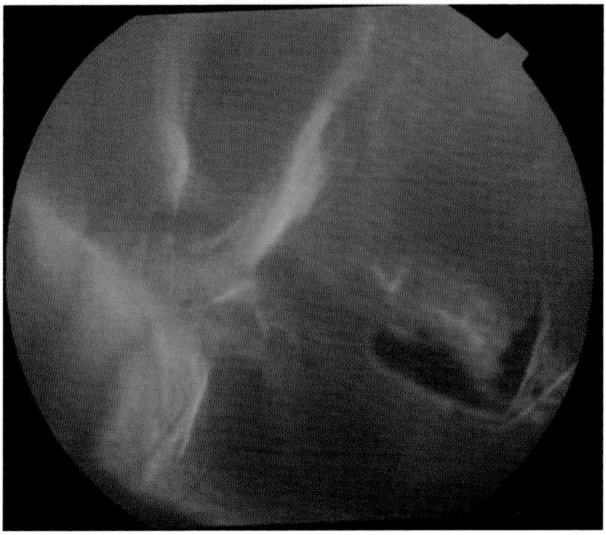

Fig. 6: Fundus photograph right eye—typical horse shoe tear with retinal detachment

Giant Retina Tear

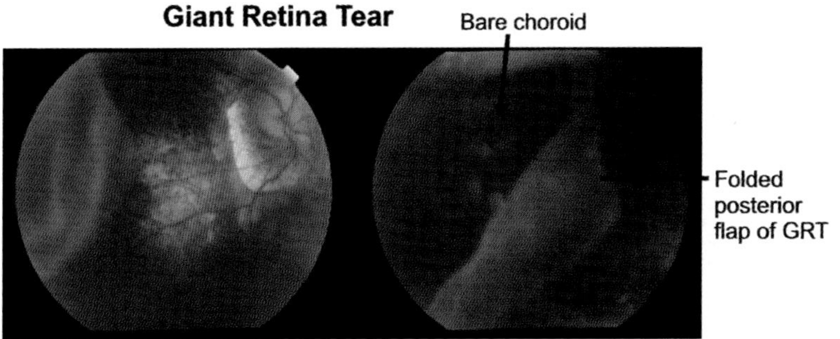

Fig. 7: Myopia with temporal GRT-note the folded posterior flap of GRT early vitreous surgery is recommended because of high chances of PVR

Recurrent RD

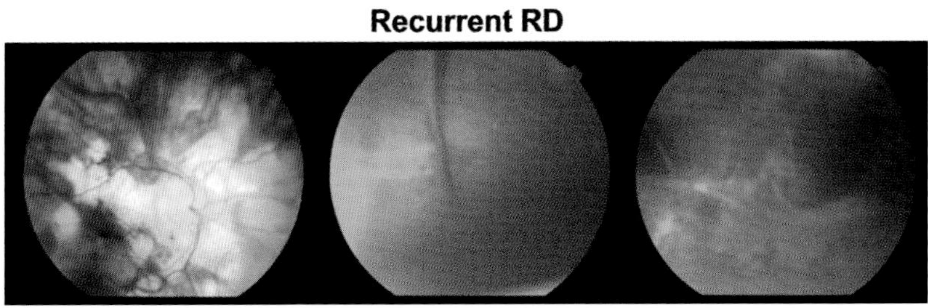

Fig. 8: Right eye of a high myopic patient after VR surgery with silicon oil macula is on. Inferior retina is off with PVR changes

b. Flashes (photopsia)
c. Decrease in vision
d. Visual field defects-late symptom of RD.

While symptoms of photopsia and floaters are not helpful in locating the position of the retinal tear or detachment, the visual field defect is very specific for locating the retinal detachment.

Ocular Evaluation

a. Visual acuity
b. Slit lamp biomicroscopy
    - Anterior segment is usually normal
    - Vitreous may show signs of pigment or tobacco dust (i.e., Shafer sign).
c. Applanation tonometry—IOP is usually low
d. Retinal evaluation
    - Indirect ophthalmoscopy with the use of scleral depression is the definitive means of diagnosing RD and definitively identify the location of the retinal tear.
    - Retinal detachment gives a milky, lackluster appearance with undulating retinal folds.
    - Detachment will not change position with changes in body posture, however it may shift and then return to its original orientation with quick eye movements
    - Associated findings may include posterior vitreous detachment and preretinal or vitreal hemorrhage. Retinal pigment epithelial hyperplasia may be noted in cases of long-standing retinal detachment (pigment demarcation line).

During retinal evaluation attention should be paid to:
a Extent of detachment
b. Number, size and location of retinal breaks
c Peripheral retinal degeneration, particularly lattice
d. Proliferaitve Vitreo Retinopathy changes.

INVESTIGATIONS

- Usually no ocular investigations are required.
- US B scan is indicated if media is hazy because of vitreous hemorrhage to ascertain condition of retina.

Management

- An acute onset rhegmatogenous detachment that involves or threatens the macula should be repaired within 24-48 hours

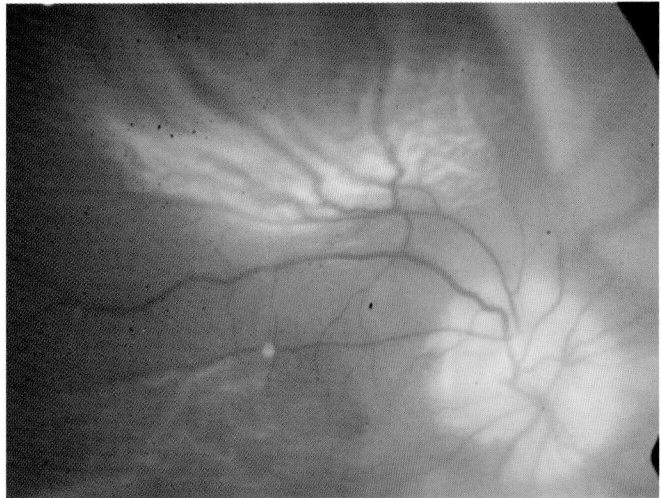

Fig. 9A: Right eye-retinal is off

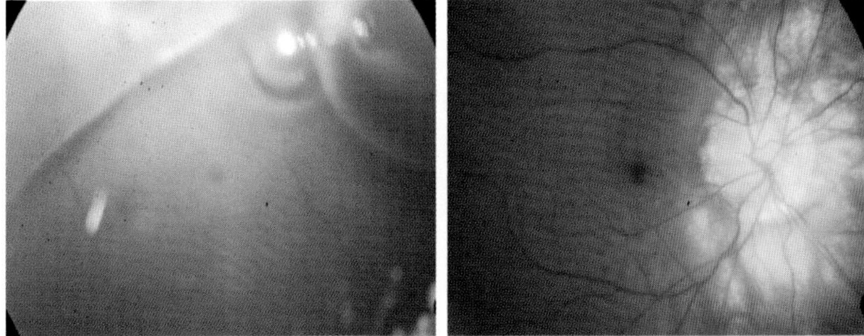

Fig. 9B: Postscleral buckling and C3F8 gas injection-retina on

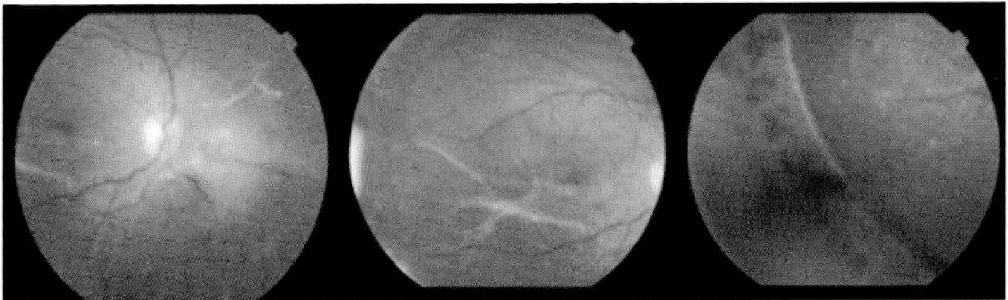

Fig. 10: Fundus photograph right eye—postvitrectomy. Note attached retina with subretinal gliotic bands with buckle effect with old laser marks

- Chronic or long-standing RRDs requiring treatment should be addressed within one to two week of diagnosis.
- While small retinal breaks or atrophic holes may be managed with laser photocoagulation or cryopexy, true retinal detachments require surgical repair.

Treatment Options for RRD

- Scleral buckling procedures
- Pneumatic retinopexy
- Vitrectomy with intraocular silicone oil tamponade/Gas tamponade.

Scleral Buckling

Principles of Surgery

a. Precise localization of all the retinal breaks
b. Creation of a chorio-retinal adhesion around the retinal break
c. Placement of scleral buckle to relieve vitreo-retinal traction on the break and
d. Drainage of subretinal fluid externally.

Pneumatic Retinopexy

- An intravitreal gas bubble (usually perfluoropropane, 0.2-0.3 cc C3F8) serves to reattach the retina
- Indicated for treating smaller, superiorly located detachments
- Cryopexy is performed at the site of the break and then the gas is injected into the vitreal cavity
- Careful eye and head positioning are important postoperatively to ensure resolution.

Vitrectomy

Indications

- Hazy media
- Posterior retinal breaks
- Multiple breaks 360 degree
- Retinal breaks not identifiable on indirect ophthalmoscopy
- Advanced PVR
- Giant retinal tear.

Intraoperative Complications

There are a number of intraoperative complications which may compromise the surgical objectives of the retinal detachment repair. The common complications are:

- Iatrogenic retinal break

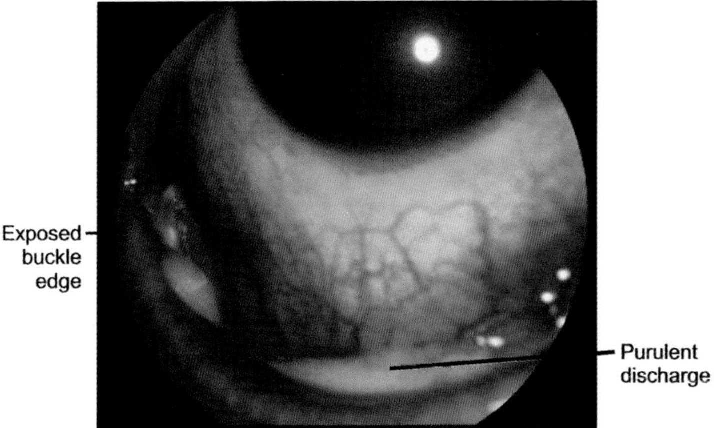

Fig. 11: External photograph-Buckle extrusion with infection

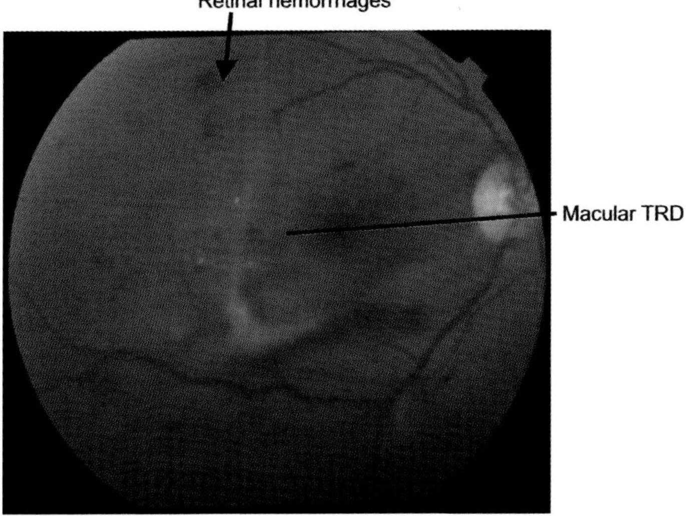

Fig. 12: Fundus photo right eye with PDR-fibrovascular proliferation just inside the inferotemporal arcade giving traction over macula

- Sub retinal hemorrhage
- Vitreous hemorrhage
- Retinal incarceration
- Central retinal artery occlusion.

Postoperative Complications

a. Recurrent detachment
b. Choroidal detachment

c. Glaucoma
d. Buckle exposure/infection
e. Endophthalmitis
f. Macular pucker.

PROGNOSIS

The anatomic and visual success rates of retinal detachment repair have gradually improved over the past decades as a result of:

a. Improved surgical techniques
b. Availability of improved materials
c. Better understanding of the pathophysiology of retinal detachments.

Anatomic Success

With the current techniques about 90% of retinal detachments can be successfully reattached with one or more operations.

Functional Success

The visual results of retinal detachment repair are variable depending on duration of retinal detachment, status of macula, age of the patient and associated features like choroidal detachment and presence of proliferative vitreo retinopathy.

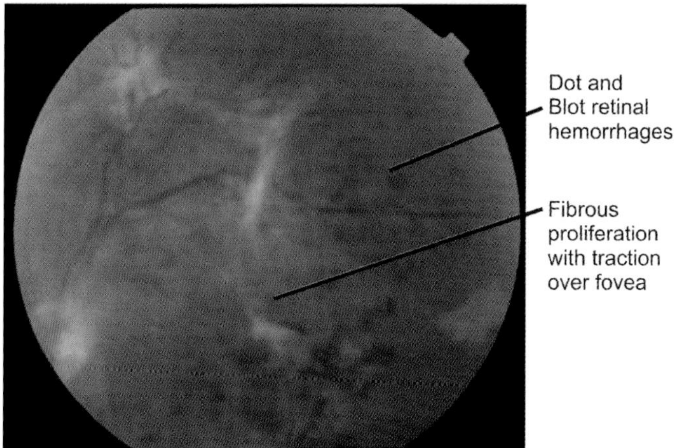

Fig. 13: Fundus photo left eye-PDR with macular TRD

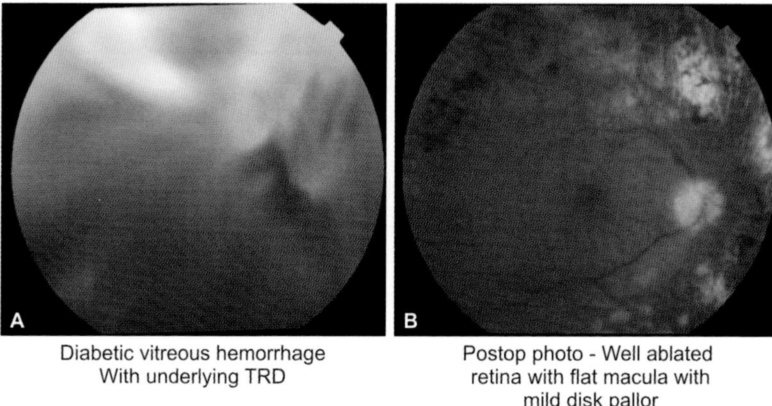

Figs 14A and B: Diabetic TRD with vitreous hemorrhage: (A) diabetic vitreous hemorrhage with underlying TRD, (B) postoperative photo—well ablated retina with flat macula with mild disk pallor

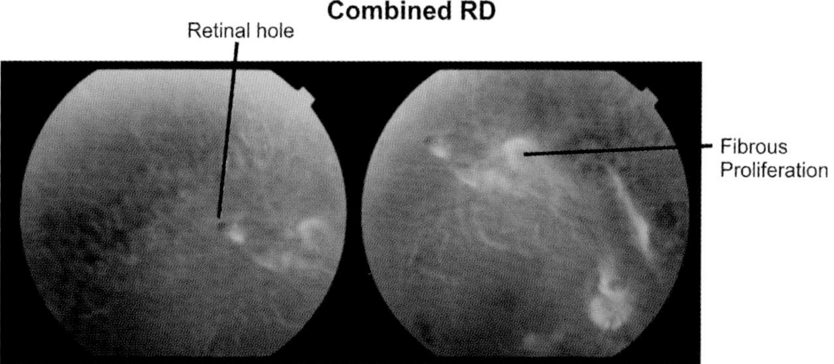

Fig. 15: A case of lasered diabetic retinopathy-dry fibrous proliferation along superotemporal arcade with a tiny hole at its edge leading to combined RD

TRACTIONAL RD

CAUSES

- Proliferative Diabetic Retinopathy (PDR)
- Retinopathy of Prematurity (ROP)
- Penetrating trauma
- Proliferative sickle retinopathy
- PVR
- Retinal venous occlusions.

ETIOLOGY

- Fibrotic scaffolding of the vitreous along proliferative vascular networks which induce strong anterior tractional forces through vitreal shrinkage.
- These forces induce the sensory retina to separate from the underlying RPE.

RETINAL EVALUATION

- Detachment has a concave configuration.
- The subretinal fluid is shallower than in RRD and often does not extend to the ora serrata.
- The highest elevation of the retina is at site of vitreoretinal traction.
- Retinal mobility is severely reduced, and shifting fluid is absent.

SYMPTOMS

- TRDs are often slow and insidious
- In peripheral TRDs , patient is either asymptomatic or has visual field defect progressing slowly and may become stationary for months or years.
- If the macula becomes involved, the patient will experience a drop in vision.

DIFFERENTIALS

- Exudative RD
- Rhegmatogenous RD
- Central retinal vein occlusion
- Branch retinal vein occlusion
- Proliferative diabetic retinopathy
- ROP.

Imaging Studies

In eyes with vitreous hemorrhage, a B-scan ultrasound is a useful adjunct to evaluate the presence or absence of retinal detachment.

Management

- Timing of surgical intervention depends on the underlying cause and extent of the TRD
- For example, A patient with TRD secondary to PDR that does not threaten the macula should be monitored closely
- The main surgical goal in these cases is to relieve vitreoretinal traction
- In certain cases, with further traction, small breaks may occur causing a combined TRD-RRD. In these cases, the surgical goal is to identify all the breaks and to close them in addition to the relief of vitreoretinal traction.

Principles of Surgery

- A scleral buckle is used in cases of combined RDA core vitrectomy
- Identifying posterior hyaloid face and relieving all vitreoretinal traction by segmentation and delamination
- Delamination refers to the separation of the retina from the extraretinal proliferation.
- Segmentation refers to cutting of the fibrovascular tissue bridge into small separate islands of tissue.
- Intraocular bleeding to be monitored closely. Diathermy to active neovascular fronds or laser photocoagulation to flat vascular proliferation may be necessary.
- Intravitreal bevacizumab 1 week before vitreous surgery is a useful preoperative adjunct in vitrectomy for PDR. Bevacizumab seems to reduce the bleeding associated with the segmentation and delamination of fibrovascular membranes.

Complications

- Retinal redetachment
- Vitreous hemorrhage
- Phthisis bulbi.

PROGNOSIS

- Visual prognosis depends on the underlying cause of TRD.
  - Anatomical success rates for retinal reattachment surgery for PVR are from 75-90% of eyes
  - The results after ROP surgery are very poor but better than the natural history (no light perception).
  - Visual recovery in PDR cases after vitrectomy is variable with 40% patients achieving visual acuity of better than 6/24. Also rebleed is seen in upto 30% patients after vitreous surgery.

EXUDATIVE RD

PATHOPHYSIOLOGY

- When there is an increase in the inflow of fluid or a decrease in the outflow of fluid from the vitreous cavity that overwhelms the normal compensatory mechanisms, fluid accumulates in the subretinal space leading to an exudative retinal detachment.
- Abnormal reinal blood vessels which leak profusely or a broken blood-retinal barrier, increase the inflow of fluid into the vitreous cavity leading to exudative RD.
- Abnormally thick sclera, as seen in nanophthalmos, decreases the outflow of fluid.
- Damage to the RPE prevents the pumping action of fluid.

SYMPTOMS

- Pain (e.g., uveitis or scleritis)
- Red eye (e.g., uveitic pathologies)
- Decrease in vision or visual field defect
- White pupil (leukocoria).

SIGNS

- The anterior segment may show signs of inflammation
- Bullous retinal detachment with smooth surface without any retinal folds with shifting subretinal fluid. In chronic cases, deposition of hard exudates may be seen. Dilated telangiectatic vessels may be seen.

CAUSES

Inflammatory

- Vogt-Koyanagi-Harada syndrome
- Scleritis
- Sympathetic ophthalmia
- Vasculitic entities (eg, Wegener granulomatosis rheumatoid arthritis)
- Other uveitic conditions (e.g. toxoplasmosis, cytomegalovirus retinitis)
- Dengue fever
- Orbital pseudotumor.

Exudative RD

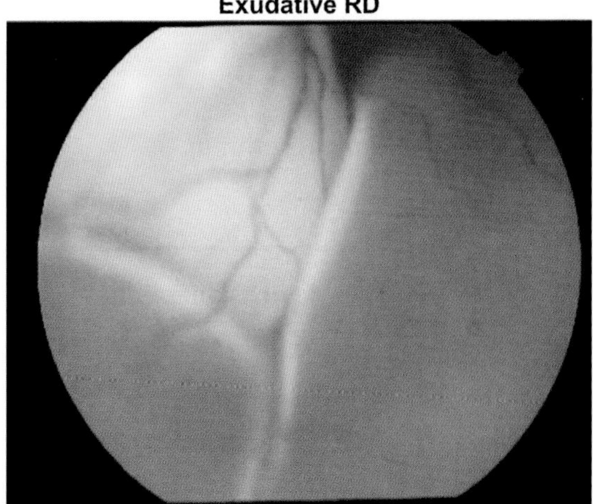

Fig. 16: Choroidal melanoma with exudative retinal detachment

Idiopathic

- Coat's disease
- Central serous chorioretinopathy
- Uveal effusion syndrome.

Congenital

- Nanophthalmos
- Familial exudative vitreoretinopathy.

Neoplastic

- Choroidal melanoma
- Choroidal hemangioma
- Choroidal nevus
- Choroidal metastases
- Retinoblastoma
- Primary intraocular lymphoma.

Iatrogenic

- Excessive laser photocoagulation
- Scleral buckling.

Vascular Factors

- Hypertension
- Eclampsia
- Exudative age-related macular degeneration.

DIFFERENTIAL DIAGNOSIS

All the above mentioned causes to be kept as differentials.

INVESTIGATIONS

Tailored approach based on clinical presentation.

Laboratory Tests

- VDRL
- Antineutrophil cytoplasmic antibodies
- Rh factor.

Fundus Fluorescein Angiography

Identifying areas of leakage in central serous chorioretinopathy, Vogt-Koyanagi-Harada syndrome, and Coats disease.

US B Scan

Indications

- Hazy media.
- To detect choroidal thickness, choroidal detachment and scleral thickness
- To detect the presence or absence, the size, location and internal character of choroidal masses.

MANAGEMENT

The management of exudative retinal detachments is directed towards treating the underlying condition.

- Infectious etiologies should be treated with antibiotics
- Inflammatory conditions, such as scleritis and Vogt-Koyanagi-Harada syndrome, should be treated with anti-inflammatory agents.

- Tumors need to be treated accordingly with radiation, chemotherapy, cryotherapy or laser photocoagulation.

INFERENCE

- Rhegmatogenous RD requires an emergent approach to achieve satisfactory anatomical and visual outcome, especially in RDs that threaten the fovea or of recent onset.
- Inflammatory retinal detachments usually are treated medically.
- Tractional retinal detachments in diabetics should be handled when fovea is involved or threatened to be involved. The main surgical goal in all these cases is to relieve vitreoretinal traction.

Exudative Retinal Detachment

Hsi Kung Kuo (Taiwan)

INTRODUCTION

There are three types of retinal detachment (RD): rhegmatogenous, tractional, and exudative. The pathogenesis of the former two types of RD come from preretinal factors, either vitreous or epiretinal membrane. The causes of exudative RD come from retina or subretinal structure.

PATHOGENESIS OF EXUDATIVE RETINAL DETACHMENT

Exudative RD may occur in a variety of diseases in which fluid leaks and accumulates under the retina. The causes of exudative RD include

1. Uveitis: Vogt-Koyanagi-Harada diseases, sympathetic ophthalmia, toxemia of pregnancy associated RD, posterior scleritis. The unusual causes reported had ocular-CNS lymphoma, syphilis, pars planitis, relapsing polychondritis.
2. Malignant tumor: choroidal metastasis, choroidal melanoma, retinoblastoma.
3. Benign tumor: choroidal hemangioma, retinal hemangioma, retinal astrocytic hamartoma.
4. Others: Coat's disease, bullous central serous chorioretinopathy, idiopathic.

VOGT-KOYANAGI-HARADA (VKH) SYNDROME

INTRODUCTION

VKH syndrome is an idiopathic autoimmune disease against melanocytes causing inflammation of melanocyte-containing tissue such as the uvea, ear, skin and meninges. It is a bilateral granulomatous panuveitis. The clinical course can be divided to acute stage and recurrent, chronic stage. Pan-uveitis with exudative retinal detachment is a unique picture of acute stage. For the recurrent, chronic cases, it would present with anterior uveitis and mild posterior uveitis.

CLINICAL SIGNS AND SYMPTOMS

1. Anterior uveitis
2. Posterior uveitis: disc edema and yellow-white exudates at the level of the RPE with serous detachment in the posterior pole during active inflammatory stage. The extent of RD depends on the severity of the disease and associated with the prognosis. Diffused RPE degeneration with sunset-glow picture at the late stage.
3. Extraocular symptoms and signs: headache, aseptic meningitis, tinnitis are common at the early stage. Skin and hair depigmentation might present later.

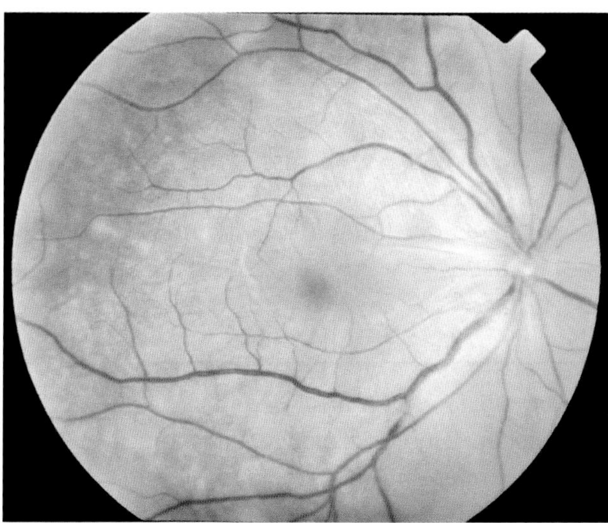

Fig. 1: Acute stage of VKH syndrome. Disc edema, yellow-white exudates at the level of the RPE and serous detachment in the posterior pole

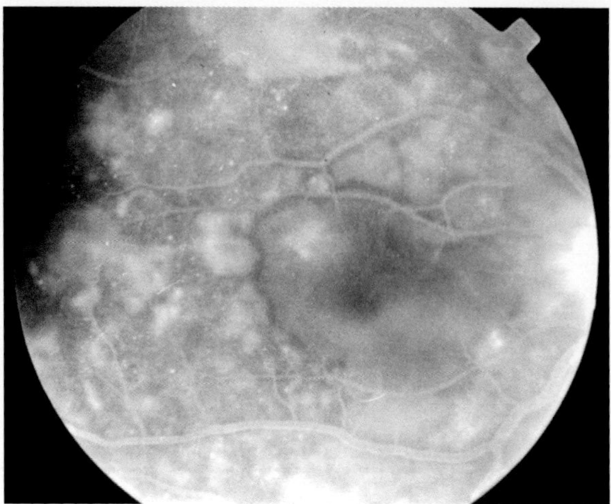

Fig. 2: FA of acute stage of VKH syndrome. Multifocal hyperfluorescent spots with the dye pooling at the RD areas

INVESTIGATIONS

1. Fluorescein angiography (FA): Multifocal hyperfluorescent spots at the RPE level with the dye pooling at the RD areas.
2. CSF analysis: Pleocytosis with predominant lymphocytes. The test is only necessary for the case with meningitis sign.

DIFFERENTIAL DIAGNOSIS

The classic ocular and extraocular presentations are enough for the diagnosis. Sympathetic ophthalmia and toxemia associated RD have almost the same ocular presentation. Ocular surgery history and pregnancy with eclampsia signs can differentiate these entities. Optic neuritis/neuropathy and central serous choroioretinopathy have to be ruled out at the early stage.

TREATMENT

Systemic oral or intravenous high-dose steroid is the standard treatment. The treatment is sustained for 2 months or longer depending on the response. Quick tapping might induce relapsing and poor clinical course.

INFERENCE

Early recognition and treatment can shorten the course and get a better result. About one third of cases suffered from recurrence and diffused RPE and choroids degeneration would have poor visual prognosis.

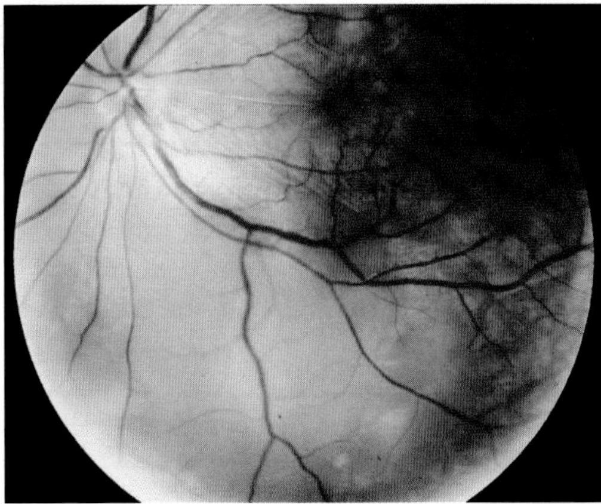

Fig. 3: Subacute stage of VKH syndrome. RPE degeneration with sunset-glow picture, inferior exudative RD

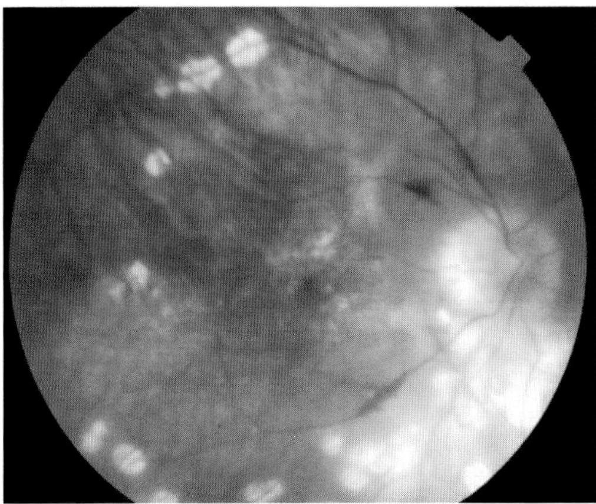

Fig. 4: Chronic stage of VKH syndrome. Diffused RPE degeneration with sunset-glow picture, scattered RPE-choroidal degeneration patches, macular degeneration

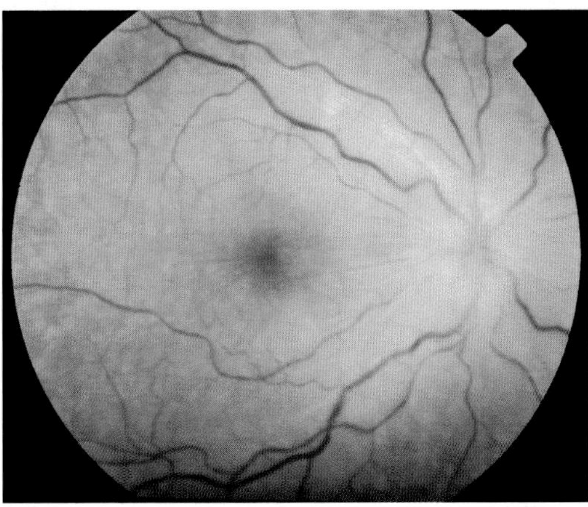

Fig. 5: VKH syndrome with disc edema. Optic neuritis or neuropathy has to be ruled out

SYMPATHETIC OPHTHALMIA

INTRODUCTION

Sympathetic ophthalmia (SO) is a granulomatous uveitis occurring after penetrating ocular trauma or ocular surgery. The traumatized eye is referred to as the exciting eye and the fellow eye is the sympathizing eye. The sympathizing eye usually develops more severe uveitis than the exciting eye.

CLINICAL SIGNS AND SYMPTOMS

The ocular presentation is similar to VKH syndrome. The course is similar to the severe form of VKH syndrome with recurrence.

INVESTIGATIONS

Fluorescein angiography: multifocal hyperfluorescent spots at the RPE level with the dye pooling at the RD areas, similar to VKH syndrome.

DIFFERENTIAL DIAGNOSIS

The classic ocular presentations and ocular trauma or surgery history are enough for the diagnosis. VKH syndrome has almost the same ocular presentation.

TREATMENT

Aggressive treatment with systemic steroid and immunosuppressants is necessary. The treatment should be maintained with slow tapering to avoid recurrence for a long time.

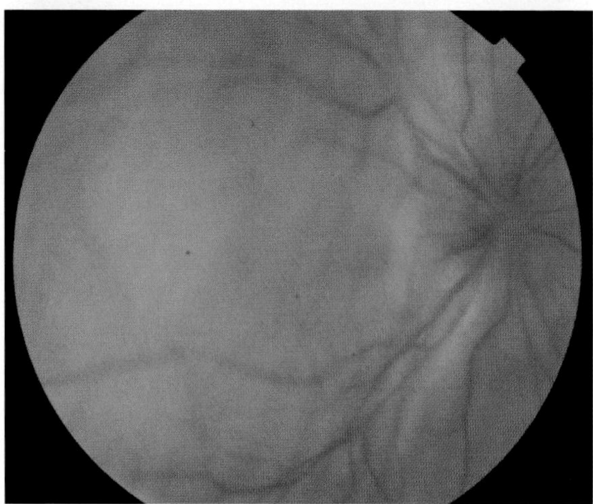

Fig. 6: Acute stage of SO in a case accepted buckling and vitrectomy (OS) 2 months ago for rhegmatogenous RD. Extensive exudative RD (OD)

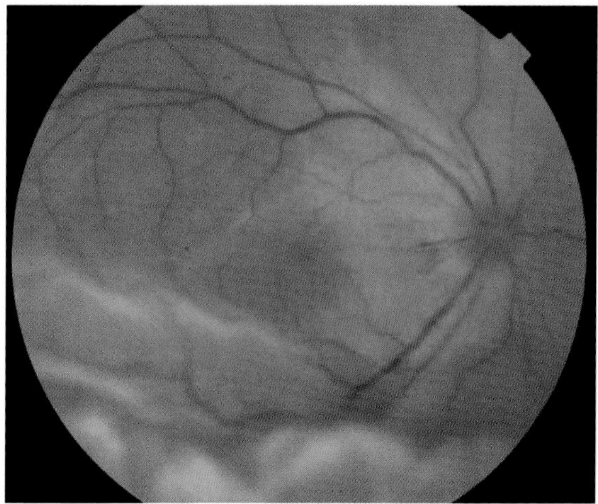

Fig. 7: After systemic steroid and cyclosporin treatment, the extent of exudative RD decreased (OD)

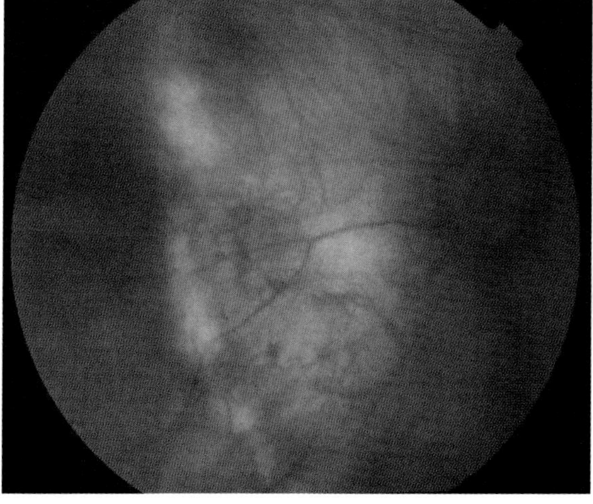

Fig. 8: One year after onset, diffused RPE degeneration and hyperplasia with sunset-glow picture (OS)

Enucleation of the blind traumatized eye in the early stage might improve the prognosis.

INFERENCE

Early recognition and aggressive treatment can get a better result. Long-term follow-up and maintained therapy are mandatory to avoid the relapsing.

TOXEMIA OF PREGNANCY ASSOCIATED RD

INTRODUCTION

Preeclampsia and eclampsia are conditions referred to as toxemia of pregnancy. Both are associated with exudative RD. The detachments are usually bilateral and bullous.

CLINICAL SIGNS AND SYMPTOMS

The major ocular presentation is exudative RD without anterior uveitis.

INVESTIGATIONS

The classic ocular and toxemia presentations are enough for the diagnosis. FA or ICG angiography is not necessary for these pregnant patients.

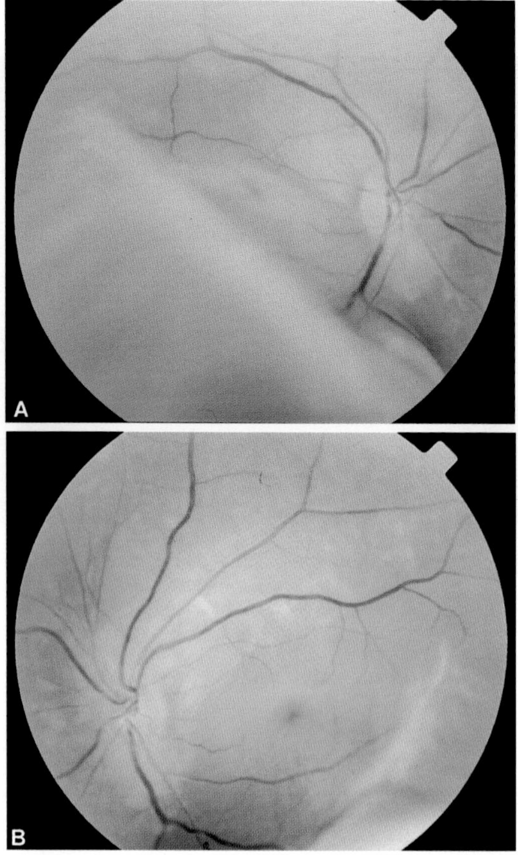

Figs 9A and B: Toxemia of pregnancy. Both eyes are associated with exudative RD

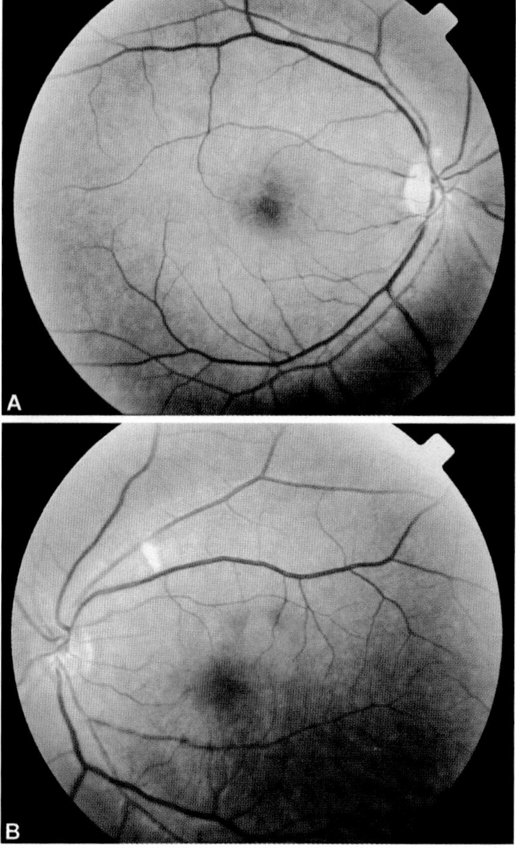

Figs 10A and B: After delivery, the RD spontaneously resolved

DIFFERENTIAL DIAGNOSIS

VKH syndrome, pregnancy associated central serous chorioretinopathy.

TREATMENT

The RD will quickly resolve after fetal delivery. For the cases in which we cannot terminate the pregnancy, systemic oral steroid can help in resolving the detachment.

INFERENCE

The disease will quickly improve after delivery. Give advise and keep close contact with obstetricians.

CHOROIDAL METASTASIS

INTRODUCTION

Metastatic tumors to the choroids are more common than primary ocular malignancies. The most frequent primary sites are lung and breast. Other less common primary sites include the gastrointestinal tract, kidney and prostrate. Prognosis depends on the nature of primary malignancy.

CLINICAL SIGNS AND SYMPTOMS

In most situations, there are creamy-white, placoid subretinal lesions at posterior pole. The lesions might be multifocal and bilateral. Sometimes, a large subretinal mass located at periphery. Exudative RD is very popular and is an important sign to differentiate from benign tumors.

INVESTIGATIONS

Fluorescein angiography shows hyperfluorescence and staining at the lesion. It also helps to find subtle lesions at clinical fundus examination. B scan shows moderately high internal acoustic reflectivity. Systemic survey and detailed history are mandatory.

DIFFERENTIAL DIAGNOSIS

Choroidal melanoma and other benign choroidal tumors need to differentiate. Orbital CT and MRI help to rule out osteoma and melanoma.

TREATMENT

Systemic chemotherapy for the primary tumor is the most important therapy. Radiotherapy and transpupillary thermotherapy are adjuvants to decrease the extent of RD and save the vision for the patient.

INFERENCE

Treatment and prognosis depend on the nature of primary malignancy and the extent of systemic metastasis.

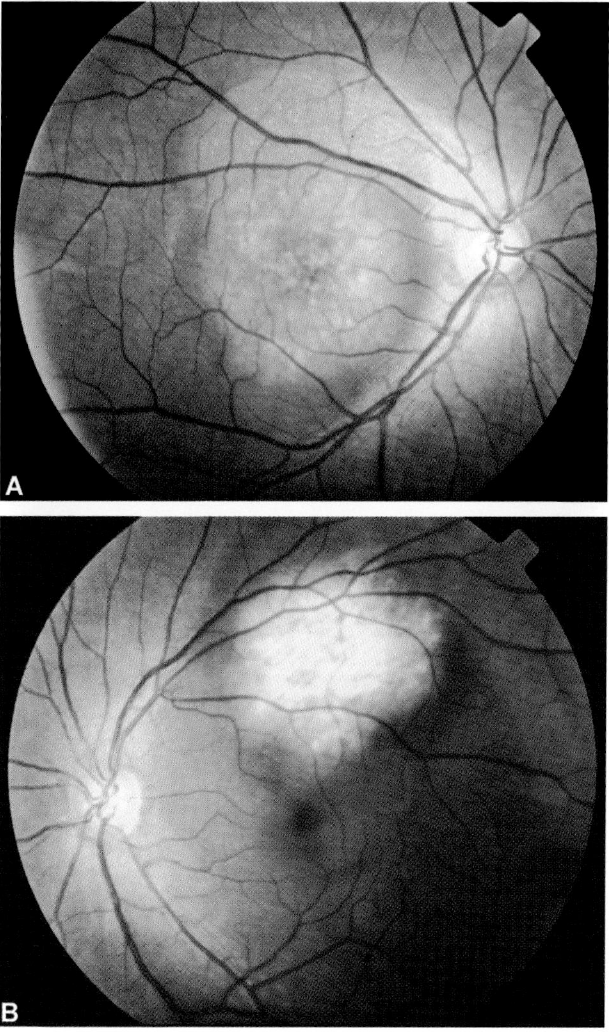

Figs 11A and B: Lung CA with choroidal metastasis (OU)

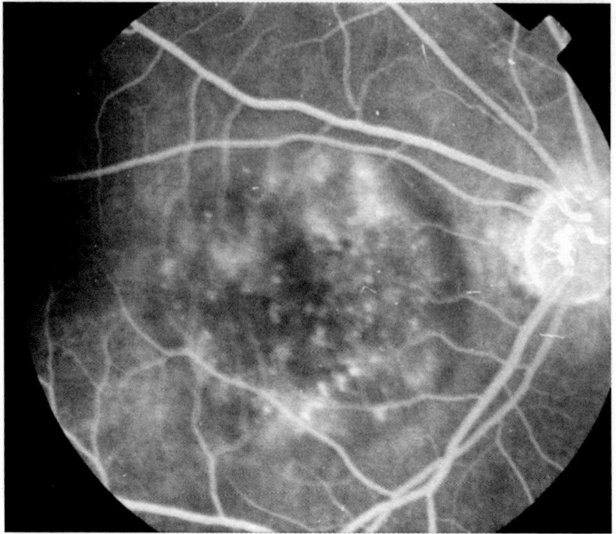

Fig. 12: Fluorescein angiography shows hyperfluorescent spots and dye staing at the lesion

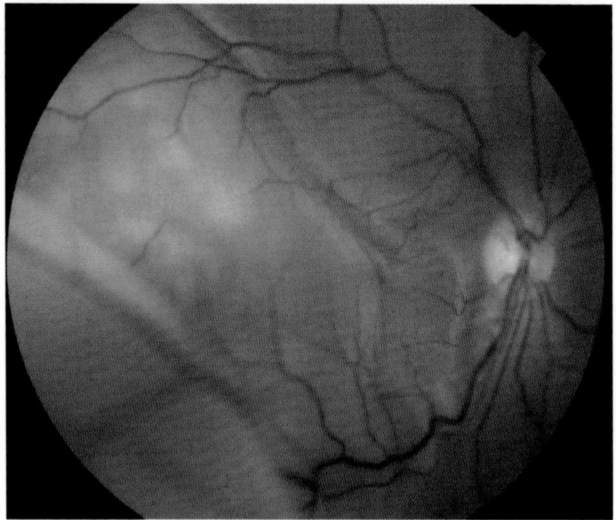

Fig. 13: Breast CA with choroidal metastasis with extensive RD (OD)

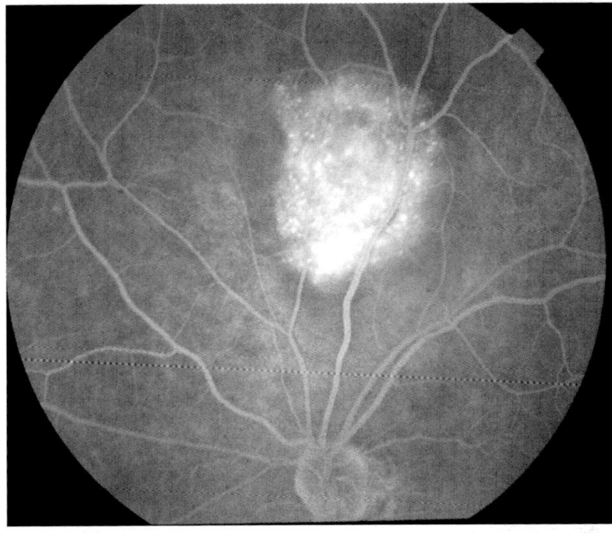

Fig. 14: Fluorescein angiography shows hyperfluorescent spots at the lesion

CHOROIDAL HEMANGIOMA

INTRODUCTION

Choroidal hemangioma can be diffuse or circumscribed. The diffused type seen with Sturge-Weber syndrome is discovered early. The circumscribed type is usually recognized in adults as a result of exudative retinal detachment and macular edema. Progressive tumor enlargement and vision deterioration are common for both types.

CLINICAL SIGNS AND SYMPTOMS

Circumscribed choroidal hemangioma is orange, oval. Exudative fluid accumulation will result macular edema and vision deterioration. At the later stage, exudative retinal detachment will be persistent.

INVESTIGATIONS

B scan shows a very high internal reflectivity but without choroidal excavation. Fluorescein angiography shows rapid early hyperfluorescence and dye staining.

DIFFERENTIAL DIAGNOSIS

Amelanotic melanoma, choroidal metastasis, and retinal hemangioma need to differentiate.

TREATMENT

Treatment is only necessary for the hemangioma with macular edema and exudative RD. Laser treatments include traditional photocoagulation, transpupillary thermotherapy and photodynamic therapy. Intravitreal injection of anti-VEGF drugs is another alternate or adjuvant.

INFERENCE

Treatment and prognosis depend on the nature of choroidal hemangioma. Diffused type had worse prognosis.

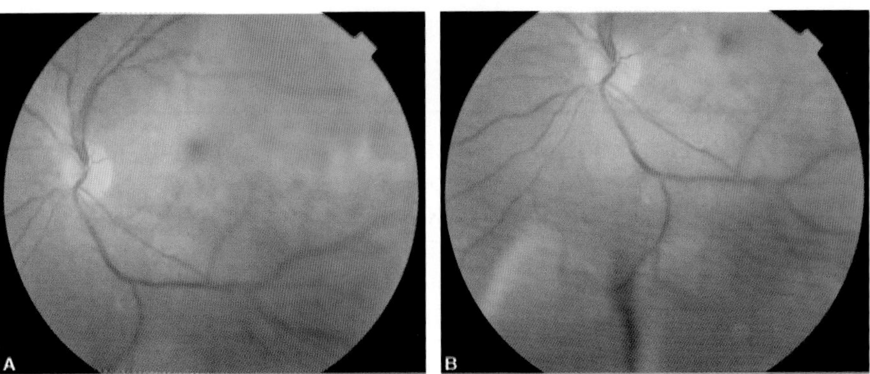

Figs 15A and B: Sturge-Weber syndrome. The diffused choroidal hemangioma at posterior pole with inferior RD

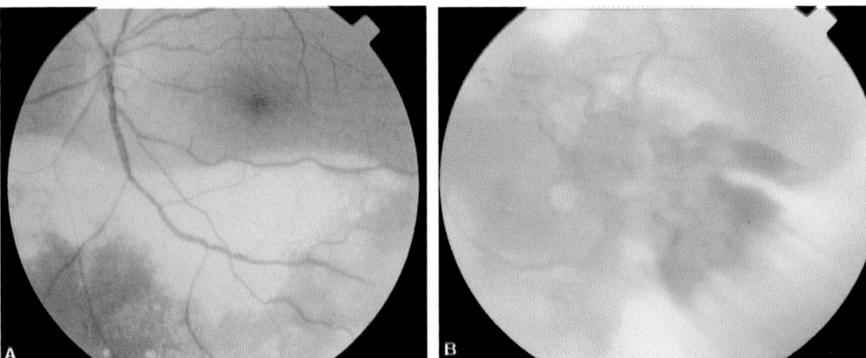

Figs 16A and B: A large retinal hemangioma at inferior periphery with inferior RD and massive exudates at margin of RD

COAT'S DISEASE

INTRODUCTION

Coat's disease is an idiopathic retinal telangiectasis with intraretinal and subretinal exudates and exudative retinal detachment. Most are male and involve one eye. It can be divided into children or adult type, depending on the age of onset.

CLINICAL SIGNS AND SYMPTOMS

Intraretinal and subretinal exudates and telangiectasis are the landmarks of the disease. The extent can be localized or diffuse. Diffused exudates accompany with exudative retinal detachment.

INVESTIGATIONS

Fluorescein angiography shows the location of vessel telangiectasis. Dye is leaking and staining at late phase.

DIFFERENTIAL DIAGNOSIS

For the infants, retinopathy of prematurity and familial exudative vitreoretinopathy need to be ruled out.

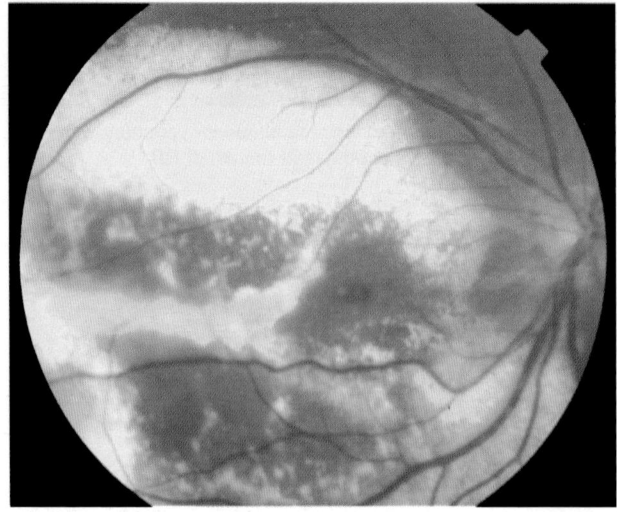

Fig. 17: Children Coat's disease.
Intraretinal and subretinal exudates at posterior pole (OD)

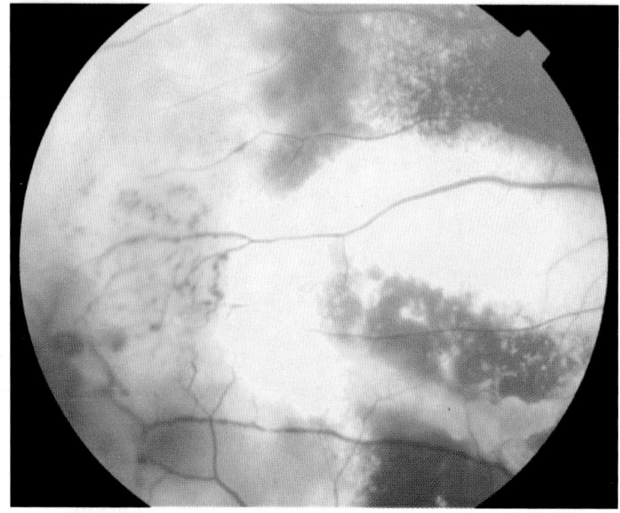

Fig. 18: Retinal telangiectasis at periphery with massive exudates (OD)

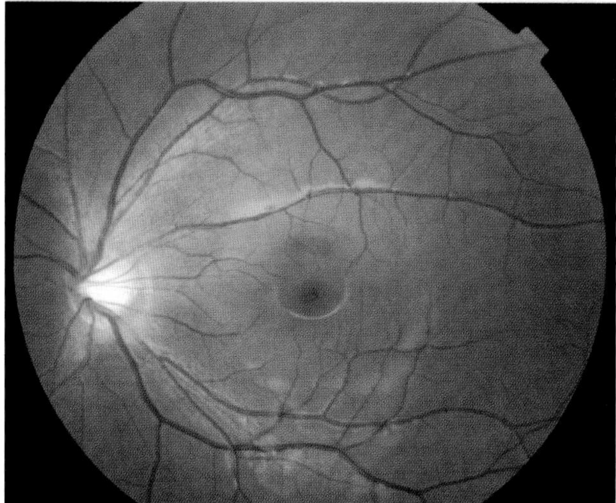

Fig. 19: The left eye is normal

TREATMENT

Laser photocoagulation and cryotherapy.

INFERENCE

Exudates are the landmarks of the disease. Fluorescein angiography can help to find the true area of telangiectasis.

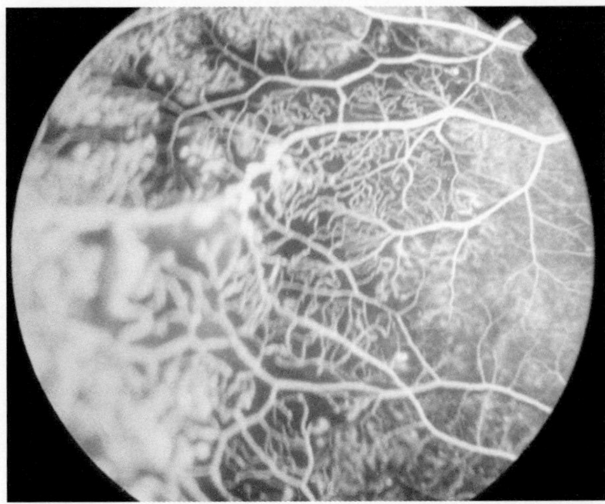

Fig. 20: FA shows retinal telangiectasis

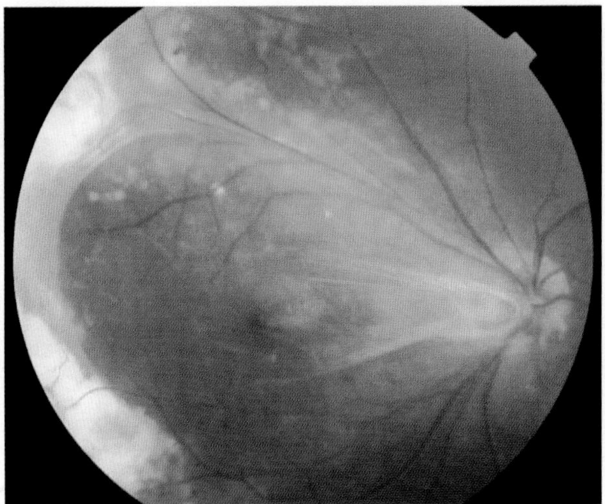

Fig. 21: After laser and cryo-therapy, exudates disappear. Macular pucker and fibrosis at previous exudates area

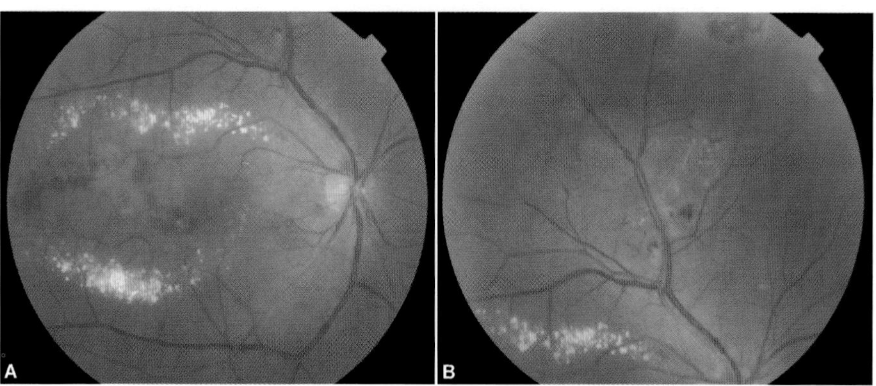

Figs 22A and B: Adult Coat's disease.
Abnormal vessels and exudates at posterior area and superior area

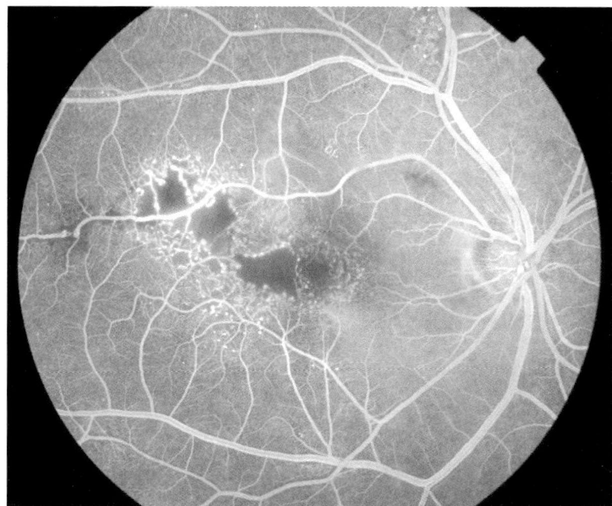

Fig. 23: FA shows nonperfusion and telangiectasis

CHAPTER

TEN

HEREDITARY RETINAL DYSTROPHIES

Supriya Dabir, Soumen Mondal, Priyanka Doctor, Nikoloz Labauri, S Natarajan (India)

- Retinitis Pigmentosa
- Stargardt's Disease and Fundus Flavimaculatus
- Vitelliform Dystrophy
- Leber's Congenital Amaurosis
- Bietti Crystalline Dystrophy
- North Carolina Macular Dystrophy
- Butterfly-shaped Pigment Dystrophy of the Fovea
- Sorsby Pseudo-inflammatory Macular Dystrophy
- Dominant Drusen
- Benign Familial Fleck Retina
- Alport Syndrome
- Dominant Cystoid Macular Dystrophy

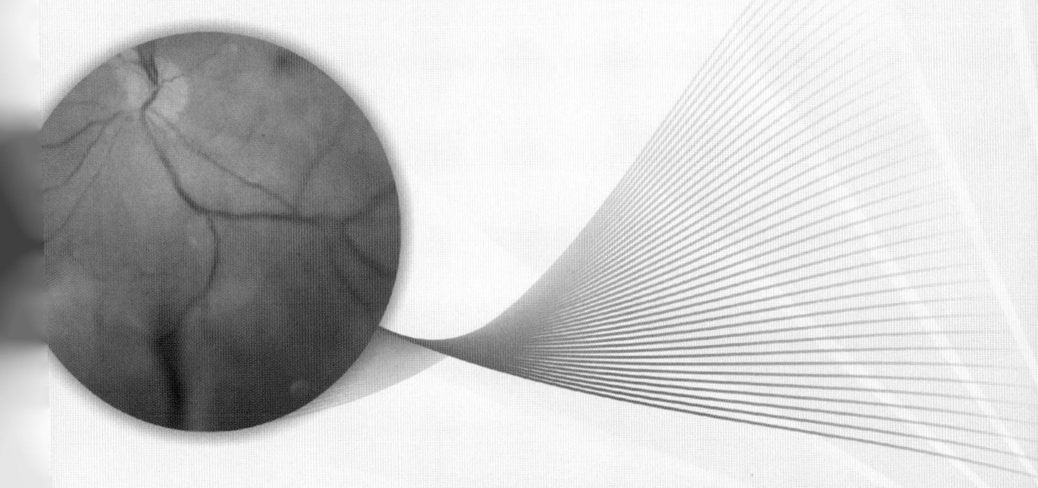

RETINITIS PIGMENTOSA

INTRODUCTION

Retinitis pigmentosa (RP) is a term used for a group of disorders characterized by inherited, progressive dysfunction, cell loss and eventual atrophy of retinal tissue.

Genetic heterogenicity is known to exist within a given hereditary pattern.[1]

Genetic types in a state in the United States were found to be 19% autosomal dominant, 19% autosomal recessive, 8% X-chromosome linked, 8% undetermined and 46% isolates with only one affected member in the family.[2]

CLINICAL SIGNS AND SYMPTOMS

The initial symptom is usually defective dark adaptation or "night blindness". Central visual acuity is usually preserved until the end stages of retinitis pigmentosa.[3]

This can however be affected if there is cystoid macular edema (CME),[4] diffuse retinal leakage[5] and retinal pigment defects in the macula.[6]

Color vision in typical RP remains good until visual acuity is 20/40 or worse. Color vision may fail early in cases where central cones appear to be abnormal from the beginning.

Myopia was found to be more common in the X-linked group. Posterior subcapsular cataracts characterized by yellowish crystalline changes within the peripheral lens cortex in the visual axis are common. All the patients have changes in the vitreous, as reported by Pruett[7] like fine colorless dust-like particles, posterior vitreous detachment; vitreous condensations and collapse of the vitreous with greatly reduced volume.

The earliest observed changes in the fundus are arteriolar narrowing, fine dust-like intraretinal pigmentation and loss of pigment from the pigment epithelium.[8] In the past the term retinitis pigmentosa sine pigmento was applied when the retina appeared normal despite documented abnormalities of photoreceptor function; however, this term is now regarded as confusing because it implies a separate disorder rather than the early stages of RP.[9] As photoreceptor deterioration progresses, there is increasing loss of pigment from the pigment epithelium with intraretinal clumping of melanin, appearing most often as coarse clumps in a "bone spicule" configuration. A golden ring or yellowish halo can be seen surrounding the disc in early RP, which is replaced by peripapillary mottling, hyperpigmentation and atrophy of the RPE as the disease progresses. Retinal vessel attenuation and waxy pallor of the optic nerve become apparent in patients with advanced RP. The cause of

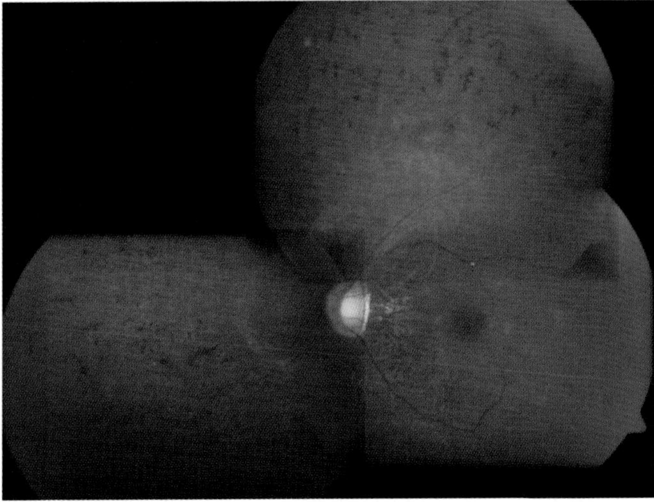

Fig. 1: Fundus photograph with arteriolar attenuation, coarse clumps in a "bone spicule" configuration and waxy pallor of the disc

the retinal vessel attenuation is unknown, but it appears to be a secondary change and not the primary disease process.[3] Other retinal changes include white dots deep in the retina at the level of the pigment epithelium. These deposits are believed to be a nonspecific manifestation of pigment epithelial degeneration and may account for the retinal appearance termed "retinitis punctata albescens," which is considered a manifestation of RP.[10]

Fishman et al reported three types of macular lesions in RP patients: atrophy of the macular area with thinning of the retinal pigment epithelium, cystic lesions or partial thickness holes within the macula with radial, inner retinal traction lines and/or various degrees of pre-retinal membranes causing a "surface wrinkling phenomenon and cystoid macular edema.[11]

Choroidal changes in advanced RP generally include loss of the choriocapillaris and eventually all but the largest choroidal vessels.

CLASSIFICATION OF RP

Subdivision Based on Inheritance Type

- Autosomal dominant RP
- Autosomal recessive RP
- X-linked recessive trait RP

Subdivision by Age of Onset

- Congenital RP
- Childhood onset RP
- Adult onset RP

Subdivision by Molecular Defect

- Genes expressed predominantly in photoreceptors or in RPE(e.g. rhodopsin)
- Genes associated with RPE and disease in other tissue (e.g. Usher syndrome)
- Genes widely expressed but for which mutations cause a retinal phenotype.

Subdivision by Fundus Appearance

- RP sine pigmento
- Retinitis punctata albescens
- RP inversus (pericentral and central RP)
- Sector RP

Systemic Associations Like Usher Syndrome

Non-progressive

1. Usher syndrome Type I
2. Usher syndrome Type II
3. Congenital adrenoleukodystrophy
4. Infantile phytanic acid storage disease.

Progressive

1. Usher syndrome Type III
2. Cockayne syndrome
3. Alstrom syndrome
4. Mitochondrial myopathy (Kearns-Sayre syndrome)
5. Refsum syndrome
6. Mucopolysaccharidoses I-H, I-H/S, I-S, II, II
7. Edwards syndrome.

TESTS OF VISUAL FUNCTION

Electroretinography

In patients with early disease the a- and b-waves generated by the photoreceptors in response to white light under dark-adapted conditions are

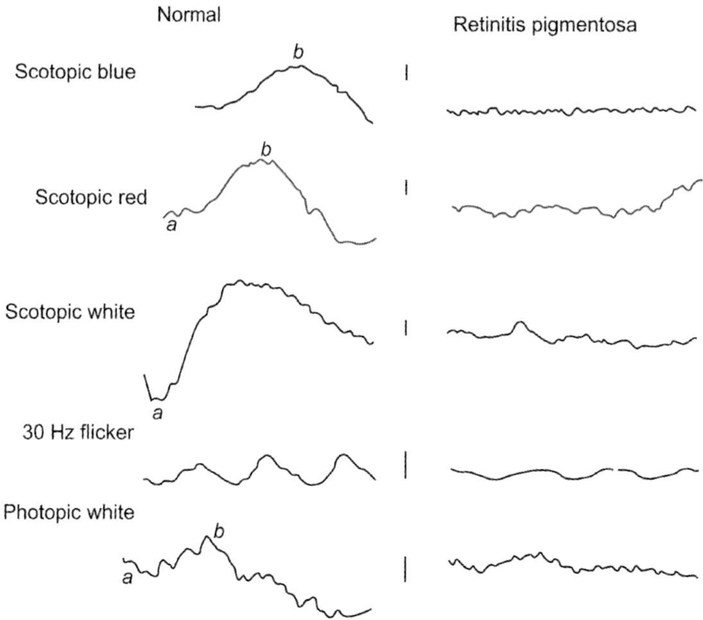

Fig. 2: ERG recordings of retinitis pigmentosa

reduced in amplitude. The above figure shows that patients with advanced RP have non-detectable rod and cone responses.[12]

The scotopic rod-dominated ERG was affected more than the photopic cone-mediated ERG in type I RP, whereas the scotopic and photopic ERGs' were more equally abnormal in type II RP.

In general, the EOG is abnormal in diffuse hereditary rod-cone degenerations of the retina.

Dark Adaptometry

Patients with RP, when tested with dark adaptometry, may show elevation of the cone segment, rod segment, or both, to a varying degree. There may be a delay in reaching a relatively good final dark adaptation rod threshold.[13]

VISUAL FIELDS

Characteristic ring scotomas are seen in the midperiphery of the visual field. It usually starts as a group of isolated scotomas in the area 20 to 25 degrees from fixation. These gradually coalesce to form a partial and then a complete ring. The outer edge of the ring expands fairly rapidly to the periphery, while the inner margin contracts slowly toward fixation. Long after the entire peripheral field is gone, there remains a small oval of intact central field.[14]

DIFFERENTIAL DIAGNOSIS

Genetic Disorders that Cause Retinal Degeneration

1. Gyrate Atrophy of Choroid and Retina
2. Choroideremia
3. Cone dystrophy
4. Lebers congenital amaurosis
5. Congenital stationary night blindness.

Drug Exposure - Thoridazine Chorioretinopathy

Infections

- Syphilis
- Rubella

TREATMENT

1. *Cataract extraction*
2. *Macular edema:* Peribulbar, oral and intraocular steroids have produced temporary reduction in CME.[15] Grover et al found oral acetazolamide was found to be more effective than topical dorzolamide.[16] Vitrectomy with inner limiting membrane peeling with gas tamponade may lead to resolution of refractory CME.
3. Vitamin A Supplements treat retinopathies associated with Vitamin A deficiency resulting from intestinal malabsorption or defective transport.
4. Lutein supplements may covey protection from oxidative damage and light induced photoreceptor cell death. Long term effects of such supplementation is unknown.
5. Docosahexaenoicacid (DHA) supplements: DHA is an abundant lipid in photoreceptors accounting for 30-40% lipids in rod outer segments. Its synthesis is impaired in few of the X-linked recessive patients and its supplementation in these patients may be beneficial.

Advances in Therapeutics

1. *Gene Therapy:* It involves replacing the mutant in "loss of function"-type disease and switching off of the disese gene in the "gain-of-function" disease. Adenoviruses have been extensively studied gene transfer vector for the eye. Intravitreal and subretinal injections of the vector have been attempted. Ribozymes, RNA enzymes, are being designed for destroying mutant mRNA in dominant disease.
2. *Growth Factors:* Injections of intravitreal and subretinal basic fibroblast growth factor have been promising.

3. *Retinal Transplantation:* This is directed at replacing abnormal RPE cells or by using immature neural cells to replace defective neuroretina. Mueller glial cells can dedifferentiate and produce new retinal neurons. Bone marrow derived stem cells can also be injected to integrate into host retina and differentiate.
4. *Artificial Retina:* Perception of light and cortical responses can be elicited in patients with advanced RP. Thus electronic prosthesis may help. Subretinal, epiretinal, optic nerve and cortical implants have been studied. Patients have reported improvement in vision, color vision and fields.

REFERENCES

1. Inglehearn CF, Jay M, Lester DH, et al. The evidence for linkage between late onset autosomal dominant retinitis pigmentosa and chromosome 3 locus D3547(C17): Evidence for genetic heterogeneity.Genomics 1990;6:168.
2. Bundey S, Crews SJ: Wishes of patients with retinitis pigmentosa concerning genetic counseling. J Med Genet 1982;19:317-18.
3. Pagon RA. Retinitis Pigmentosa. Surv Ophthalmol 1988;33:137-77.
4. Ffytche TJ. Cystoid maculopathy in retinitis pigmentosa. Trans Ophthalmoc Soc UK 1972;92:265-83.
5. Geltzer AI, Berson EL. Fluorescein angiography of hereditary retinal degenerations. Arch Ophthalmol 1969;81:776-82.
6. Hansen RI, Friedman AH, Gartner S, Henkind P. The association of retinitis plgmentosa with preretinal macular gliosis. Br J Ophthalmol 1977;6l:597-600.
7. Pruett RC. Retinitis pigmentoha. A biomicroscopical study of vitreous abnormalities. Arch Ophthalmol 1975;93:603-08.
8. Sunga RN, Sloan LL. Pigmentary degeneration of the retina: early diagnosis and natural history. Invest Ophthalmol Vis Sci 1967;6:309-25.
9. Pearlman JT, Flood TP, Seiff SK. Retinitis pigmentosa without pigment. Am J Ophthalmol 1976;81:417-19.
10. Merin S, Auerbach E. Retinitis pigmentosa. Surv Ophthalmol 1976;20:303-46.
11. Fishman GA, Fishman M, Maggiano J: Macular lesions associated with retinitis pigmentosa. Arch Ophthalmol 1977;95:798-803.
12. Berson EL. Retinitis pigmentosa and allied diseases: Applications of electroretinographic testing. International Ophthalmol 1981;4:7-22.
13. Alexander KR, Fishman GA. Prolonged dark adaptation in retinitis pigmentosa. Br J Ophthalmol 1984;68:561-69.
14. Harrington DO. The visual fields: A textbook and atlas of clinical perimetry. Saint Louis, CV Mosby 1976;172.
15. Saraiva VS, Sallum JM, Farah ME. Treatment of cystoid macular edema related to retinitis pigmentosa with intravitreal triamcinolone acetonide.Ophthalm Surg Lasers Imaging 2003;34:398-400.
16. Grover S, Fishman GA, Fiscella RG, et al. Efficacy of dorzolamide hydrochloride in the management of chronic cystoid macular edema in retinitis pigmentosa. Retina 1997;17:222-31.

STARGARDT'S DISEASE AND FUNDUS FLAVIMACULATUS

INTRODUCTION

Karl Stargardt, in Graefes Archives of Clinical and Experimental Ophthalmology in 1909 described a familial degeneration which was associated with an atrophic macular dystrophy surrounded by yellowish, ill-defined subretinal lesions.[1] Later on, in 1962, A Franceschetti introduced the term fundus flavimaculatus to characterize a fundus with yellow irregular subretinal "flecks" scattered diffusely throughout the posterior pole, and only half of the patients in his series had macular atrophy.[2] Examination of multiplex families uncovering intrafamilial presence of both Stargardt's Disease (SD) and Fundus Flavimaculatus (FFM),[3] and seemingly caused by the same gene (ABCR4 gene) on the short arm of chromosome1, it is now assumed, (not without controversy) that the two disease entities are temporally variant expressions of each other.[4]

CLINICAL SYMPTOMS AND SIGNS

As visual loss due to macular atrophy forces the patient to go for check-up, SD is detected in childhood. On the contrary, FFM is detected in adulthood, as macular atrophy is a late manifestation in FFM. So, onset of symptoms occurs in the first or second decade of life in SD and in FFM it is generally after the third decade. Bilateral symmetric gradual dimness of vision is the most common presenting symptom. Some patients with advanced disease may complain of a central scotoma.

In the initial stage, the clinical appearance of fundus can be deceptively normal. There can be loss of foveal reflex and symmetric atrophic retinal pigment epithelial changes. A tapetal reflex (beaten bronze), granularity or RPE destruction all manifests atrophy of the macula. This is accompanied by adjacent flecks. They are irregularly shaped yellow subretinal lesions varying in shape (described as round, linear, crescentic or pisciform [2]) and size (100 to 200 μm) extending as far as midperiphery. As the disease progresses the flecks disappear leaving behind RPE atrophy, and new flecks appear at a different location. In longstanding cases flecks become less yellow and pigmentations may occur. The central annular focus of atrophy may extend to the deeper layers of posterior pole resulting in extensive atrophy of the choriocapillaries.

CLASSIFICATION (FISHMAN)[5]

Stage 1: Central macular atrophy of RPE and choriocapillaris often associated with ring of flecks.

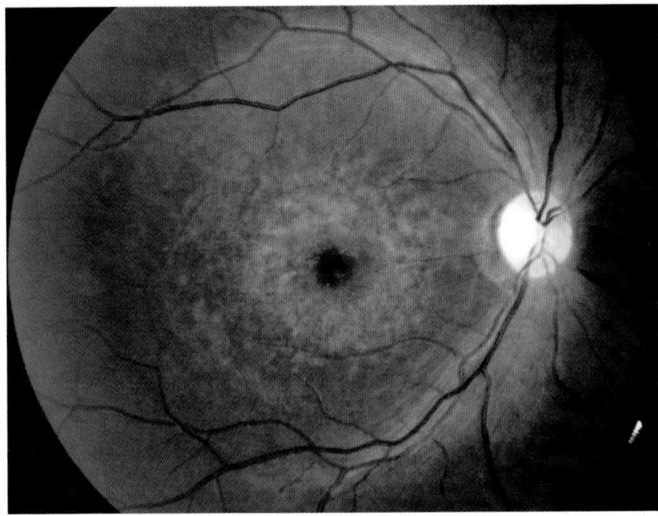

Fig. 3: Beaten bronze appearance seen in Stage 1

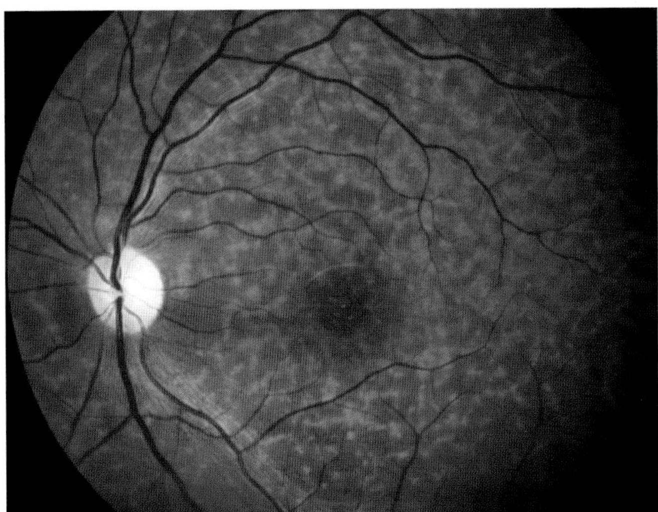

Fig. 4: Pisciform flecks seen

Stage 2: Central macular atrophy and flecks of different stages of development often extending to equator

Stage 3: Extensive fleck resorption in the posterior pole with early choriocapillaris atrophy

Stage 4: End stage; flecks completely replaced by diffuse RPE and choriocapillaris atrophy throughout the fundus.

INVESTIGATION

Autofluorescence: Hypofluorescence suggesting RPE atrophy in the area noted to have beaten metal appearance clinically and it ascertains the extent of the condition.

FFA: In early cases, central oval zone of hyperflourescence which may be surrounded by some hyperfluorescent flecks. "Choroidal silence" is often seen which is because of increased filtering action of the RPE secondary to the absorption by lipofuscin of the excitatory blue wavelength emitted by the camera during FFA.[6] As the disease progresses, there are more flecks until the entire posterior pole shows a blotchy pattern of hyperfluorescence, which may later on show confluence suggestive of widespread RPE atrophy as seen in Figure 6. In late stages, central choroidal atrophy is seen.

RETINAL FUNCTION TESTS

Visual acuity: The majority of patients with stage 1 and stage 2 Stargardt's disease maintains 20/200 or better VA at their initial and most recent visits. When fundus flecks show a notable degree of resorption, VA will decreases below 20/200.[7]

Visual fields: Initially relative central scotoma followed by absolute central scotoma.

Color vision: Mild red - green dyschromatopsia.

ERG: Early in the disease process normal photopic and scotopic response. Later on ERG amplitudes may decrease, and the degree of abnormality correlates with the clinical severity of the disease.[8]

EOG: Subnormal in most cases suggesting a diffuse disturbance in RPE function.[8]

DIFFERENTIAL DIAGNOSIS

Variants of retinitis pigmentosa: Abnormal or extinguished ERG response as opposed to SD.

Progressive Cone dystrophy: Abnormal single/flicker photopic response as opposed to SD

Vitteliform macular dystrophy:

- Chloroquine toxicity
- Familial drusen
- Bietti crystalline dystrophy.

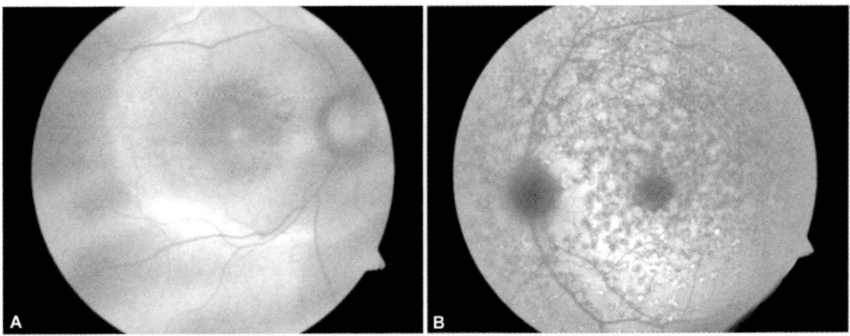

Figs 5A and B: Hypo-autofluorescence at the macula and periphery respectively

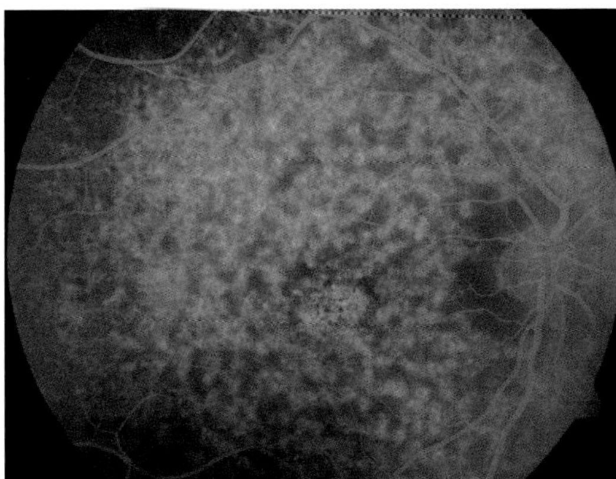

Fig. 6: Choroidal silence with hyperfluorescent flecks

TREATMENT

No known treatment. In case of considerable visual loss, low visual aids can be tried. It is mandatory to undergo genetic counseling if the patient is contemplating marriage or having children.

REFERENCES

1. Stargardt K. Ueber familiare Degeneration in der Maculagegend des Auges. Graefes Arch Clin Exp Ophthalmol 1909;71:534.
2. Franceschetti A. Uber tapeto-retinale degenerationen im kindesalter. In von Sautter H (ed): Entwicklung und Fortschritt in der Augenheilkunde. Stuttgart, Ferdinand EnkeVerlag, 1963;107-20.
3. Aaberg TM. Stargardt's disease and fundus flavimaculatus: evaluation of morphologic progression and intrafamilial co-existence. Trans Am Ophthalmol Soc 84:453-87.
4. Noble KG, Carr RE. Stargardt's disease and fundus flavimaculatus. Arch Ophthalmol; 97:1281-85.
5. Fishman GA. Fundus flavimaculatus: a clinical classification. Arch Ophthalmol 94:2061-67.
6. Eagle RC Jr, Lucier AC, BernardinoVB Jr, Yanoff M. Retinal pigment epithelial abnormalities in fundus flavimaculatus. Ophthalmology 87:1189-200.
7. Oh KT, Weleber RG, Oh DM, et al. Clinical phenotype as a prognostic factor in Stargardt disease. Retina 2004;24:254-62.
8. Deutman AF. Hereditary dystrophies of the posterior pole of the eye. Assen, Netherlands. Van Gorcum, 1971.

VITELLIFORM DYSTROPHY

INTRODUCTION

This is a clearly distinct entity among the inherited macular dystrophies. The first pedigree was presented by Best[1] and is hence also known as Best's disease. Inheritance is irregular autosomal dominant.[2] The causative gene is VMD2 and maps to chromosome 11q13. Disturbance in the fluid transport across the RPE could result in accumulation of debris between RPE and photoreceptors and between RPE and Bruch's membrane, leading to the EOG changes.[3]

CLINICAL FEATURES[3]

Visual acuity is often minimally affected and the typical vitelliform structures may be noted during routine ophthalmoscopy. Severely diminished visual acuity may occur particularly in older age groups. Occasionally, light flashes and retinal detachment may be associated. Refraction is often hyperopic with astigmatism.

The vitelliform changes are usually noted bilaterally. The evolution of vitelliform dystrophy is schematically as follows:

1. Normal fovea, EOG pathologic
2. *Previtelliform stage* — Small, round yellowish dot at the site of the foveola or a tiny honeycomb structure centrally
3. *Vitelliform stage* — The classic vitelliform structure is an egg-yellow, sometimes orange, round, slightly elevated structure surrounded by a darker border. This macular disc may measure 0.5 to 3.0 disc diameters, with a resemblance to the intact yolk of a fried egg. The disc may disappear completely, leaving a normal-appearing macula
4. *Scrambled-egg stage* — The yellowish material in the disc may disintegrate, leaving a scrambled-egg appearance. The disc may appear to rupture at a certain spot, with a decrease in visual acuity.
5. *Cyst stage* — The disc may in some cases give the appearance of a cyst
6. *Pseudohypopyon stage* — The disc may disintegrate or demonstrate syneresis, giving rise to a cyst with a fluid level, thus resembling a hypopyon.
7. *Round chorioretinal atrophy stage* — Subretinal neovascularization may occur accompanied with visual decline. Ultimately either round areas of chorioretinal atrophy or marked pigmentation may occur.

Multifocal vitelliform dystrophy — Lesions typically are manifested as sharply demarcated yellowish cysts in the macula, near the retinal vascular arcades and surrounding the optic disc. A variation in size and number (as many as 20) can be observed. Lesions may grow and merge with neighboring lesions. The evolution of the peripheral lesions may parallel the evolution of the central lesion but may also have a different time course.[4]

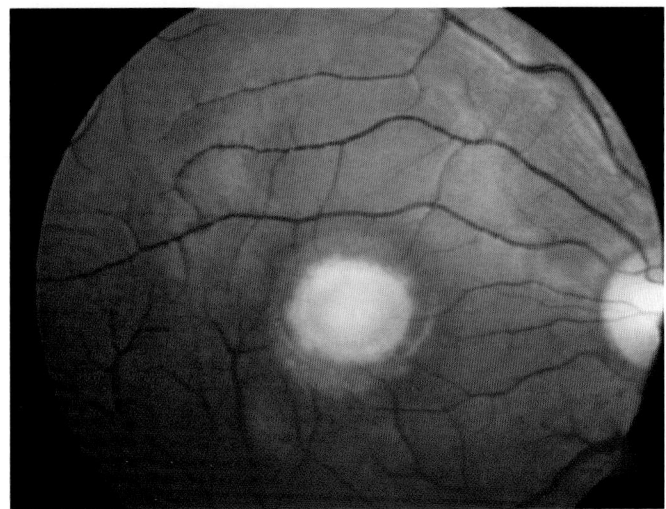

Fig. 7: Classic vitelliform stage with the egg yolk appearance at the macula

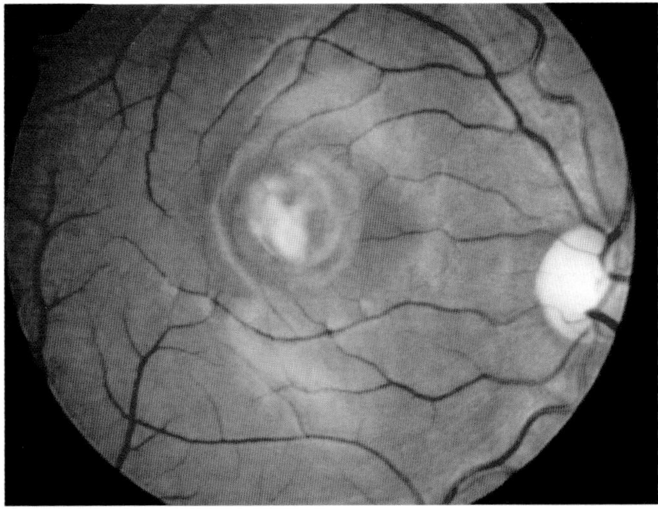

Fig. 8: Scrambled-egg stage where the yellowish material in the disk has disintegrated

Adult-onset foveomacular vitelliform dystrophy (AOFVD) is a rare macular condition that usually results in slow progressive bilateral vision loss. First described by Gass in 1974,[5] these bilateral macular lesions are usually symmetrical, one third to one half disc diameter in size, round or oval, slightly elevated grayish-yellow subfoveal lesions that occur with or without a central pigmented spot in the fovea of each eye.[5]AOFVD typically occurs in adults between the ages of 30 and 50 years old and has an autosomal dominance inheritance pattern with variable expression and incomplete penetrance.[5-7] In the early stages of the disease, patients with AOFVD are usually visually asymptomatic or have mild complaints of visual blur or metamorphopsia in one or both eyes.[5] As the disease progress, vision loss may become more drastic when the vitelliform lesion disrupts and leads to geographical atrophy similar to that seen in ARMD, or infrequently if the patient has choroidal neovascularization (CNV).

INVESTIGATIONS[3,7]

Fluorescein angiography—Hypofluorescence corresponding to the macular disc in the intact disc stage is seen as the yellowish material does not transmit choroidal fluorescence. As the disc disintegrates, areas of hyperfluorescence indicating atrophic retinal pigment epithelium become visible.

At autofluorescence imaging, areas of highly increased autofluorescence within lesions correspond with the yellow-white material as seen at ophthalmoscopy. More advanced lesions show loss of autofluorescence centrally with an increased amount of autofluorescence at the outer border of the ovoid lesion.

Color vision—As in most macular diseases, color vision is affected with a mild red-green dyschromatopsia.

ERG— is completely normal

EOG— is subnormal even in carriers and is an important diagnostic tool. The light-dark ratio is rarely higher than 1.5.

DIFFERENTIAL DIAGNOSIS[2,3,7]

Central serous chorioretinopathy, in individuals aged 20-60. It is usually unilateral, seen as a dome-shaped elevation at the macula. Hyperfluorescence with a smock-stack or inkblot pattern is noted. OCT reveals elevated neurosensory retina separated from the intact RPE by optically empty subretinal fluid and is associated with a normal EOG.

- Pigment epithelial detachment in individuals over 40 years. It is seen as a round elevated lesion, hyperfluorescent on angiography. OCT reveals elevated RPE layer without separation from photoreceptor.

- Fundus flavimaculatus in which pisciform flecks and beaten-metal appearance of the macula may be noted. Angiography is characterized by early stage: dark silent choroid and late stage: central hyperfluorescence.
- Basilar laminar drusen in which numerous, small, uniform sized, round, slightly raised, yellow subretinal lesions may be visualized with early discrete hyperfluorescence corresponding to these lesions on angiography.
- Geographic AMD is usually seen in older individuals (>60 years) bilaterally with hyperfluorescence on angiography and absence of reflective band of photoreceptor layer with enhanced reflectivity of the choroid on OCT.
- Central areolar atrophy is visualized as atrophic macula 1-3 DD in size with visible choroidal vasculature.

TREATMENT

No therapy exists for halting the progression of the disease with the possible exception of treatment of complications such as choroidal neovascularization, macular hole and retinal detachment. However, an accurate diagnosis and pedigree analysis is important for allowing the physician to perform adequate family and genetic counseling to affected patients.

REFERENCES

1. Best F. Ueber eine hereditaire Makulaaffection. Beitraege zur Vererbungslehre. Zschr Augenheilik 1905;13:199-12.
2. Spaide RF, Noble K, Morgan A, Freund KB. Vitelliform macular dystrophy. Ophthalmology. 2006;113(8):1392-400.
3. Deutman AF, Hoyng CB, van Lith-Verhoeven JJC. Macular dystrophies. In: Schachat AP, ed. Retina. Vol 2. St. Louis, MO:Mosby; 2006:1163-1210.
4. Boon CJ, Klevering BJ, den Hollander AI, Zonneveld MN, Theelen T, Cremers FP, Hoyng CB. Clinical and genetic heterogeneity in multifocal vitelliform dystrophy. Arch Ophthalmol. 2007;125(8):1100-06.
5. JDM Gass, A clinicopathologic study of a peculiar foveomacular dystrophy, Trans Am Ophthalmol Soc 1974;72:139-56.
6. GA Epstein, MF Rabb, Adult vitelliform macular degeneration diagnosis and natural history, Br J Ophthalmol 1980;64(10):733-40.
7. Youssri AI, Miller JW. Best's macular dystrophy. Int Ophthalmol Clin. 2001 Fall;41(4):165-71. Review.

LEBER'S CONGENITAL AMAUROSIS

INTRODUCTION

Leber's congenital amaurosis (LCA) is a clinically and genetically heterogeneous disorder characterized by severe loss of vision at birth. It was first described by Theodor von Leber in 1869[1] and is the earliest and most severe form of all the inherited retinal dystrophies responsible for congenital blindness[2] Its incidence is 2-3 per 100 000 births.[1,3,4]

CLINICAL FEATURES

The currently recognized (although still debated) criteria for a diagnosis of LCA are the ones proposed by De Laey in 1991.[5]

- Onset of blindness or poor vision (appearing early in the first year of life, before 6 months of age);
- Sluggish pupillary reactions;
- Roving eye movements/nystagmus;
- Oculo-digital signs (eye poking, eye rubbing, eye pressing, etc.);
- Extinguished or severely reduced scotopic and photopic electroretinogram (ERG);
- Absent or abnormal VEPs;
- Variable fundus (for example, normal, marbled, albinotic with pigmentation).

In addition to these ocular symptoms a series of symptoms has been variably described that includes: neurodevelopmental delay, mental retardation, associated systemic anomalies.

INVESTIGATIONS

The specific hallmark of LCA is seen in the ERG, which, in this disease, is extinguished or severely reduced in both the scotopic and photopic components.

Autosomal recessive inheritance is commonly found and six genes with disparate functions have been implicated in LCA.

Neuroradiological studies - the only consistent finding is hypoplasia of the cerebellar vermis, which can be seen in 10% of infants affected by LCA.[6,7] Electroencephalography reveals epileptiform abnormalities on EEG.

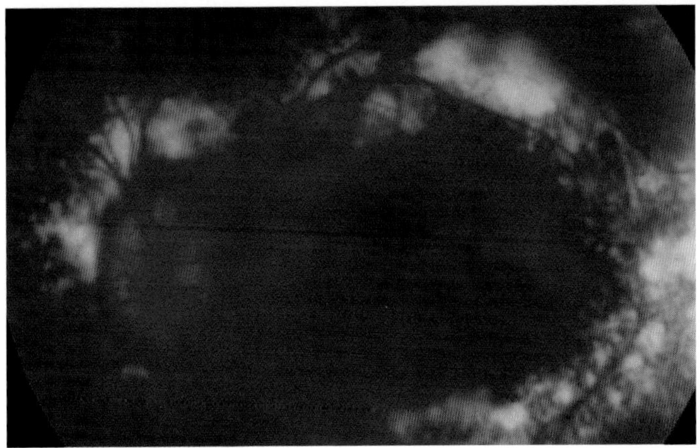

Fig. 9: Multiple hard exudates all over the posterior pole as a fundus variant in LCA

DIFFERENTIAL DIAGNOSIS[8]

Differential Diagnosis of the Ocular Phenotype of LCA Without a Syndrome

	Features	*Tests*	*Inheritance*
LCA		ERG-not detectable	AR, rare AD
Complete achromatopsia	Striking photoaversion and blepharospasm	ERG-non-detectable or absent cone response, D15, FM 100-absent color vision	AR
Blue cone monochromatism	less severe photoaversion and blepharospasm	ERG-non-detectable or absent cone response, D15, FM 100-tritanopia	XR
Complete CSNB	High myopia, good central day vision	ERG-absent rod responses, normal cone ERG, electronegative ERG	XR,AR,AD
Incomplete CSNB	High myopia, good central day vision	ERG-absent rod responses, abnormal cone ERG, electronegative ERG	XR,AR,AD
Oculo Cutaneous Albinism	Iris transillumination, blond fundus, foveal hypoplasia , hyperopia with oblique astigmatism		AR

Differential Diagnosis of the Ocular Phenotype of LCA Associated With A Syndrome

Syndrome	*Features*
Bardet-Biedl syndrome	Polydactyly, mental retardation, obesity, retinitis pigmentosa, kidneys often abnormal
Alstrom syndrome	Cone-rod dystrophy, hearing loss, obesity, diabetes mellitus, cardiomyopathy
Abetalipoproteinemia	Rod-cone degeneration, celiac syndrome, ataxia, demyelination, steatorrhea, RBC acanthocytosis
Peroxisomal disorders	Malformation syndrome, hypotonia, liver failure, kidney failure, brain malformations, leopard spot retinopathy, Urine testing for very long chain fatty acids
Batten disease	Neurodegeneration, Bull's eye maculopathy. Rectal, conjunctival biopsy
Senior-Loken syndrome	Nephrophthisis
Saldino-Mainzer syndrome	Phalangeal cone shaped epiphyses of hand, ataxia
Joubert syndrome	Agenesis of cerebellar vermis, hypoplasia of corpus callosum, neonatal tachypnea
Lhermitte-Duclos syndrome	Macrocephaly, seizures

TREATMENT

Various lines of investigation are currently open. These include retinal and stem cell transplantation, drug therapies (for patients with normal but inactive retina) and gene therapy.

INFERENCE

LCA is a highly heterogeneous disorder in which much remains to be clarified. In particular, an adequate classification is yet to be developed and the differences between the various clinical forms need to be established, as does the relationship between these and the genetic subtypes, in order to devise therapies for this disorder.

REFERENCES

1. T Leber , Über Retinitis pigmentosa und angeborene Amaurose. Graefes Arch Klin Exp Ophthalmol 1869;15:1-25.
2. I Perrault, JM Rozet S. Gerber, et al., Leber congenital amaurosis. Molec Genet Metab 1999;68:200-08.
3. JR Heckenlively, SG Foxman, ES Parelhoff , Retinal dystrophy and macular coloboma. Documenta Ophthalmologica 1988;68:257-71.
4. J Schuil, FM Meire, JW Delleman , Mental retardation in amaurosis congenital of Leber. Neuropediatrics 1998;29:294-97.
5. JJ De Laey, Leber's congenital amaurosis. Bull Soc Belge Ophthalmol 1991;241:41-50.
6. EW Harris, Leber's congenital amaurosis and RPE65. Int Ophthalmol Clin 2001;41:73-82.
7. B. Nickel, CS Hoyt , Leber's congenital amaurosis. Is mental retardation a frequent associated defect?. Arch Ophthalmol 1982;100:1089-92.
8. Lambert SR, Taylor D, Kriss A. The infant with nystagmus, normal appearing fundi, but an abnormal ERG. Surv Ophthalmol. 1989;34(3):173-86. Review.

BIETTI CRYSTALLINE DYSTROPHY

INTRODUCTION

Bietti crystalline dystrophy is a very rare condition, which predominantly affects males. Inheritance may be either X-linked or autosomal recessive.

CLINICAL SIGNS AND SYMPTOMS

It is characterized by the deposition of crystals in the peripheral cornea and retina. Presentation is in the third decade of life with progressive visual loss.

SIGNS IN CHRONOLOGICAL ORDER

- Yellow-white crystals scattered throughout the posterior fundus.
- Localized atrophy of the RPE and choriocapillaris at the posterior pole.
- Diffuse atrophy of the choriocapillaris.
- Gradual confluence and expansion of the atrophic areas into the retinal periphery.

INVESTIGATION

ERG and EOG are subnormal.

TREATMENT

No known treatment is available.

INFERENCE

Prognosis is variable, because the rate of disease progression differs in individual cases.

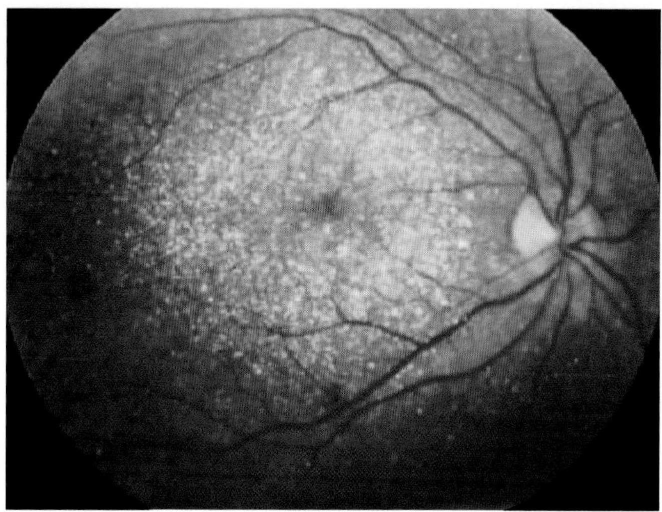

Fig. 10: Bietti crystalline dystrophy

NORTH CAROLINA MACULAR DYSTROPHY
SYNONYM: LEFLER-WADSWORTH-SIDBURY DYSTROPHY

INTRODUCTION

In 1971, Lefler and colleagues described an autosomal dominant foveal dystrophy found in 25 of 70 members of a family spanning four generations. By 1974, this pedigree had been expanded to include 545 individuals spanning seven generations; 130 were studied ophthalmoscopically, and 50 were found to be affected by the dystrophy. As this pedigree has been traced back to a family originating in North Carolina, it is now referred to as North Carolina macular dystrophy.

CLINICAL SIGNS AND SYMPTOMS

The dystrophy develops during the first year of life, and the foveal lesions were thought to progress throughout childhood to reach their final stage by late puberty. The final visual acuity is also reached by late puberty. Marked variations are noted in the final stage achieved by different siblings. Some individuals have foveal lesions arresting at an early or intermediate stage, whereas the lesions of others progress to a final atrophic stage.

Ophthalmoscopically, the Macular Changes can be Divided into Three Stages

Stage 1: Scattered drusen and pigment dispersion within the fovea Visual acuity is usually 20/20, and central or paracentral scotomas are not present. Fluorescein angiography reveals transmission defects within the fovea corresponding to the drusen.

Stage 2: Confluent drusen with or without pigment clumping within the central macula. RPE atrophy and partial choroidal atrophy may be seen The visual acuity is usually in the 20/50 range, and small central or paracentral scotomas may be present. Fluorescein angiography shows a more confluent pattern of transmission defects with no evidence of dye leakage or pooling.

Stage 3: Choroidal atrophy. Total RPE and choriocapillary atrophy of the fovea, parafovea, or entire macula may develop.

Visual acuity is usually in between 20/50 to 20/200. Large central or paracentral scotomas are present. The foveal lesion is always moderately severe before any decrease in visual acuity occurs. Thereafter, the decrease in visual acuity closely parallels the severity of the foveal lesion. Likewise, the

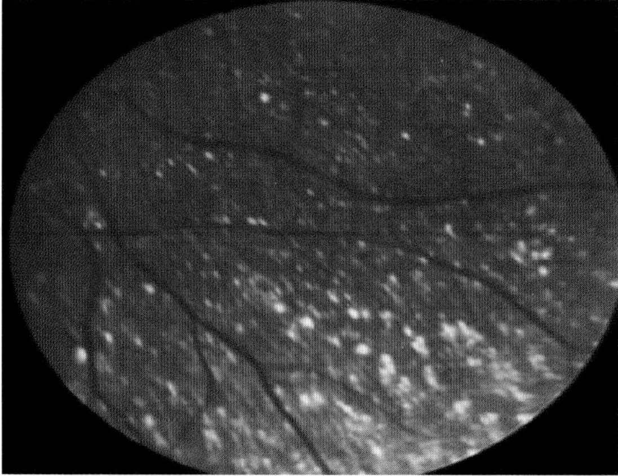

Fig. 11: Grade 1 of North Carolina macular dystrophy

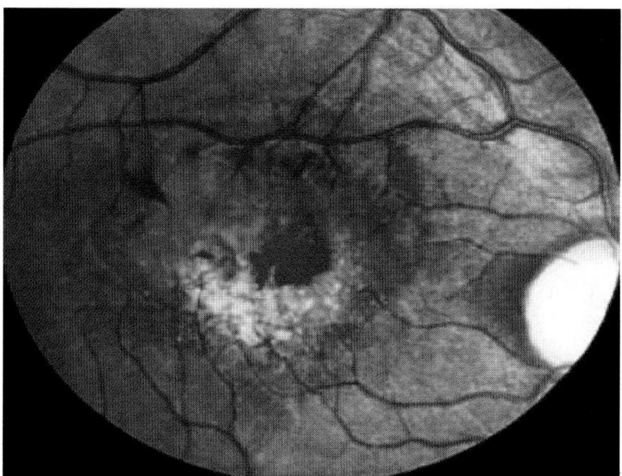

Fig. 12: Exudative maculopathy in Grade 2 North Carolina macular dystrophy

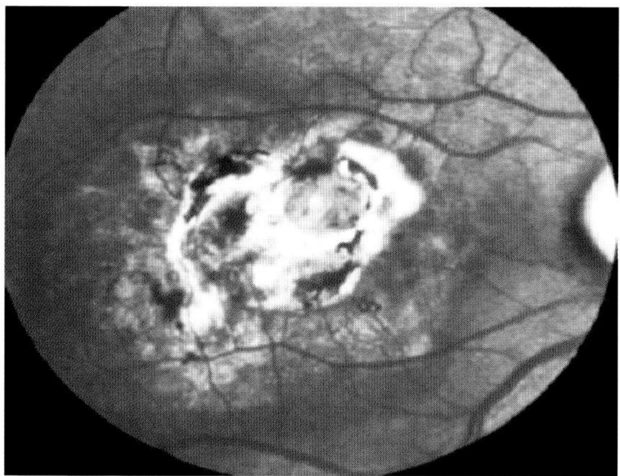

Fig. 13: Subretinal scarring in North Carolina macular dystrophy

size and development of central scotomas correspond closely to the stage and size of the foveal lesions.

INVESTIGATION

The ERG and EOG are normal, as are dark adaptometry and color vision testing.

DIFFERENTIAL DIAGNOSIS

The differential diagnosis includes dominant progressive foveal dystrophy (dominant Stargardt's), familial drusen, central areolar choroidal dystrophy, and congenital macular colobomas.

TREATMENT

There is no known therapy for this dystrophy.

INFERENCE

Small in 1989 reexamined 22 members of the original family and reported that only 1 patient demonstrated progression of macular disease. Gass, who examined two families with this entity who originated from North Carolina, also emphasized the generally stationary nature of this dystrophy.

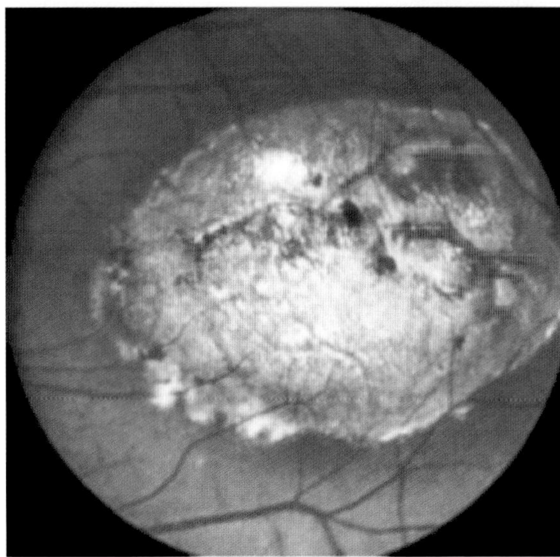

Fig. 14: Grade 3 of North Carolina macular dystrophy

BUTTERFLY-SHAPED PIGMENT DYSTROPHY OF THE FOVEA

INTRODUCTION

Deutman and associates in The Netherlands in 1970 first described this autosomal dominant dystrophy with a peculiar pigmentary pattern in the central macula.

CLINICAL SIGNS AND SYMPTOMS

This disorder manifests itself in the second to fifth decades and is accompanied by normal or only slightly decreased vision between 20/20 to 20/25. The predominant feature of this dystrophy is the presence of a bilaterally symmetric reticular pattern of pigmentation (the so-called butterfly-shape) within the central macula, which is best seen with fluorescein angiography. Pigment stippling in various configurations and drusen-like changes may also be noted in the peripheral retina.

INVESTIGATION

Fluorescein angiography demonstrates a reticular hypofluorescent pattern corresponding to the areas of hyperpigmentation with no obvious hyperfluorescence or dye leakage. In cases in which the pigmented structures are barely visible on fundus examination, the lesions can be seen clearly on fluorescein angiography, a characteristic shared by all the pattern dystrophies of the retinal pigment epithelium.

The ERG is normal, while the EOG may demonstrate abnormal values, suggesting a more widespread disturbance of the retinal pigment epithelium than is appreciable ophthalmoscopically. Dark adaptometry and color testing are normal, while visual field studies may reveal a relative central scotoma with normal peripheral fields.

DIFFERENTIAL DIAGNOSIS

The clinical findings, however, suggest a primary dystrophy of the retinal pigment epithelium. Butterfly-shaped pigment dystrophy of the fovea, as well as pattern dystrophy of the pigment epithelium of Marmor and Byers, foveomacular vitelliform dystrophy: adult type, dominant slowly progressive macular dystrophy of Singerman-Berkow-Patz, macroreticular dystrophy, fundus pulverulentus, the reticular dystrophies of Benedikt-Wernerand of Kingham-Fenzl-Willerson-Aaberg, and autosomal dominant dystrophy of the retinal pigment epithelium of O'Donnell-Schatz-Reid-Green demonstrate remarkably similar characteristics, both clinically and pathophysiologically.

TREATMENT

No known treatment is available.

INFERENCE

Prognosis is generally good, although a minority of patients may develop visual impairment.

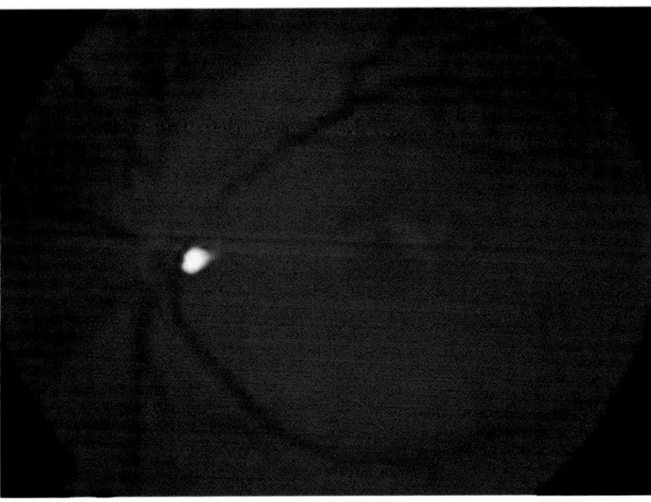

Fig. 15: Butterfly dystrophy

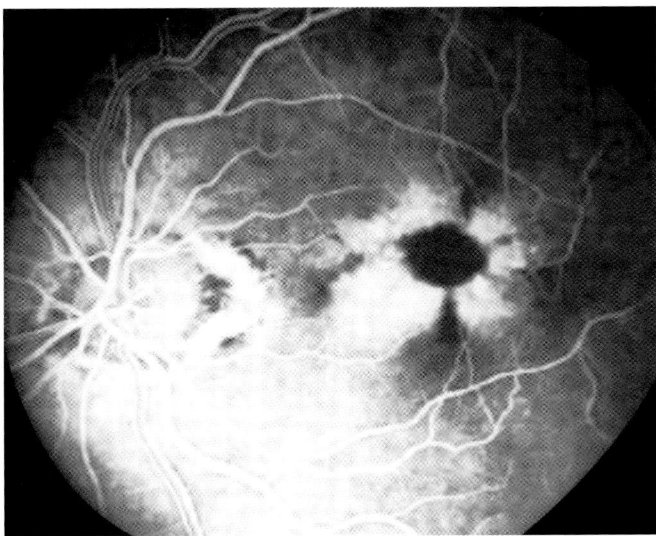

Fig. 16: Fluorescein angiography shows reticular hypofluorescent pattern corresponding to the yellow and yellow-gray deposition material with pigment epithelial transmission leading to a hyperfluorescence pattern

SORSBY PSEUDO-INFLAMMATORY MACULAR DYSTROPHY

INTRODUCTION

Sorsby pseudo-inflammatory macular dystrophy, which is also referred to as hereditary hemorrhagic macular dystrophy, is a very rare but serious condition. Inheritance is autosomal dominant.

CLINICAL SIGNS AND SYMPTOMS

Presentation is during the second and fourth decades with initially unilateral impairment of central vision and metamorphopsia.

Signs are yellow-white, confluent spots located along the arcades and nasal to the optic disc.

INVESTIGATION

ERG is normal.

DIFFERENTIAL DIAGNOSIS

Age-related macular degeneration

TREATMENT

No known treatment is available.

INFERENCE

Prognosis is poor due to the development, during the fifth decade of life, of exudative maculopathy and subsequent subretinal scarring similar to that seen in age-related macular degeneration.

Fig. 17: Early Sorsby pseudo-inflammatory macular dystrophy showing confluent spots along the arcades

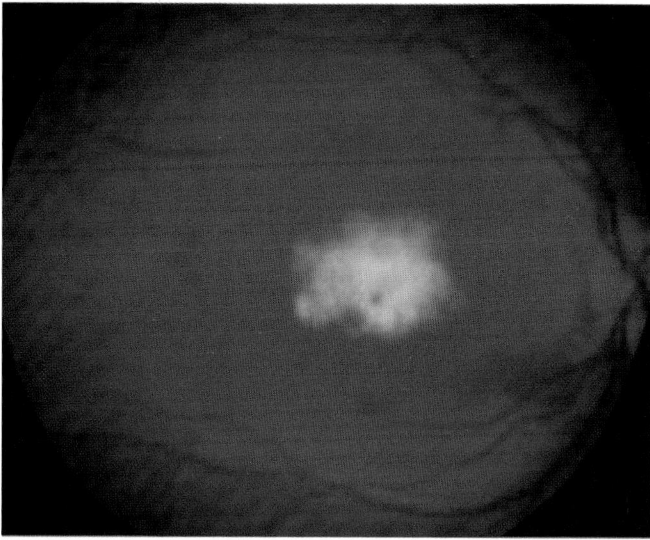

Fig. 18: Exudative maculopathy in Sorsby pseudo-inflammatory macular dystrophy

DOMINANT DRUSEN

A spectrum of disease characterized by dominantly inherited drusen, it is variously named as Doyne's honeycomb dystrophy, Mallatia Levantinese, Hutchinson-Tay choroiditis, Holthouse-Batten superficial chorioretinitis or familial drusen.

SYMPTOMS AND SIGNS

Initially, no symptoms. Later, decrease in visual acuity and metamorphopsia.

Affected persons present in the second and third decade with drusens in the fundus and have a history of conditions affecting several generations. These sharply delineated drusens are distributed in the macula and around the optic nerve head with a nasal predominance (pathognomonic of familial drusens[1]). There is a halo of drusen surrounding the foveola. Later these spots coalesce and retina shows atrophic RPE. In late stages, oval white plaques surrounding the discs are characteristic findings in this dystrophy.

FLUORESCEIN ANGIOGRAPHY

In the arterial phase sharply defined fluorescent spots are seen corresponding to lesions observed during ophthalmoscopy. Also RPE atrophy is revealed by window defects. Occasionally, large drusens (hyaline bodies consisting a large mass) may not show hyperfluorescence. No leakage is seen in the late phases.

RETINAL FUNCTION TESTS

Diminution of visual acuity is rarely seen before 40 years. In advanced cases there may be central scotoma. Mild red-green dyschromatopsia in HRR test is seen. Dark adaptation and ERG are usually normal. EOG is normal at initial stages but may be subnormal later on, depending upon the extent of involvement.[2]

REFERENCES

1. Deutman A, Jansen LMAA: Dominant drusen of Bruch's membrane. In Deutman A ed. The hereditary dystrophies of the posterior pole of the eye. Assen, The Netherlands: van Gorcum; 1971.
2. Deutman A, Hoyng CB, van Lith-Verhoeven. Macular Dystrophies. In Ryan SJ ed. Retina Vol II 3th Edn. 2006:1190-93.

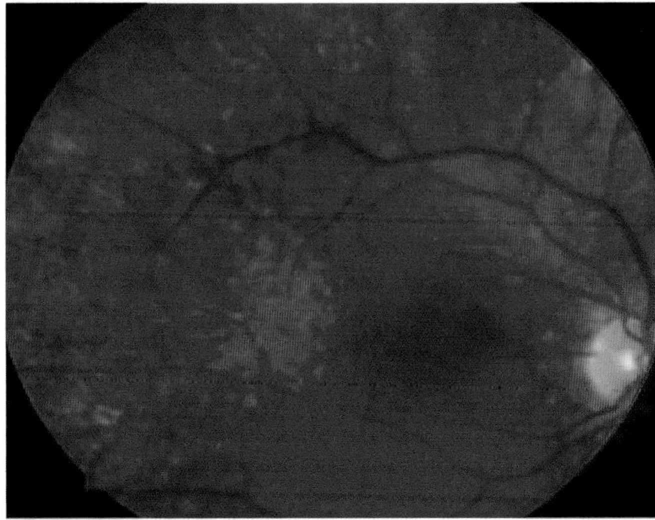

Fig. 19: Sharply delineated drusens are distributed in the macula and around the optic nerve head

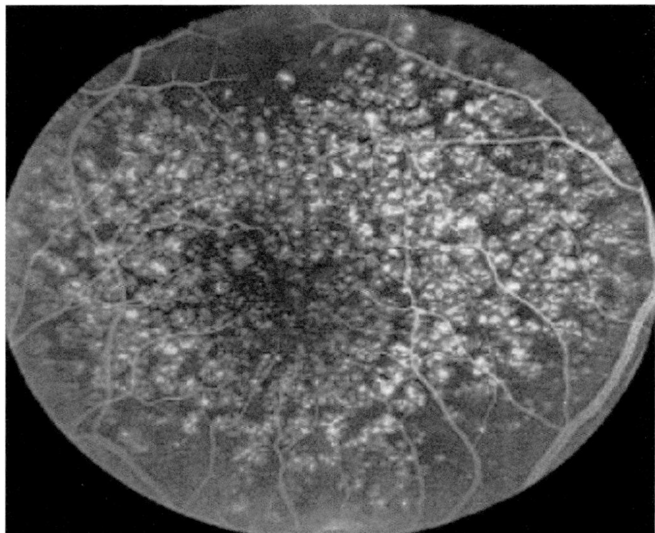

Fig. 20: FFA of familial drusen

BENIGN FAMILIAL FLECK RETINA

INTRODUCTION

Benign familial fleck retina is a rare autosomal recessive disorder which is asymptomatic and, therefore, usually discovered by chance.

CLINICAL SIGNS AND SYMPTOMS

Widespread, discrete, yellow-white, flecks at the level of the RPE, which spare the fovea.

The flecks have variable shapes and extend to the far periphery.

INVESTIGATION

ERG is normal

DIFFERENTIAL DIAGNOSIS

Differential Diagnosis of Fundus Flecks

Benign Familial Fleck Retina

Differences — Shape of flecks is highly variable: many are larger and spare the macula.

Alport Syndrome

Differences — Macular flecks are pale and punctate; periphery flecks are confluent.

Early North Carolina Macular Dystrophy

Differences — Flecks at the macula are smaller and tightly packed together.

Fundus Albipunctatus

Differences — Flecks are punctate and spare the macula.

Basal Lamina Drusen

Differences — flecks are more numerous, smaller and more subtle.

TREATMENT

No known treatment is available.

INFERENCE

Prognosis is excellent.

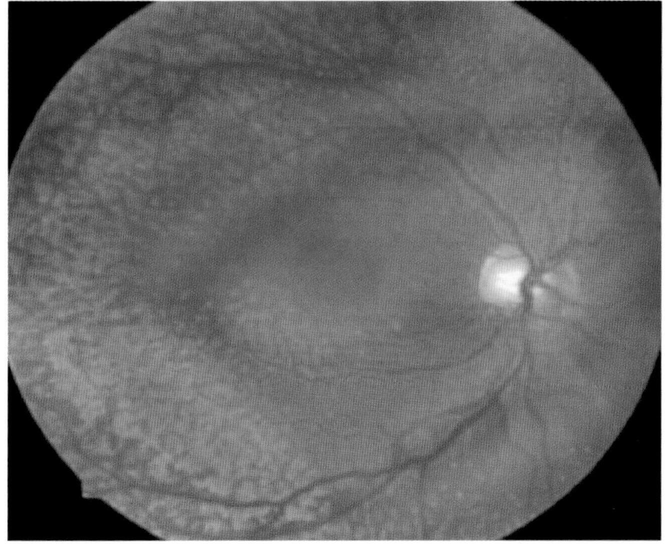

Fig. 21: Central lesions, which spare the fovea in benign familial fleck retina

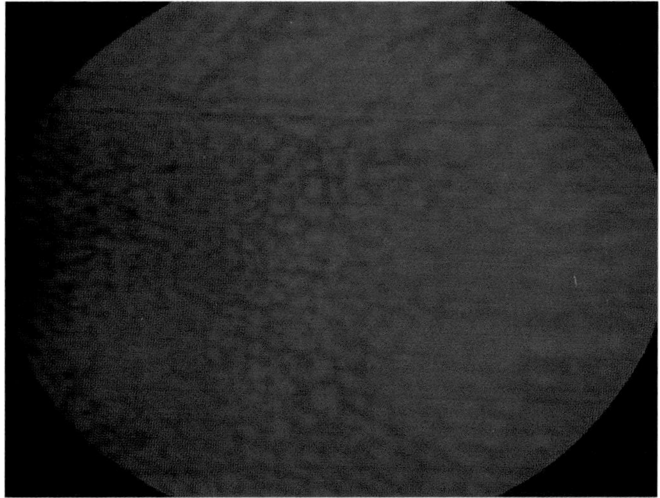

Fig. 22: Peripheral lesions in benign familial fleck retina

ALPORT SYNDROME

INTRODUCTION

Alport syndrome is a rare abnormality of glomerular basement membrane which is characterized by chronic renal failure and sensorineural deafness. Inheritance is X-linked dominant.

CLINICAL SIGNS AND SYMPTOMS

Scattered, pale, yellow, punctate flecks at the macula with normal visual acuity.
- Larger flecks, some of which may be confuent, are seen at the periphery.

INVESTIGATION

ERG is usually normal.

TREATMENT

No medical treatment is available.

INFERENCE

Prognosis is excellent because the retinal changes are innocuous.

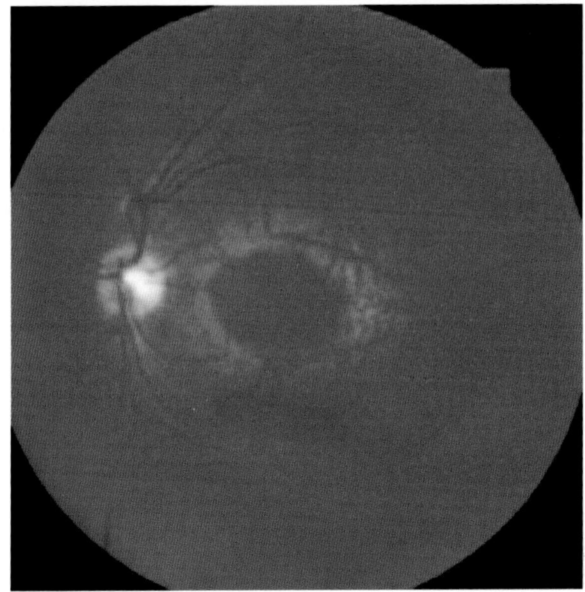

Fig. 23: Macular flecks in Alport syndrome

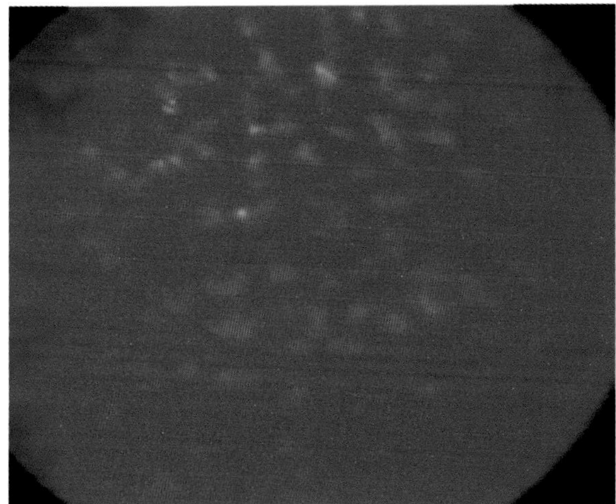

Fig. 24: Larger peripheral flecks in Alport syndrome

DOMINANT CYSTOID MACULAR DYSTROPHY

INTRODUCTION

Reports from the Netherlands indicate that cystoid macular edema can be inherited as an autosomal dominant trait. An additional report describes an affected Greek family.

CLINICAL SIGNS AND SYMPTOMS

Dominantly inherited cystoid macular edema is characterized by an early onset in the first and second decades with a prolonged course of macular cystoid change and progressive loss of central vision. Hyperopia from + 2.00 to + 10.00 D is frequently seen along with hypopigmentation within the central macula. Macular atrophy is a fairly prominent finding late in the disease. Occasionally, a bull's-eye pattern of atrophic change may be seen. Vitreous cells, strands, and veils, and peripheral retinal pigmentary disturbances ranging from a slight hyperpigmentation and depigmentation to the formation of bone spicule changes have also been reported. Late in the disease, vision may be reduced to the 20/200 to finger counting range and a relative-to-absolute central scotoma may be present.

INVESTIGATION

Fluorescein angiography reveals leakage from perifoveal capillaries with dye pooling in a cystoid pattern. Later in the disease, transmission defects are seen in areas of RPE atrophy. In some cases, fluorescein leakage from optic disc capillaries has also been noted.

The ERG has been normal in all patients studied to date. The EOG and results of dark adaptometry, however, are subnormal in most, but not all, patients. The subnormal EOG would indicate widespread dysfunction of the retinal pigment epithelium. Color testing usually shows mild-to-moderate deuteran-tritan defects.

DIFFERENTIAL DIAGNOSIS

The pathogenesis and prevalence of this dystrophy are as yet undetermined. The condition should be differentiated from other hereditary retinal disorders that are associated with cystoid macular edema, especially retinitis pigmentosa (rod-cone dystrophy), and dystrophies characterized by the presence of foveal retinoschisis (which may be mistaken for cystoid macular edema) such as X-linked juvenile retinoschisis and familial foveal retinoschisis.

TREATMENT

No known treatment is available.

INFERENCE

Prognosis is poor because the disease is progressive with the eventual development of pericentric pigmentary changes and a decline of visual acuity to counting fingers.

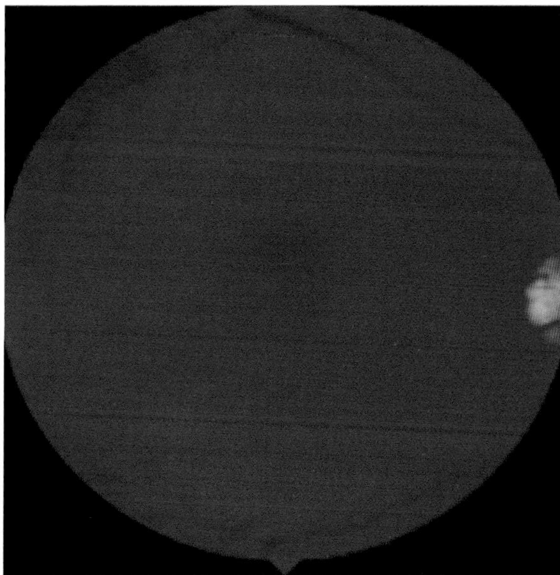

Fig. 25: Dominant cystoid macular edema

CHAPTER
ELEVEN

EALES DISEASE

Rajpal Vohra, Ashok Garg (India)

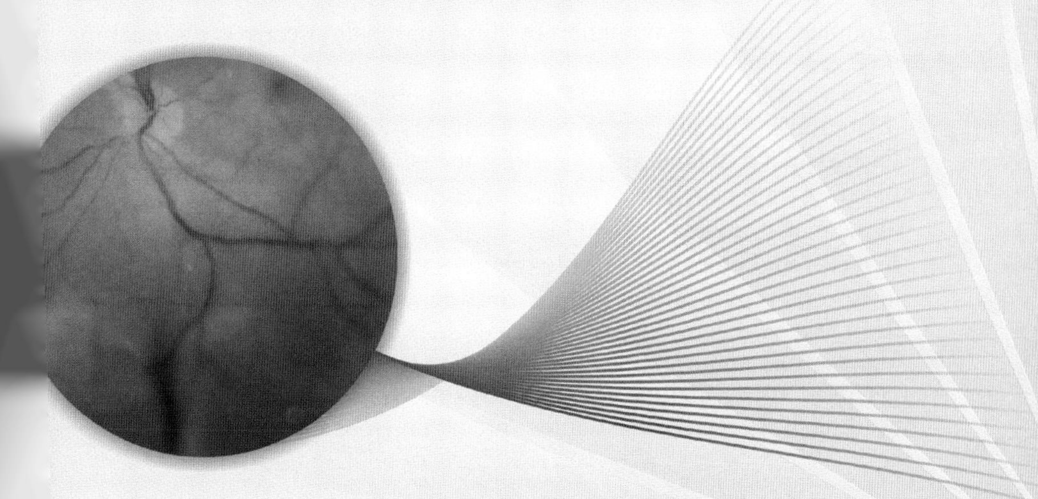

INTRODUCTION

- Eale's disease is an idiopathic inflammatory venous occlusion that primarily affects the peripheral retina of adults.
- Eale's disease predominantly affects the healthy young adults. It is a male predominance disease.
- Peak age of onset of symptoms is 20-30 years.
- Initially patients complain of symptoms in only one eye, however eventually between 70-80% of patients develop bilateral involvement though he extent of retinal involvement may not be to the same extent.
- The etiopathogenesis of Eale's disease is ill understood to date.
- Eale's disease is recognized as primary vasculitis of unknown etiology occurring in young adults.

CLINICAL SIGNS AND SYMPTOMS

- Eale's disease is characterized by retinal phlebitis, peripheral nonperfusion and retinal neovascularization.
- Most patients symptoms include vitreous hemorrhage such as small specs. Floaters, cobwebs, blurring or decrease of visual acuity. While others have blurring of vision associated with retinal vasculitis but without vitreous hemorrhage.
- Signs and symptoms of inflammation (retinal phlebitis) occur at varying times in the course of disease but are less common in the late stage.
- Most patients with Eale's disease develop varying degree of peripheral retinal non perfusion. Intraretinal Hemorrhages often appear first in the affected area followed by an increase in vascular tortuosity.
- Neovascularization is observed in 80% of patients with Eale's disease. The new vessels can form either on the disc (NVD) or elsewhere on the retina (NVE). The NVE is however more common than NVD.

INVESTIGATIONS

- Complete fundus examination by direct ophthalmoscopy is essential for both eyes.
- Fundus examination in the early stages of the disease reveals venous dilatation in the periphery with tortuosity and discontinuity of veins. Perivascular exudates are seen along the peripheral veins.
- Bleeding from neovascularization is common, usually recurrent and is one of the major causes of visual loss.
- In recurrent bleeding the fundus shows evidence of old blood with signs of fibrous organization, retinitis proliferans or even tractional retinal detachment.
- The vascular abnormalities at the junction between the perfused and non perfused zones include microaneurysms, veno-venous shunts venous beading and even hard exudates and cotton wool spots.

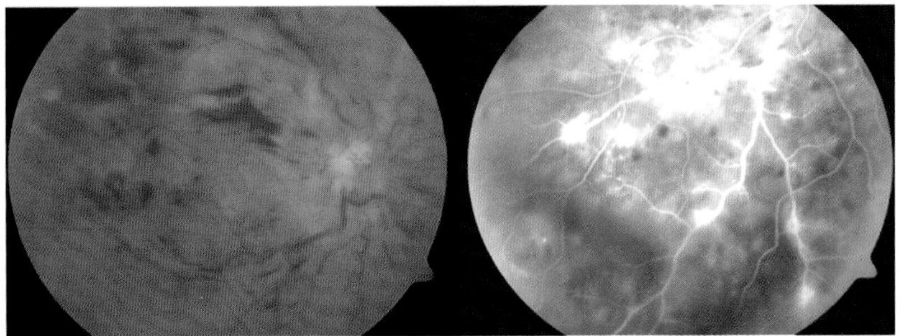

Fig. 1: Eale's disease

- Idiopathic peripheral vasculitis
- Prime suspect-M tuberculosis
- Difficult to prove conclusively

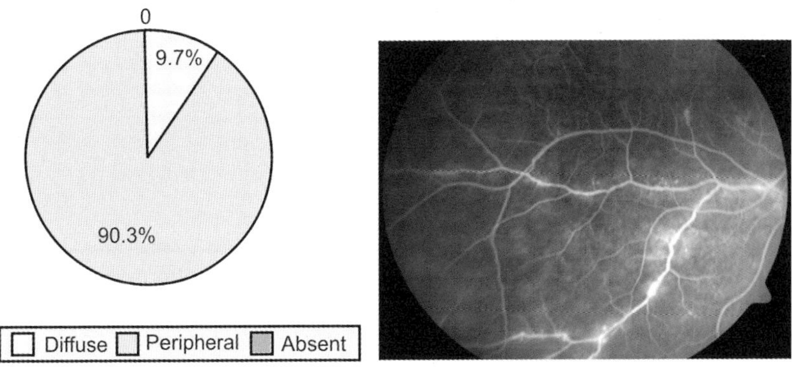

Fig. 2: Healed vasculitis

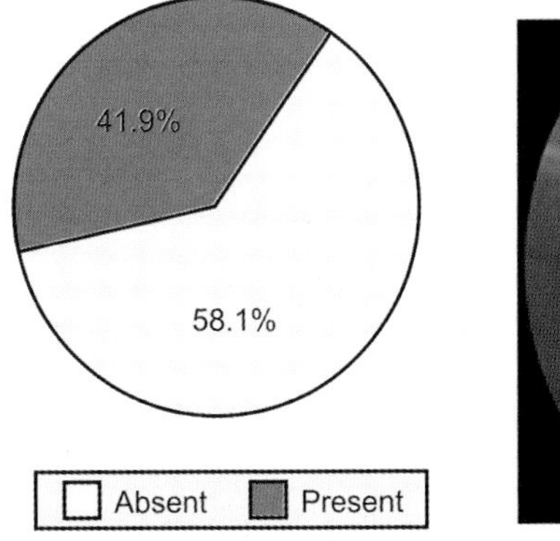

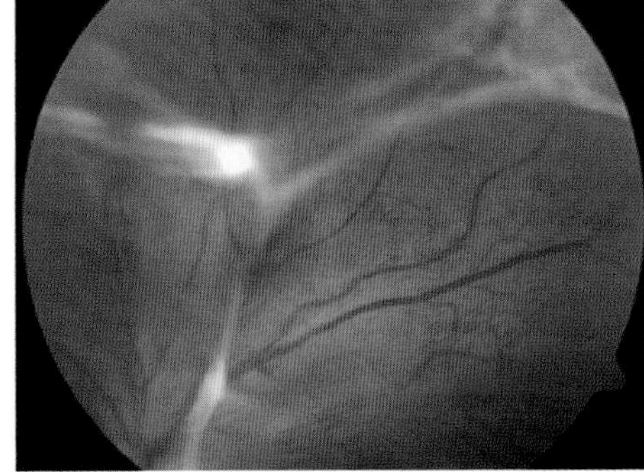

Fig. 3: Tractional bands

- Fluorescein angiography is vital in Eale's disease. Active vasculitis is characterized by staining of the vessel wall or even Frank extravasation. Inflammation of the venous segment results in various degree of obstruction to the venous flow.
- Venous stasis consequent to venous obstruction is manifested by engorged tortuous vein distal to the obstruction, engorgement of the capillary bed, microaneurysms and retinal edema.
- Fluorescein angiography also helps in monitoring the regression and disappearance of new vessels during treatment and follow-up.
- Following subsidence of the venous inflammation, the dye leakage and later the dye staining stops.

DIFFERENTIAL DIAGNOSIS

- Papillitis or papilledema
- Behcet disease
- Diabetes mellitus
- Infectious mononucleosis
- Hypertension
- Multiple sclerosis
- Acute retinal necrosis
- Viral infection specially CMV retinitis.

TREATMENT

- The treatment of Eale's disease is mainly symptomatic and is aimed at reducing retinal perivasculitis and associated vitritis, reducing the risk of vitreous hemorrhage from new vessels on to retina by retinal ablation and surgical removal of non-resolving vitreous hemorrhage/or vitreous membranes.
- The present day modalities of treatment are confined to corticosteroids, photocoagulation with or without anterior retinal cryoablation (ARC) and vitrectomy at various stages of the disease process.
- Corticosteroids forms the mainstay of treatment for cases with active perivasculitis. Oral and periocular steroids have been advocated. Initially high dose of oral steroids prednisolone 2 mg/kg body weight are given, gradually tapering off as the vasculitis begins to subside.
- Periocular depot steroids are given as deep posterior sub-Tenon injection in active retinal vasculitis (Hydrocortisone or depomedrol).
- Antitubercular treatment (ATT) is also given in a select group of patients who presents with active phlebitis with massive infiltration, nodule formation.
- Complete obliteration of segments of vein. The ATT regimen usually includes two drugs (Rifampicin 450 mg and Isoniazid 300 mg once daily for a period of nine months.
- Recently low dose Methotrexate therapy has been advocated to decrease the fibrovascular proliferation.

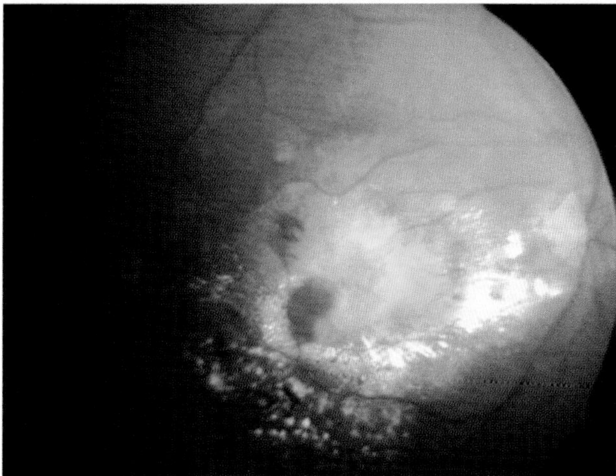

Fig. 4: Vitreous hemorrhage

- Photocoagulation is the treatment of choice in the proliferative stage of this disease. The main purpose is the prevention of hemorrhages that occur from the proliferations and aneurysmal dilations of blood vessels.
- Argon Green Laser is most commonly used. The Red Krypton Laser (647 mm) is useful in creating cases in which media opacities may preclude effective Argon Laser Penetration.
- Laser photocoagulation can be delivered through a slit-lamp, binocular indirect ophthalmoscope or by endolaser probe. Green Argon dye laser burns of 200-500 micrometer diameter and 0.1 second duration are used.
- Anterior retinal cryoablation is now a days used to decrease anterior segment neovascularisation leading to intractable glaucoma. ARC is done under direct visualization using indirect ophthalmoscope technique.
- Pars plana vitreous surgery restores vision by removing the unresolved blood and vitreous membranes. The main indications for vitrectomy include unresolving vitreous hemorrhage, tractional retinal detachment involving posterior pole, multiple vitreous membranes, etc.

PROGNOSIS

With the advent of new therapies in recent time which can control fibrovascular proliferation in conjunction with systemic steroids, a new hopes has arisen for Eale's disease patients. The prognosis is coming good in recent time.

CHAPTER TWELVE

TUMORS

- **TUMORS**
  Debraj Shome, Ashok Garg (India)
  - Retinoblastoma
  - Retinal Capillary Hemangioma
  - Retinal Cavernous Hemangioma
  - Vasoproliferative Tumor of the Retina
  - Retinal Astrocytoma
  - Choroidal Melanoma
  - Solitary Choroidal Hemangioma

- **CHOROIDAL METASTASIS**
- **CHOROIDAL HEMANGIOMA**
  Hsi Kung Kuo (Taiwan)

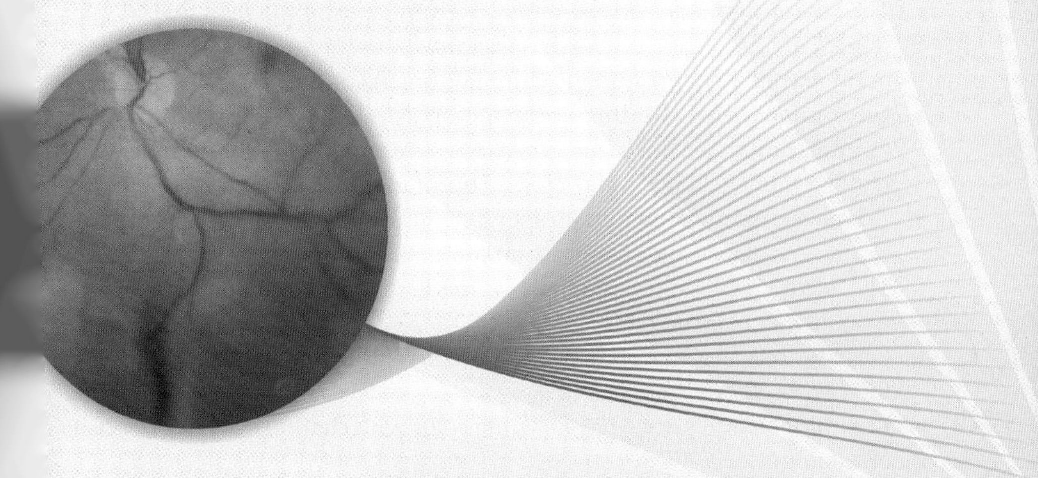

Tumors

Debraj Shome, Ashok Garg (India)

RETINOBLASTOMA

INTRODUCTION

- Retinoblastoma is the most common primary Intraocular malignancy of infancy and childhood.
- Retinoblastoma represents the phenotype expression of an abnormal or absent tumor suppressor gene known as the retinoblastoma gene (RBI).
- It is second only to malignant melanoma of the uvea as the most common malignancy of the eye.
- There is no predisposition for retinoblastoma by race or gender. Both eyes are affected equally.
- The incidence of retinoblastoma worldwide ranges from 1 in 14000 Live birth to 1 in 34000.
- A substantial proportions of cases of retinoblastoma are hereditary arising through germ-line mutations in tumor suppressor genes.
- The incidence peaks in the first year of life and declines gradually with age thereafter.

CLINICAL SIGNS AND SYMPTOMS

- Initially there may be little or no signs or symptoms hence public awareness and regular eye checkups are essential to catch the disease at an early stage of presentation.
- The tumor first starts in the retina (Neural layer of the eye) and in later stages, involves the entire eye and spreads to the orbital structures and brain and finally spreading to different organs of the body.
- Most infants and children with retinoblastoma are referred for ocular examination at a later stage when physician detects an abnormal while papillary reflex (Leukocoria), crossed eyes (strabismus) or decreased vision.
- Advanced tumor present with spontaneous hyphema, pseudo-hypopyon, secondary glaucoma or chronic inflammation.
- The accuracy of clinical diagnosis is made with indirect ophthalmoscopy when the ocular media is clear.
- Early lesions appear as flat, transparent or slightly white placoid tumor in the neurosensory retina.
- As tumor enlarges, they have a white color with chalky, fleck like deposits of calcium.

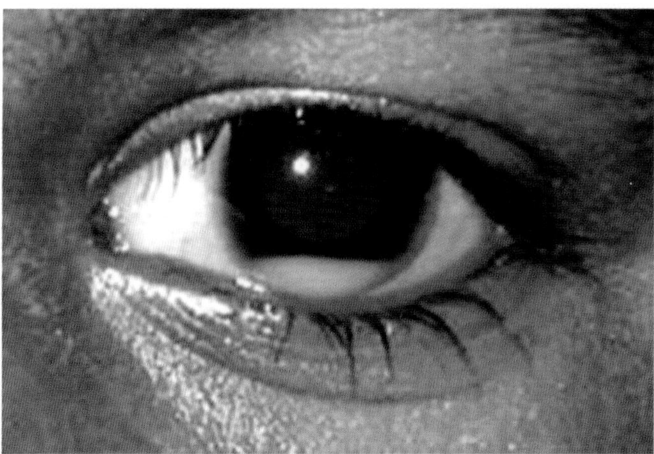

Fig. 1: Pseudohypopyon due to retinoblastoma cells

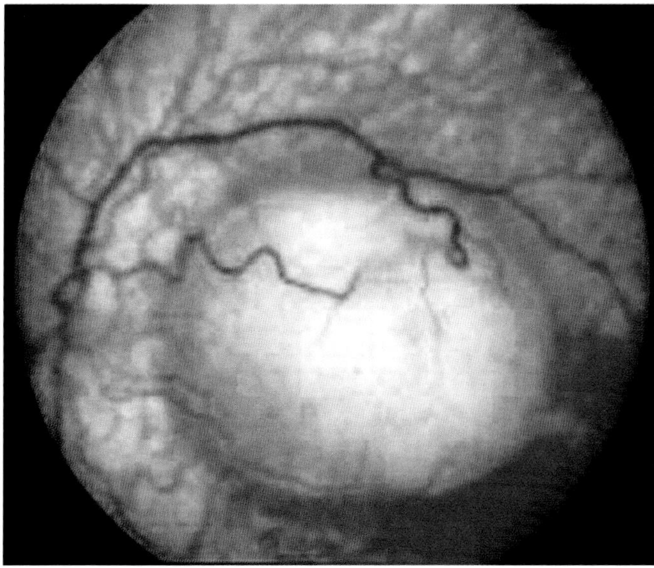

Fig. 2: Color fundus photograph of the left eye showing early macular retinoblastoma

- Growth is either endophytic (into the vitreous) or exophytic (under the neurosensory retina) or combined.
- If vitreous hemorrhage obscures the fundus view, ultrasonography and computed tomography are indispensable in the workup. Calcium within the tumor is highly characteristic of retinoblastoma and usually is easily demonstrable by both methods.

DIFFERENTIAL DIAGNOSIS

Diagnosis of retinoblastoma requires differentiation from other causes of leukocoria. These are as follows:

- Congenital cataract may be hereditary or may result from other conditions like congenital rubella, galactosemia and intraocular infections
- Anomalous optic disk
- Coat's disease
- Congenital corneal opacity
- Coloboma of choroid and optic disk
- Persistant hyperplastic primary vitreous
- Developmental retinal cyst
- Retinal glaucoma
- Hematoma under retinal pigment epithelium
- High myopia with advanced chorioretinal degeneration
- Juvenile retinoschisis
- Toxocara canis
- Medullation of nerve fibers layer
- Metastatic Endophthalmitis
- Norrie's Disease
- Retinal detachment due to choroidal or vitreous hemorrhage
- Vitreous hemorrhage
- Oligodendroglioma of the retina
- Retinal dysplasia
- Retinopathy of prematurity (ROP)
- Secondary glaucoma
- Rhegmatogenous retinal detachment
- Tapetiretinal degeneration
- Microophthalmia
- Ocular Toxoplasmosis
- Traumatic chorioretinitis
- White with pressure sign
- Trisomy 13.

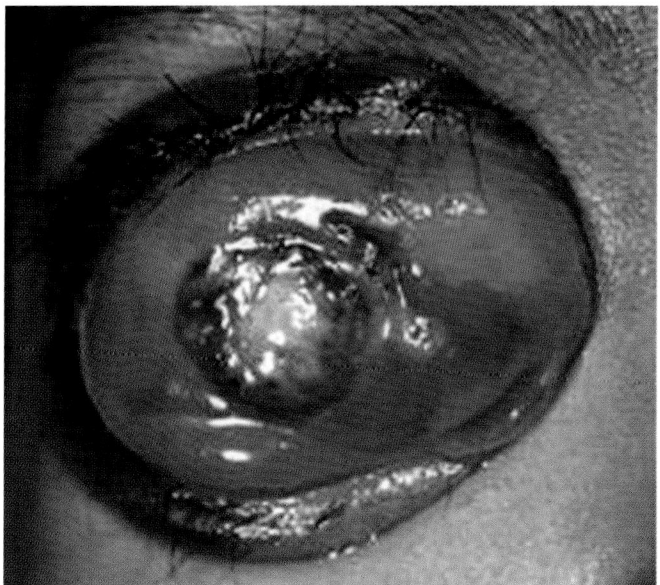

Fig. 3: Orbital retinoblastoma

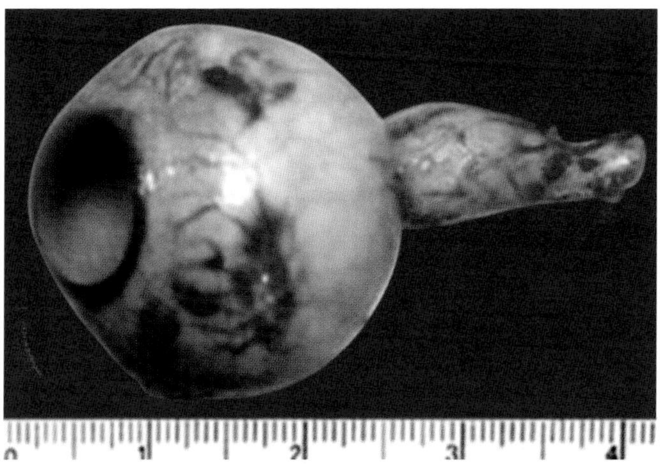

Fig. 4: Enucleated eyeball with enlarged optic nerve suggestive of nerve involvement with tumor

INVESTIGATIONS

The diagnosis of retinoblastoma is best made using indirect ophthalmoscopy. Other investigations to be performed are:

- Ocular ultrasonography.
- Fluorescein angiography.
- Computerised photographic imaging.
- Computed tomography.
- Magnetic resonance imaging.
- Calcium within the tumor is highly characteristic of retinoblastoma and is easily demonstrable by ultrasonography and computed tomography.
- Computed tomography is also helpful in excluding orbital extension and in demonstrating pineal tumor.

TREATMENT

- Early diagnosis and recent advances in management have improved the prognosis of this potentially fatal tumor significantly.
- Survival rate has improved to nearly 95% in last decade.
- It is very important to recognize the other causes of white papillary reflex (leukocoria) before starting definitive treatment of RB.
- The most important factor that must be considered in the treatment are the tumor size, number, location and laterality, condition of other eye, threat of metastasis, risk for second malignant neoplasms and systemic status of the patient. The latest international classification is given at the end of this clinical condition.

Treatment modality currently available as classified as:

a. Focal therapy like cryotheraphy, tanspupillary therapy and laser photocoagulation.
b. Local therapy like external beam radio therapy and enucleation.
c. Systemic therapy like chemotheraphy.

Cryotherapy

It involves freezing the tumor leading to ischemic necrosis of tumor. It is performed for small equatorial or peripheral retinoblastoma measuring upto 4 mm in basal diameter and 2 mm in thickness.

Complications include:

- Transient serous retinal detachment
- Retinal tear
- Pre-retinal fibrosis
- Rhegmatogenous retinal detachment.

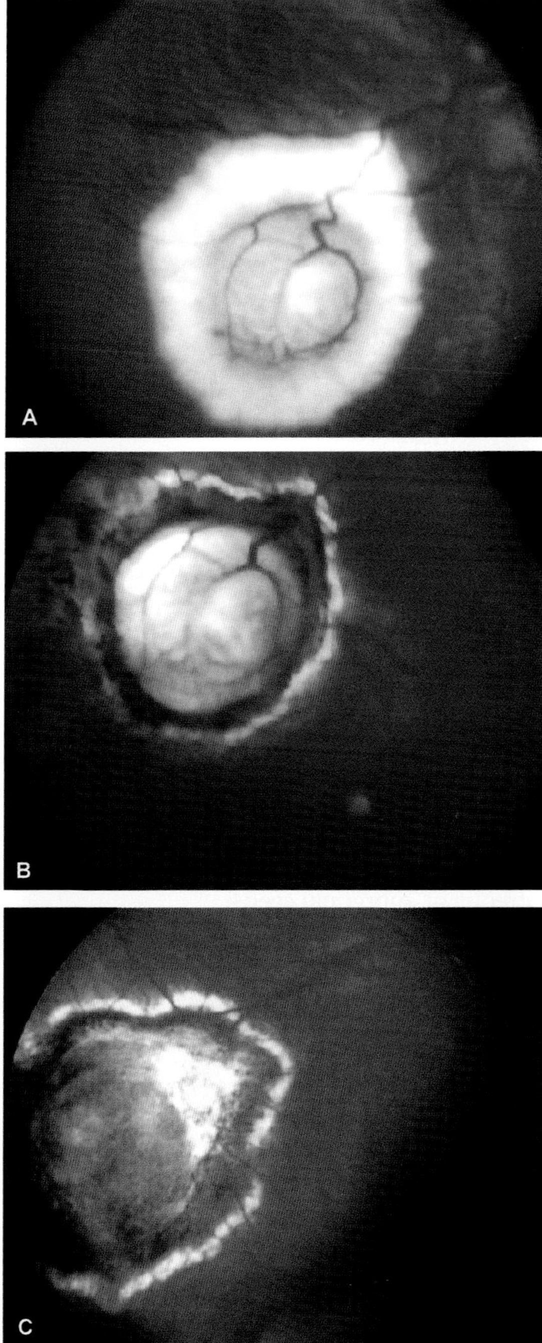

Figs 5A to C : TTT in retinoblastoma (tumor is heated till it turns subtle gray)

Laser Photocoagulation

This modality of managing RB has been sidelined with the advent of thermotherapy as laser involves destruction of retina and retinal pigment epithelium.

- This is usually done for small posterior tumors 4 mm in basal diameter and 2 mm or less in thickness.

Complications includes:

- Vascular occlusion
- Retinal traction
- Transient serous retinal detachment
- Retinal hole.

Transpupillary Thermotherapy (TTT)

TTT is the delivery of heat using infrared radiation. The goal is to reach a subcoagulative temperature range of 40-60° Celsius thus sparing retinal vessels of photocoagulation.

- TTT using infrared radiation from a semiconductor diode laser has become a standard practice. It is specially useful in treating lesions at the macula.
- The large spot adapted indirect ophthalmoscope, operating microscope with a laser delivery system or trans-scleral route using a diopexy probe can be used to deliver it.
- TTT alone can be used for small tumors measuring upto 4 mm in basal diameter and 2 mm in thickness. However its major application is an adjunct to chemoreduction.
- TTT alone is highly effective for relatively small retinoblastomas without associated vitreous or subretinal seeds.

The chief complications of TTT are:

- Focal iris atrophy.
- Peripheral focal lens opacity.
- Retinal traction.
- Retinal vascular occlusion.
- Transient serous retinal detachment.

Brachytherapy Plaque

Retinoblastoma is a radiosensitive tumor. In brachytherapy, a radioactive implant is placed on the sclera over the base of the tumor to irradiate the tumor transclerally. The goal is to deliver a radiation dose of 4000-5000 cGy to the apex of the tumor selectively without irradiating the remaining ocular structures.

- The Radioactive materials used commonly are 125 Iodine and 106 Ruthenium.

- Plaque brachytherapy can be performed as primary or as secondary treatment. It is generally reserved for the tumors less than 16 mm in diameter and 8 mm in thickness ideally situated > 3 mm from the optic nerve and fovea.
- The radiation associated problems of papillopathy and retinopathy usually become clinically manifest at above 18 months after irradiation.
- Custom design of plaques have reduced the incidence of radiation induced complications.

External Beam Radiotherapy (EBRT)

- EBRT was conventionally indicated for moderately advanced unilateral or bilateral retinoblastoma.
- Currently EBRT is indicated in eyes where chemoreduction and/or local therapy have failed and in rare conditions where chemotherapy is contraindicated due to poor systemic status.
- EBRT is also used as a standard adjunct following enucleation in patients with retinoblastoma with gross or histopathological involvement beyond the optic nerve transaction, sclera infiltration and orbital extension.

Enucleation

- About a decade ago primary enucleation was standard procedure in majority of unilateral retinoblastoma. However the advent of chemotherapy has changed this radical managemnt of retinoblastoma. Enucleation is thus the second or third line of management and is reserved for patients who fail focal therapy, Chemotherapy and EBRT. However tumors where there characteristics are not visualized are primarily managed by by enucleation.
- Minimum manipulation surgical technique should be necessarily practiced. Optic nerve head should be examined carefully postenucleation for thickening, suggestive of tumor involvement.
- Nonintegrated orbital implants like PMMA or silicon or biointegrated implants like hydroxypatite or porous polyethylene promotes orbital growth, provides better cosmeses and enhances prosthetic motility.

Orbital Exenteration

It is usually done for orbital recurrence after the child has received the maximum dose of radiation and chemotherapy.

Chemotherapy

- With the advent of chemotherapy, radical methods of management like enucleation have been shifted to second and third place. The introduction of newer chemotherapy protocols has dramatically improved the prognosis for life, eye salvage and residual vision.

- Chemotherapy can be local or systemic. Local chemotherapy is under Phase III clinical trials. The role of systemic chemotherapy in the management of retinoblastoma includes Chemoreduction, adjuvant chemotherapy and treatment of metastasis.

Systemic Chemotherapy Drugs and Disk Schedules

Standard Chemotherapy

Vincristine 0.05 mg/kg on day 1 of chemotherapy
Etoposide, 5 mg/kg on days 1 and 2 of chemotherapy
Carboplatin, 18.6 mg/kg on day 1 of chemotherapy

High Dose Chemotherapy

Vincristine 0.025 mg/kg on day 1 of chemotherapy
Etoposide, 12 mg/kg on day 1 and 2 of chemotherapy
Carboplatin, 28 mg/kg on day 1 of chemotherapy

Periocular Chemotherapy

- One of the main concern in systemic chemotherapy is that Chemotherapeutic agents may not be able to penetrate the blood retinal barrier. The other route suggested to the deliver chemotherapy locally thereby allowing transscleral penetration of drugs and high intraocular concentrations.
- Carboplatin administered subconjunctivally has been shown to be efficacious in the management of retinoblastoma specially in the presence of vitreous seeds as it can penetrate the sclera and achieve effective concentrations in the vitreous cavity. However response may be short lived with tumor recurrences.

Follow-up Schedule

- The usual protocol is to schedule the first examination 3-6 weeks after the initial therapy. In cases where chemoreduction therapy has been administered, the examination should be done every 3 weeks with each cycle of chemotherapy.
- Patients under focal therapy are evaluated and treated after every 4-8 weeks until complete tumor regression.
- Following tumor regression, follow up examination should be done 3 monthly for the first year, 6 monthly for three years or until the child attains 6 years of age and yearly thereafter.

PROGNOSIS

- Early detection and recent advances in the management of retinoblastoma along with customized multispeciality management for individual patient have yielded gratifying outcomes in terms of preservation of life, salvage of the eye and optimal residual vision.

INTERNATIONAL CLASSIFICATION (NEW)

Group	*Quick reference*	*Specific features*
A.	Small tumor	RB < 3 mm
B.	Larger tumor Macula Juxtapapillary Subretinal fluied	RB > mm or • Macular RB location [< 3mm to foveola] • Juxtapapillary RB location [< 1.5 mm to the disk] Additional subretinal fluid < 3 mm from margin.
C.	Focal seeds	RB with : • Subretinal seeds < 3 mm from RB • Vitreous seeds < 3 mm from RB • Both subretinal and Vitreous seeds <3 mm from RB.
D.	Diffuse seeds	RB with: • Subretinal fluid > 3 mm from RB • Subretinal seeds > 3 mm from RB • Vitreous seeds > 3 mm from RB • Both subretinal and vitreous seeds > 3 mm from RB.
E.	Extensive RB	Extensive RB occupying > 50% of the globe or • Neovascular glaucoma • Opaque media from hemorrhage in anterior chamber, vitreous or subretinal space. • Invasion of postlaminar optic nerve, choroid (> 2 mm), sclera, orbit and anterior chamber. • Pthisis bulbi post RB • Orbital cellulitis due to aseptic tumor necrosis.

RETINAL CAPILLARY HEMANGIOMA

INTRODUCTION

- Retinal capillary hemangioma (RCH) are benign angiomatous hamartomas of the retina composed of expansive capillary networks with in the matrices of interstitial cells.
- They may be located in the peripheral retina or associated with the optic disk and may be accompanied by potentially life threatening systemic condition like Von-Hippel - Lindau syndrome.
- About 50% of occurrences are bilateral or with multiple angiomas in the same eye, implying a genetic etiology.

CLINICAL SIGNS AND SYMPTOMS

- The clinical appearance of RCHs varies according to its location in the retina, its size and the degree of the accompanying exudative changes.
- The peripheral retina is a more common location for RCHs.
- RCHs are associated with dilated feeder arteries and enlarged, tortuous draining veins.
- With time, RCHs enlarge, becoming bright orange red masses sometimes greater than 8 mm in size with progressive exudation of fluid and lipid into the retina.
- Loss of vision is usually due to cystoid macular edema, serous retinal Detachment, hard exudates and tractional retinal detachment.

INVESTIGATIONS

- Funduscopic examination and workup for decreased visual acuity shall help in making the diagnosis.
- Initial ophthalmoscopic appearance of peripheral capillary hemangiona (The Von-Hippel tumor) is subtle; a red or grayish dot no larger than a diabetic microaneurysm. Afferent and efferent vessels may be normal to slightly dilated but later they show fine tortuosity or focal telangiectasia.
- The Appearance of Endophytic and Exophytic Juxtapapillary capillary hemangioma is quite different.
- Endophytic hemangiomas are well circumscribed, bright red sessile tumor that lie on the surface of and partially obscure the optic disk. These tumors may give rise to surface neovascularization, traction and exudation.
- Exophytic Juxtapapillary lesions appear as a diffuse, graying thickening that obscures the border of the optic disk often without prominent vascular channels. Intraretinal exudates are often present.

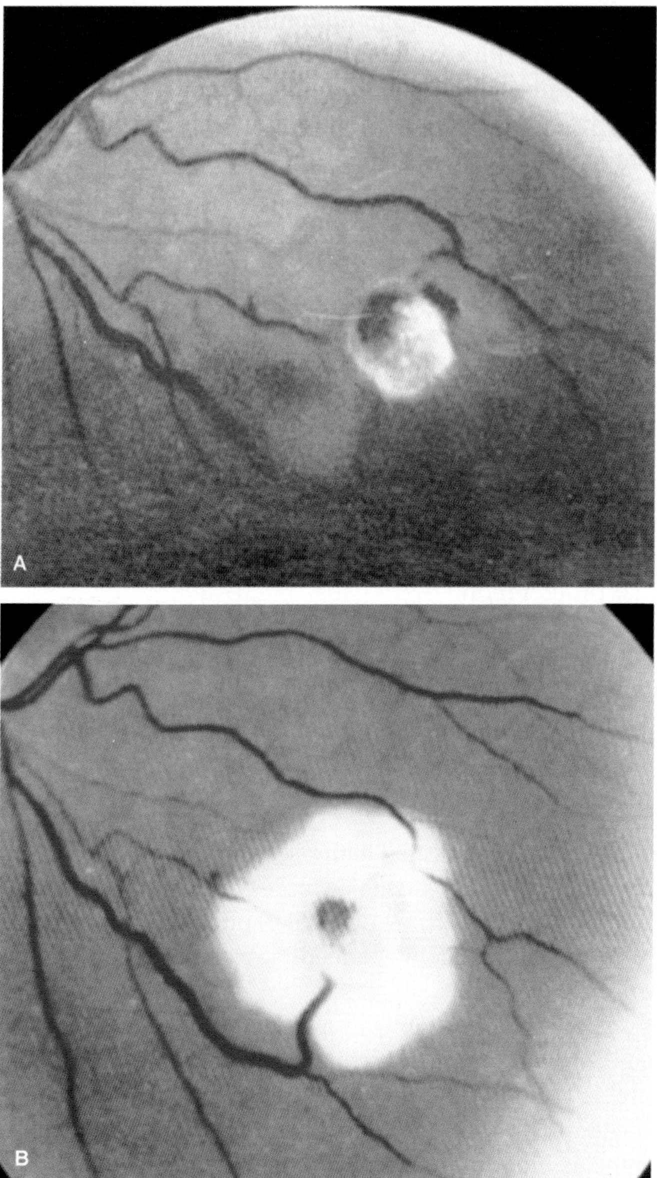

Figs 6 A and B: Retinal capillary hemangioma

- Steroscopic fluorescein angiography. Show early filling of a vascular intraretinal mass with a variable degree of leakage and late edema.
- Ultrasonography optical coherence tomography. Color fundus Photography, MRI, Blood tests, Genetic testing are other investigations which can be performed.

DIFFERENTIAL DIAGNOSIS

These lesions may be confused with:
- Papilledema
- Papillitis
- Choroiditis
- Choroidal neovascularization
- Choroidal hemangioma
- Malignant melanoma
- Vitreous hemorrhage
- Exudate
- Fibroglial proliferation
- Coat's disease
- Neurofibromatosis
- Retinitis pigmentosa
- Inflammatory conditions

TREATMENT

- Periperal RCHs may be treated with laser photocoagulation or cryotherapy. Laser photocoagulation tends to be more effective on smaller tumors with less exudation (that are 1.5 mm or smaller) photocoagulation can be applied directly to the tumor or to the feeder artery or a combination of both techniques can be used.
- Recently photodynamic therapy has been reported to induce occlusion of Juxtapapillary and peripheral retinal capillary hemangimos. Cryotherapy is preferable to photocoagulation when the retinal capillary hemangioma is located anterior with sub retinal fluid that might reduce laser energy uptake and is more than 3.0 mm in diameter. In general cryotherapy is effective for RCH up to 4.5 mm in size.
- RCHs that are larger than 4 mm show a poor response to cryotherapy and laser photocoagulation. Such tumors are treated successfully with plaque radiotherapy.
- Low dose external beam radiotherapy may be option in cases refractory to other modes of treatment.

PROGNOSIS

- RCHs tumors may remain asymptomatic for a long period.
- Visual loss results from intraretinal exudation, macular edema, surface neovascularization and its consequences or epiretinal membrane formation.

RETINAL CAVERNOUS HEMANGIOMA

INTRODUCTION

- Cavernous hemangioma of the retina is a rare vascular hamartoma.
- The tumor is composed of clumps of dark intraretinal aneurysms that demonstrate a characterstic "Cluster of grapes" appearance.
- It is usually unilateral and rarerly increases in size.
- Patients with this hamartoma also may have hemangiomas involving the skin and nervous system.
- It has an autosomal dominant pattern of inheritance.

CLINICAL SIGNS AND SYMPTOMS

- Retinal cavernous hemangiomas are composed of cluster of saccular aneurysms filled with dark blood. The aneurysms range in size from microaneruysm to a half disk diameter.
- The typical tumor is isolated, 1-2 disk diameters in size and resembles an intraretinal cluster of grapes.
- The clinical appearance can be quite variable with the wide distribution over the entire fundus or following the course of a major vein.
- Often a white or gray fibroglial membrane covers the surface of the tumor. The adjacent retinal blood vessels appear unaffected by the tumor.
- Retinal cavernous hemangiomas are symptomatic when they are located in or adjacent to the macula.
- Visual acuity can be decreased both on the basis of tumor location as well as amblyopia.
- Cavernous hemangiomas can cause simultaneous subretinal, intraretinal and preretinal hemorrhage.

INVESTIGATIONS

- Fluorescein angiography may show autofluorescence of the gray white epiretinal membrane overlying the tumor. The aneurysms will slowly fill and often incompletely upto 30 minutes after dye injection.
- The plasma-erythrocytic separation often seen on clinical examination is dramatically demonstrated in the later phases of the angiogram.
- In certain cases when diagnosis is made difficult by vitreous hemorrhage ultrasonography is required.
- A scan shows a high initial spike and high internal reflectivity while B-scan shows an irregular surface, large internal acoustic density and absence of choroidal excavation.

DIFFERENTIAL DIAGNOSIS

- Retinal teleangiectasis
- Coat's disease
- Lebers miliary aneurysms
- Von Hippel's disease
- Racemose hemangioma.

TREATMENT

- As cavernous hemangiomas rarely increase in size or cause lipid exudation or severe vitreous hemorrhage, these tumors generally do not require treatment.
- Photocoagulation or cryotherapy have been advocated if vitreous haemorrhage occurs.

PROGNOSIS

As cavernous hemangiomas rarely increases in size and are generally asymptomatic the prognosis is good.

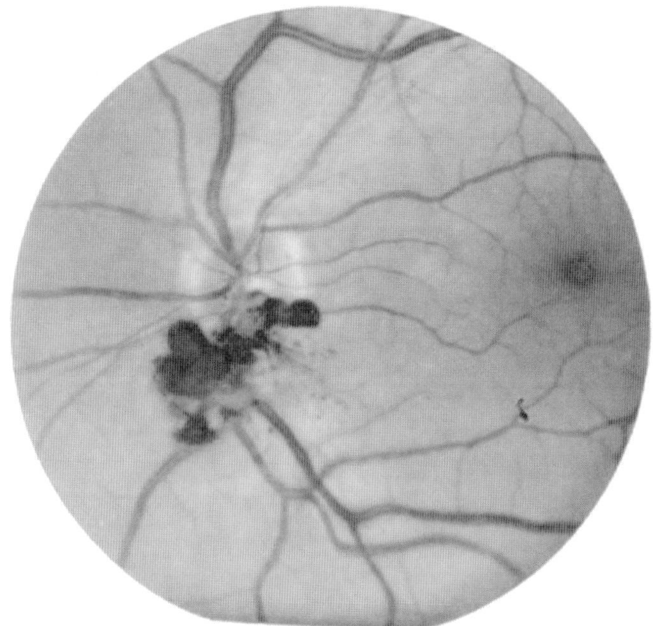

Fig. 7: Retinal cavernous hemangioma

VASOPROLIFERATIVE TUMOR OF THE RETINA

INTRODUCTION

These are solitary tumors commonly involves the inferotemporal of inferior quadrants of the retina.

- These may occur without any antecedent cause and may be associated with prior retinitis pigmentosa, Coat's disease, familial exudative vitreoretinopathy and toxoplasma scars.
- These tumors may be multiple or diffuse tumors.
- The pathogenesis of these lesions is unclear.

CLINICAL SIGNS AND SYMPTOMS

These tumors appear as solitary mass lesions with minimally dilated feeder vessels associated with intraretinal and subretinal exudation and hemorrhage, secondary retinal detachment, RPE hyperplasia, macular edema and vitreous hemorrhage.

INVESTIGATIONS

Fluorescein angiography shows early filling and later leakge and dilated feeder vessels.

DIFFERENTIAL DIAGNOSIS

- Racemose hemangioma
- Retinal telangiectasia
- Capillary hemangioma
- Neurofibromatosis.

TREATMENT

- If progressive exudation causes loss of vision, cryotherapy, photocoagulation, plaque brachytherapy may be required.
- Epiretinal proliferation may need vitreous surgery.

PROGNOSIS

- Good

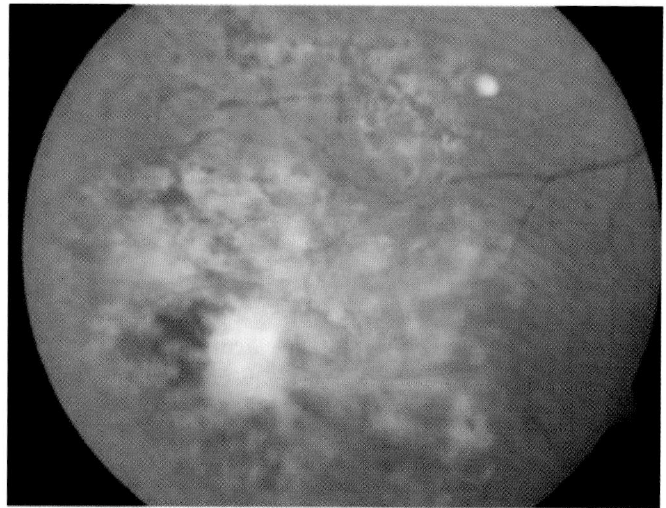

Fig. 8: Vasoproliferative tumor of the retina

RETINAL ASTROCYTOMA

INTRODUCTION

- Retinal astrocytoma of the retina rarely occurs.
- It may appear as isolated lesions and are commonly seen in patients with tuberous sclerosis which is one of the phacomatosis.
- Retinal astrocytoma is of autosomal dominant inheritance with new mutations in about 50% of cases.
- It is characterized by the triad of mental retardation, epilepsy and adenoma sebaceum skin lesions.

CLINICAL SIGNS AND SYMPTOMS

- Retinal lesions arise from the inner layers and can be single or multiple.
- These are usually present at or near the optic nerve head although they may be present in periphery also.
- The tumor may be small and flat or modular and well circumscribed with the size ranging from 0.5 to 1 mm in diameter.
- Early tumors may appear semitranslucent but in later stage they become more dense white color and the occurrence of multiple areas of calcification with in the tumor may give it a mulberry like appearance.

INVESTIGATIONS

- Fluorescein angiography and color fundus photography alongwith ophthalmoscopy are recommended for the diagnosis of the disease.

DIFFERENTIAL DIAGNOSIS

- Retinoblastoma
- Hyaline bodies.

TREATMENT

Generally treatment is not required as the lesions are usually asymptomatic and show only a minimal tendency to grow.

PROGNOSIS

- Good

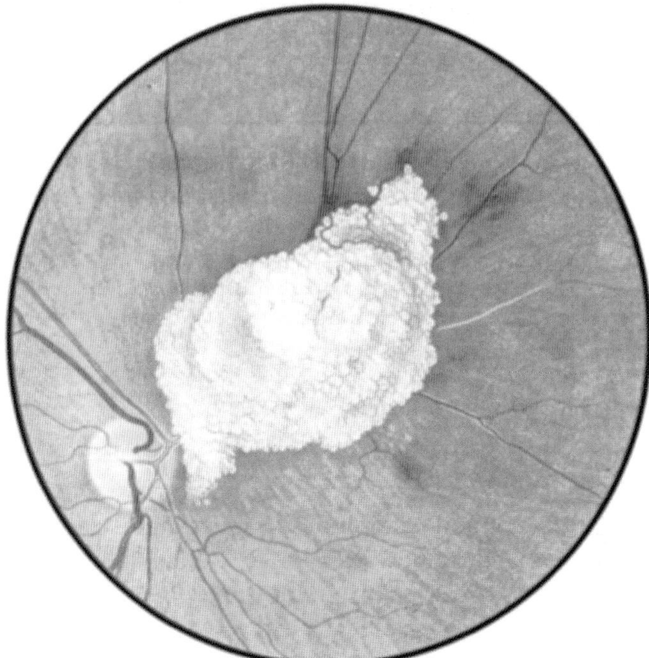

Fig. 9: Retinal astrocytoma of larger size

CHOROIDAL MELANOMA

INTRODUCTION

- Choroidal (uveal) melanoma is the leading primary eye malignant tumor.
- It arises either from a uveal nevus or may arise de novo without a pre-existing lesions.
- It often strikes without symptoms and carries a risk of spread via metastasis to the liver, lung and skin.
- The average age of patient with choroidal melanoma is about 50 years.
- Patients with ocular or oculodermal melanosis are at increased risk of choroidal melanoma.

CLINICAL SIGNS AND SYMPTOMS

- The tumor is usually unilateral and clinical features are variable.
- A typical melanoma is characterized by pigmented, elevated, oval shaped mass. The color of tumor is usually brown although it may appear as dark brown or black or may be amelanotic.
- When tumor grows it break through the Bruch's membrane and appear as mushroom shaped mass giving rise to exudative detachment of the retina.
- Other associated features of choroidal melanoma can be choroidal folds, subretinal or intraretinal hemorrhage, hard yellow exudation, vitreous hemorrhage, secondary glaucoma, cataract and posterior uveitis.

INVESTIGATIONS

- The diagnosis of uveal melanoma is best made using Indirect ophthalmoloscopy by expert clinician familiar with ocular tumors.
- Noninvasive ancillary testing include transillumination, ocular ultrasonography. Fluorescein angiography, Indocyanine green angiography, ultrasound biomicroscopy, color Doppler imaging and P32 testing. Fine needle biopsy may be employed for difficult cases that pose a diagnostic dilemma.
- Visual field examination, computed tomography and magnetic resonance imaging are other investigations which are of value in clinching diagnosis.

DIFFERENTIAL DIAGNOSIS

- Retinal detachment
- Metastatic tumor of choroid
- Exudative ARMD
- Choroidal detachment

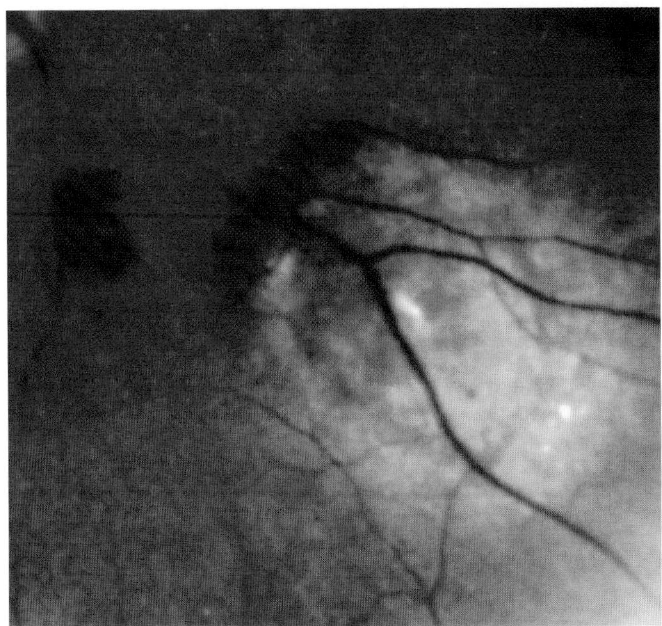

Fig. 10: Choroidal melanoma

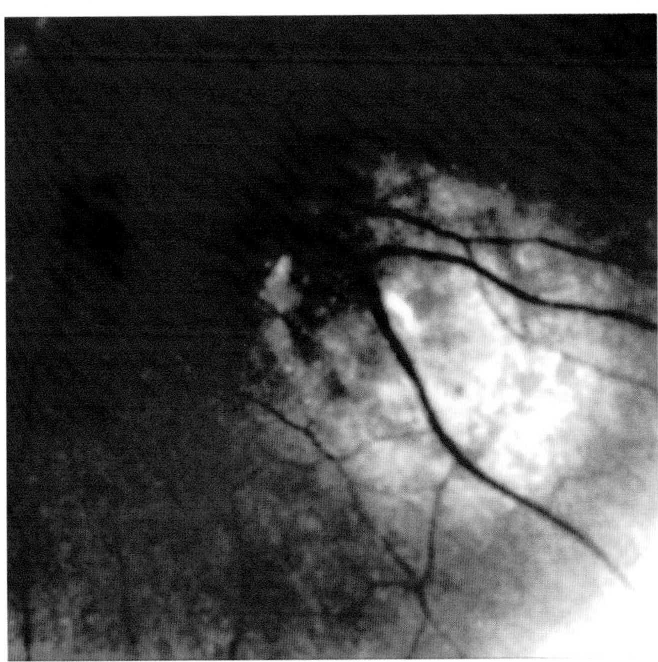

Fig. 11A

- Choroidal hemangioma
- Large choroidal nevus.

TREATMENT

Tumor growth pattern is a factor in the therapeutic decision if there is diffuse melanoma or if there is extraocular extension, enucleation is of choice but radiation therapy can be employed for less extensive disease. Based on COMS classification the therapeutic opinions for medium sized choroidal melanomas are:

- Plaque radiation therapy.
- External beam, charged particle radiation therapy.
- Local eye wall resection.
- Combined therapy with ablative laser coagulation or transpupillary thermotherapy (TTT) to supplement plaque treatment.
- Photocoagulation.
- Transpupillary Thermotherapy (TTT)
- Encucleation
- Chemotherapy and immune therapy regimens (using melanoma vaccine).
- Laser photocoagulation has a limited role to play in the treatment of choroidal melanomas.
- Therapeutic options for large choroidal melanomas.
- Radiation therapy plus enucleation
- Enucleation.

PROGNOSIS

- It depends upon on cell type. Spindle a cell tumors have the best prognosis and those composed of epitheloid cells have the worst prognosis.
- Tumor size – large tumors have a worse prognosis than small tumors.
- Diffuse tumors have worst prognosis.
- If Bruch's membrane is ruptured than prognosis is not favorable.
- Patient over the age of 65 years have worst prognosis.
- Extrascleral extension carries a poor prognosis.

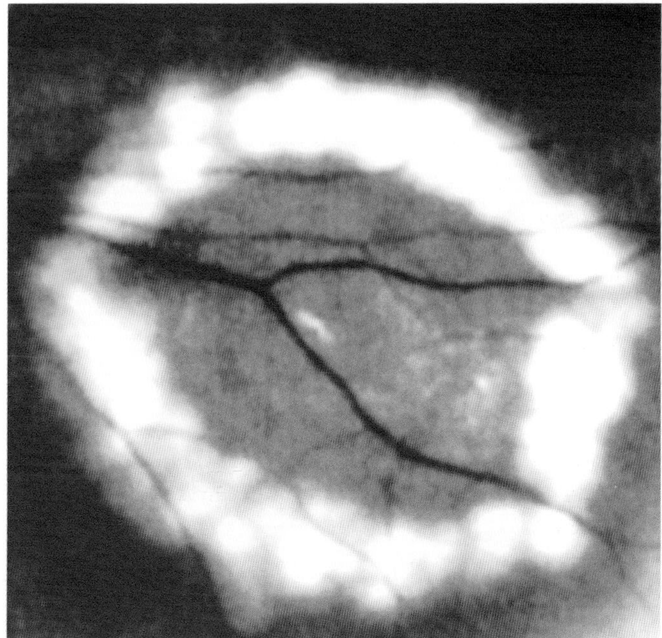

Fig. 11B

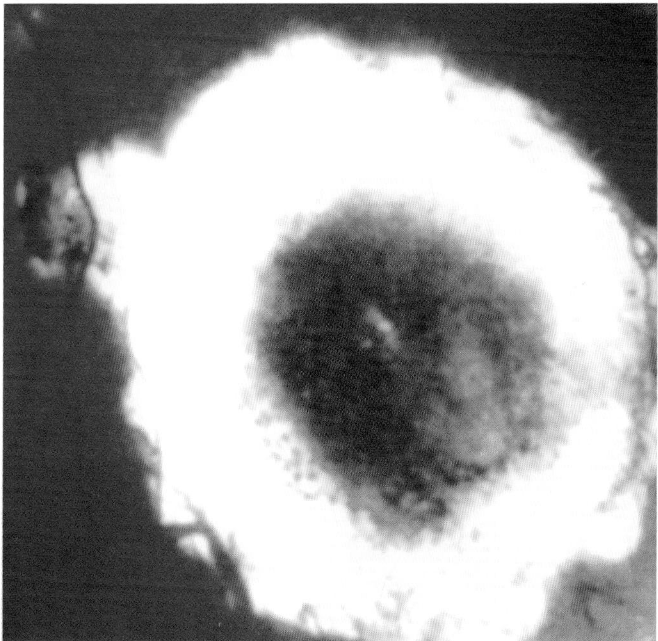

Fig. 11C

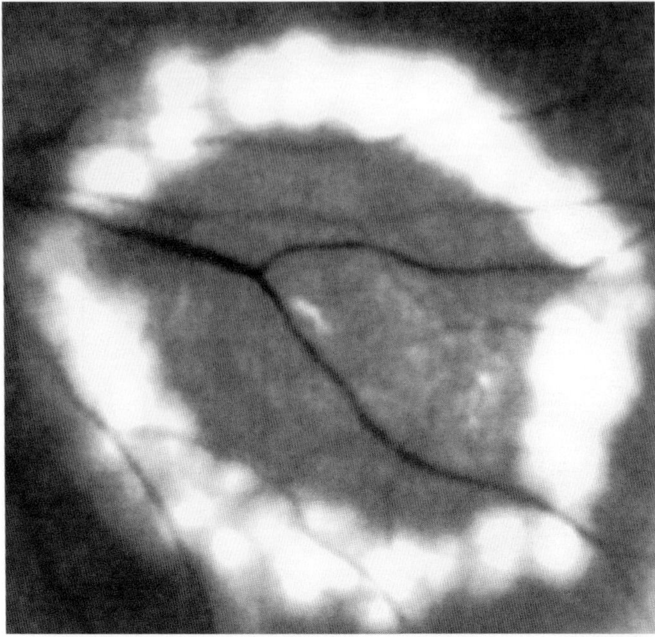

Fig. 11D

Figs 11 A to D: Photocoagulation with argon and krypton laser in choroidal melanoma

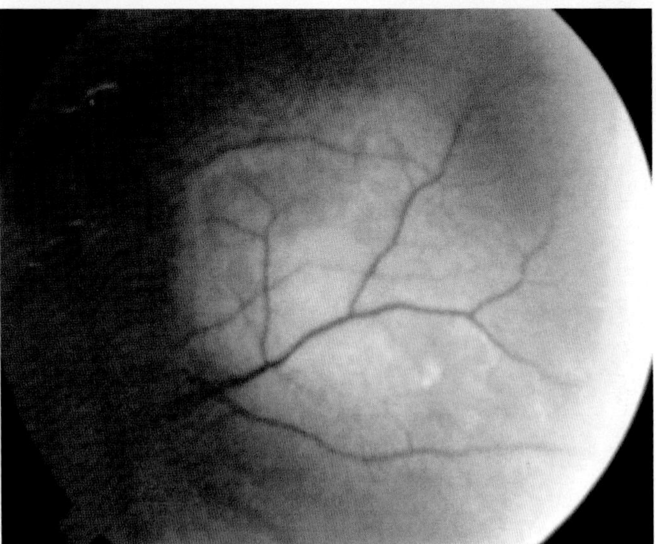

Fig. 12A

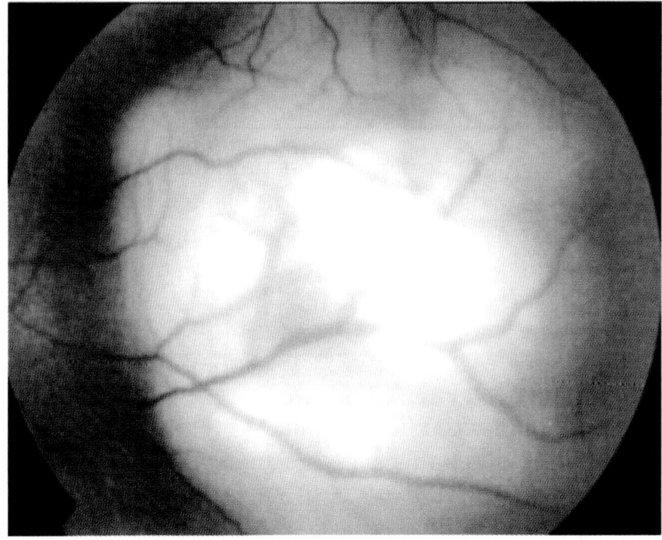

Fig. 12B

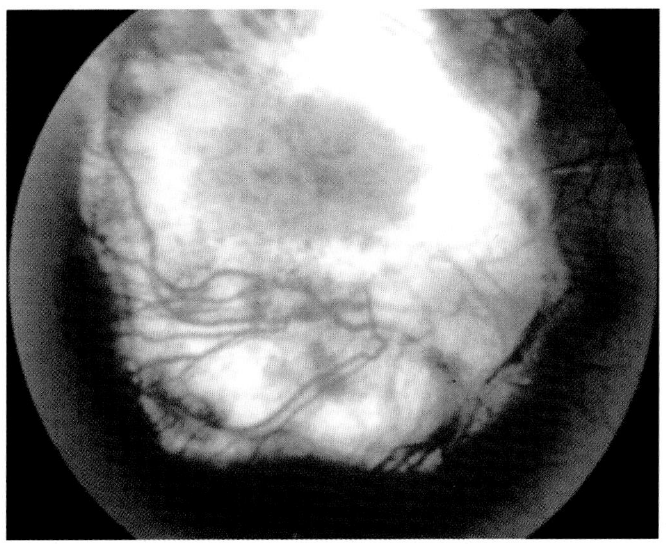

Fig. 12C

Figs 12 A to C: Transpupillary thermotherapy in choroidal melonoma

SOLITARY CHOROIDAL HEMANGIOMA

INTRODUCTION

- Choroidal hemangiomas are benign and may be circumscribed or diffused.
- Circumscribed choroidal hemangiomas are usually unifocal and unilateral while diffuse hemangiomas are commonly associated with sturge weber syndrome and may be bilateral.

CLINICAL SIGNS AND SYMPTOMS

- Choroidal hemangiomas typically appears as a dome shaped or placoid red orange lesion most commonly situated at the posterior pole.
- Frequent secondary changes include non-rhegmatogenous retinal detachment, cystoid degeneration and pigment epithelium mottling of the overlying retina.
- A useful clinical sign is blanching of the lesion with pressure on the globe.
- Choroidal hemangiomas can cause decrease in vision and photoreceptor loss.

INVESTIGATIONS

- Ultrasonography.
- A scan shows a high initial spike with high internal reflectivity. B scan shows an oval or placoid lesion with a sharp. Anterior border and acoustic solidity.
- Fluorescein angiography usually shows up the large choroidal vessels during the prearterial or arterial phase with late staining of the tumor and cystoid spaces in the retina.

DIFFERENTIAL DIAGNOSIS

- Amelanotic choroidal melanoma
- Metastatic tumor

TREATMENT

- Laser photocoagulation has been advocated in the management of choroidal hemangioma associated with exudative retinal detachment.
- Both Argon Laser and Dye Yellow Laser can be used in the treatment.
- If there is no secondary retinal detachment than there is no indication for treatment.
- Low dose external beam radiotherapy has also been used in the management of refractory tumors.

PROGNOSIS

Prognosis in choroidal hemangioma without exudative retinal detachment is good. However, prognosis in hemangiomas with ERD is gaurded.

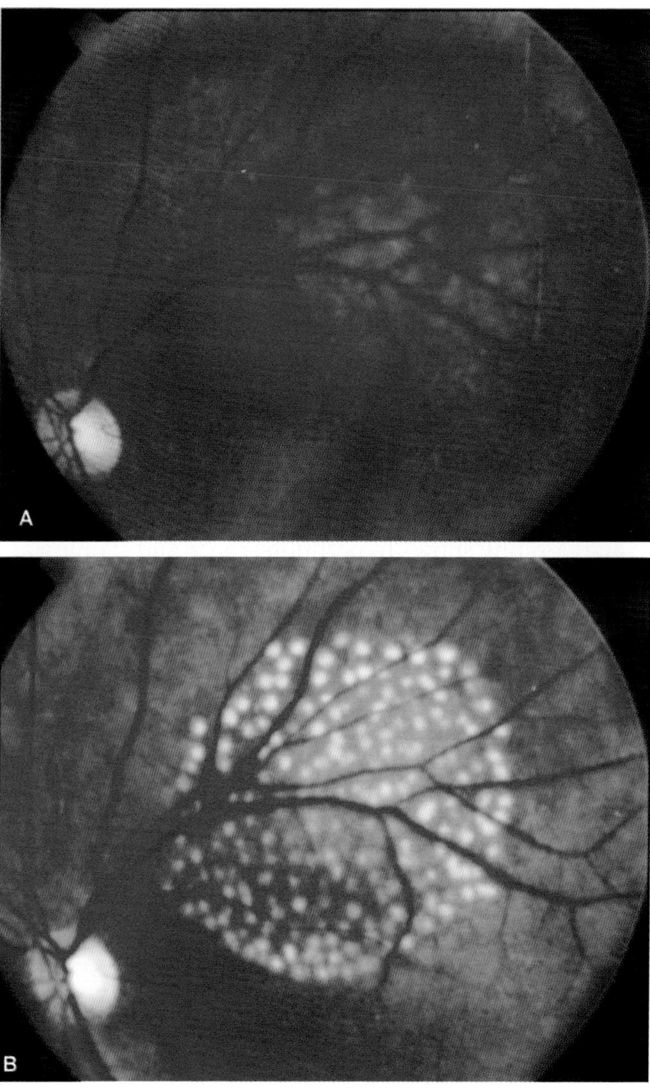

Figs 13A and B: Choroidal hemangioma

Choroidal Metastasis

Hsi Kung Kuo (Taiwan)

INTRODUCTION

Metastatic tumors to the choroids are more common than primary ocular malignancies. The most frequent primary sites are lung and breast. Other less common primary sites include the gastrointestinal tract, kidney and prostrate. Prognosis depends on the nature of primary malignancy.

CLINICAL SIGNS AND SYMPTOMS

In most situations, there are creamy-white, placoid subretinal lesions at posterior pole. The lesions might be multifocal and bilateral. Sometimes, a large subretinal mass located at periphery. Exudative RD is very popular and is an important sign to differentiate from benign tumors.

INVESTIGATIONS

Fluorescein angiography shows hyperfluorescence and staining at the lesion. It also helps to find subtle lesions at clinical fundus examination. B scan shows moderately high internal acoustic reflectivity. Systemic survey and detailed history are mandatory.

DIFFERENTIAL DIAGNOSIS

Choroidal melanoma and other benign choroidal tumors need to differentiate. Orbital CT and MRI help to rule out osteoma and melanoma.

TREATMENT

Systemic chemotherapy for the primary tumor is the most important therapy. Radiotherapy and transpupillary thermotherapy are adjuvants to decrease the extent of RD and save the vision for the patient.

INFERENCE

Treatment and prognosis depend on the nature of primary malignancy and the extent of systemic metastasis.

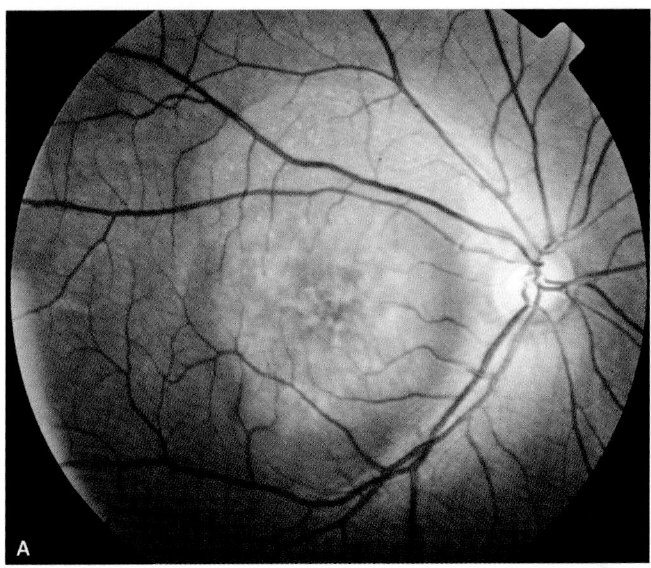

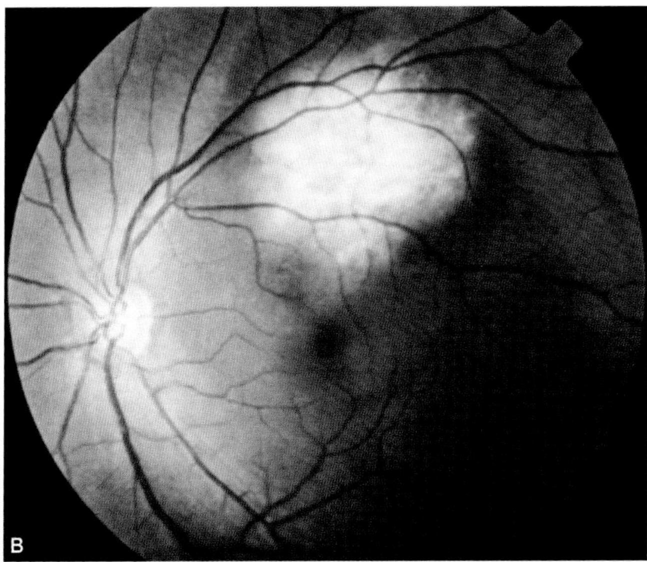

Figs 1A and B : Lung CA with choroidal metastasis (OU)

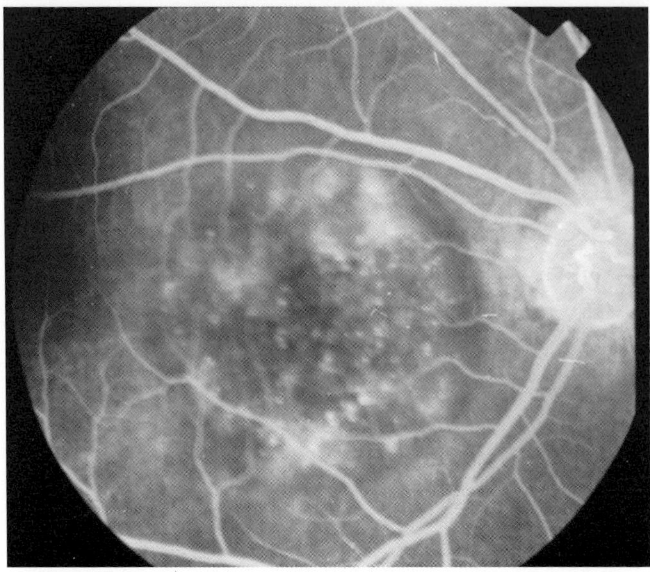

Fig. 2 : Fluorescein angiography shows hyperfluorescent spots and dye staining at the lesion

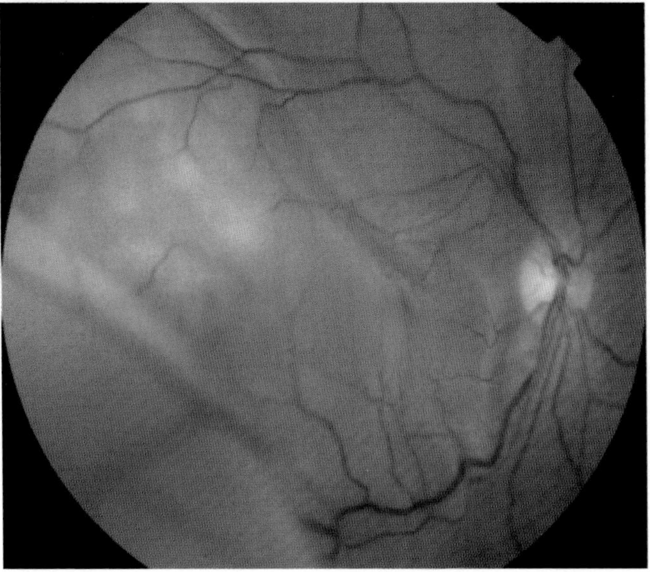

Fig. 3 : Breast CA with choroidal metastasis with extensive RD (OD)

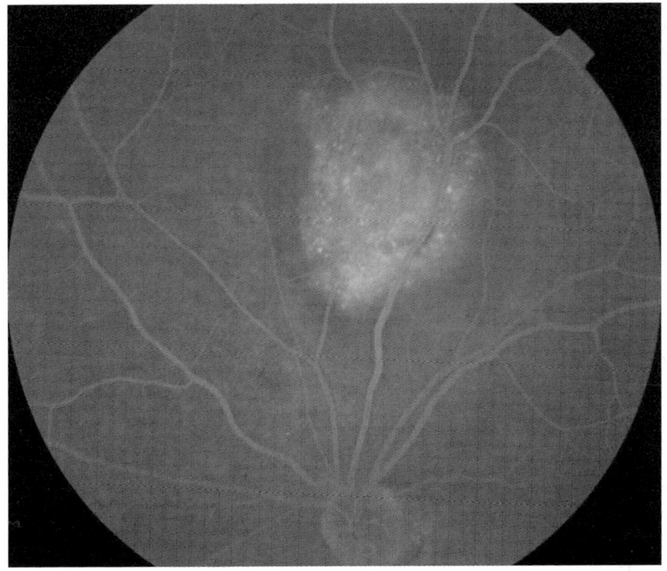

Fig. 4 : Fluorescein angiography shows hyperfluorescent spots at the lesion

Choroidal Hemangioma

Hsi Kung Kuo (Taiwan)

INTRODUCTION

Choroidal hemangioma can be diffuse or circumscribed. The diffused type seen with Sturge-Weber syndrome is discovered early. The circumscribed type is usually recognized in adults as a result of exudative retinal detachment and macular edema. Progressive tumor enlargement and vision deterioration are common for both types.

CLINICAL SIGNS AND SYMPTOMS

Circumscribed choroidal hemangioma is orange, oval. Exudative fluid accumulation will result macular edema and vision deterioration. At the later stage, exudative retinal detachment will be persistent.

INVESTIGATIONS

B scan shows a very high internal reflectivity but without choroidal excavation. Fluorescein angiography shows rapid early hyperfluorescence and dye staining.

DIFFERENTIAL DIAGNOSIS

Amelanotic melanoma, choroidal metastasis, and retinal hemangioma need to differentiate.

TREATMENT

Treatment is only necessary for the hemangioma with macular edema and exudative RD. Laser treatments include traditional photocoagulation, transpupillary thermotherapy and photodynamic therapy. Intravitreal injection of anti-VEGF drugs is another alternate or adjuvant.

INFERENCE

Treatment and prognosis depend on the nature of choroidal hemangioma. Diffused type had worse prognosis.

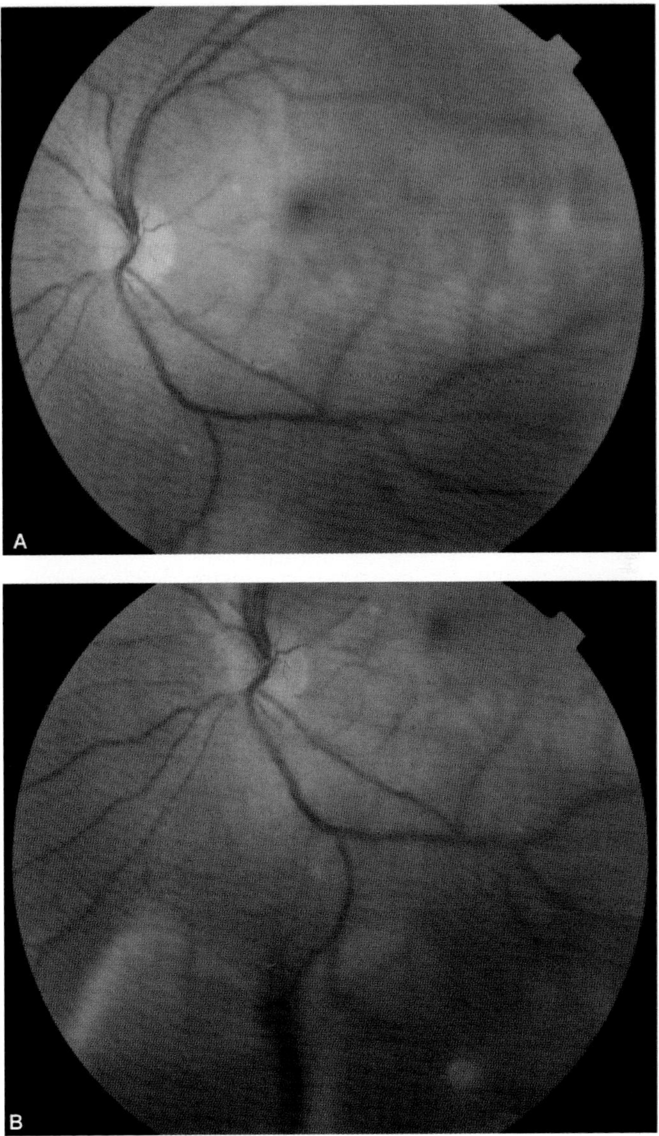

Figs 1A and B: Sturge-Weber syndrome. The diffused choroidal hemangioma at posterior pole with inferior RD

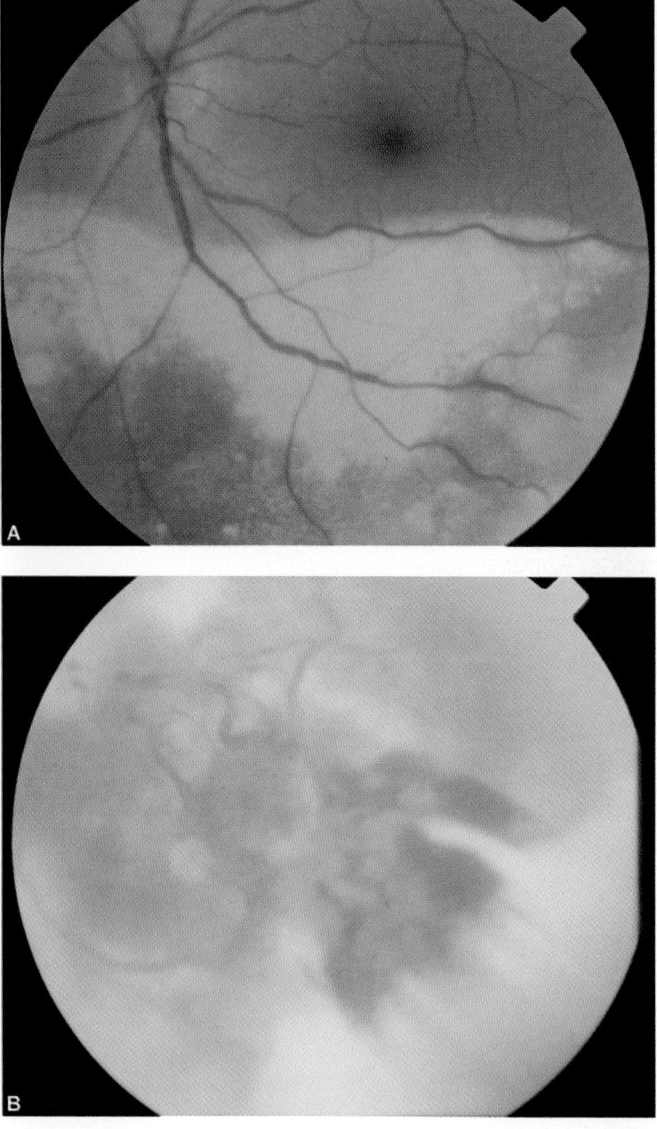

Figs 2 A and B: A large retinal hemangioma at inferior periphery with inferior RD and massive exudates at margin of RD

CHAPTER
THIRTEEN

TRAUMA

Neeraj Sanduja, Rupesh Aggarwal, Ajay Aurora (India)

- **BLUNT TRAUMA**
  - Vitreous Hemorrhage
  - Retinal Tear or Detachment
  - Commotio Retinae
  - Choroidal Rupture
  - Macular Hole
  - Avulsed Optic Nerve
  - Scleral Rupture

- **PENETRATING TRAUMA**
  - Post-traumatic Endophthalmitis
  - Retained IOFB
  - Sympathetic Ophthalmia

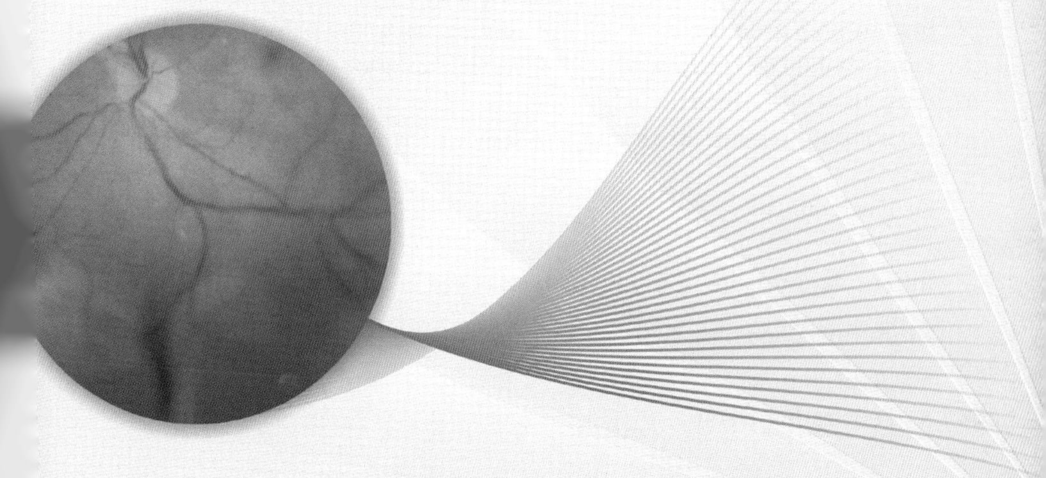

INTRODUCTION

Ocular trauma is the cause of blindness or partial loss of vision in more than half a million people worldwide.

It is regarded as the most important cause of monocular blindness in the USA. About one quarter of all serious eye injuries are related to activities in the workplace.

The goals of the initial evaluation:

Recognition of Emergent Conditions

1. Life-threatening injuries
2. Emergent ocular conditions (appropriate emergency treatment can be started)
   a. Chemical injuries
   b. Central retinal artery occlusion (CRAO)

Recognition of the Complete Extent of Ocular Involvement

EVALUATION OF A PATIENT WITH POSTERIOR SEGMENT OCULAR TRAUMA

History

- Age
- Occupation
- Brief history of accident—Type of injury and when
- Specific symptoms
- Prior condition of eyes

Slit-lamp Examination of Anterior Segment

Step-by-step examination from the lid margins to the palpebral, bulbar, and tarsal conjunctiva, followed by the cornea, anterior chamber, iris, lens, and vitreous is performed.

Do not put pressure on a traumatized eye

BCVA

Ocular motility

PUPIL

Intraocular pressure—Should not be checked in cases with open globe injury.

Posterior Segment Trauma

- Blunt trauma
- Penetrating trauma.

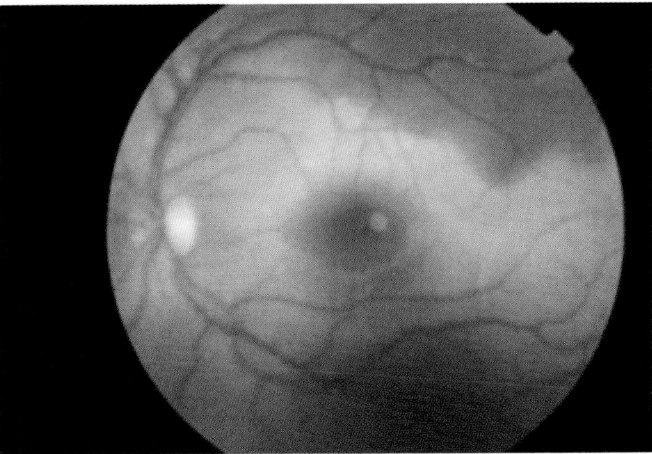

Fig. 1: Fundus photo left eye-4 hours after injury with a cricket ball Berlin's edema. Note retinal whitening at macula

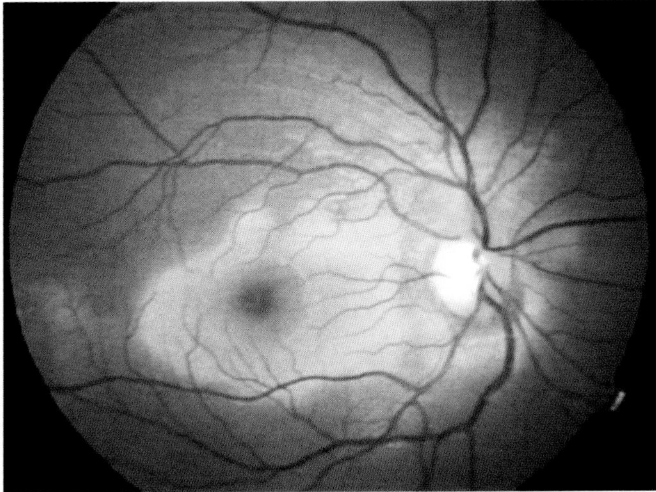

Figs 2: Berlin's edema

BLUNT TRAUMA

Manifestations

- Vitreous hemorrhage
- Retinal tear or detachment
- Commotio retinae
- Choroidal rupture
- Macular hole
- Avulsed optic nerve
- Scleral rupture.

VITREOUS HEMORRHAGE

- Source:
  - Damaged blood vessel of ciliary body, retina or choroids
  - Retinal dialysis or giant retinal tear
  - Scleral rupture
- Management:
  - Bedrest with elevation of head
  - Frequent F/U, repeat U/S to rule out retinal detachment
  - Observe for 2 weeks to clear
  - By 2 weeks posterior vitreous detachment takes place and also choroid is not congested ,thereby vitreoretinal surgery becomes easy
  - If no clearing by 2 weeks, vitrectomy to clear vitreous hemorrhage and treating any retinal dialysis or GRT if present.

COMMOTIO RETINAE

- Damage to outer retinal layers caused by shock waves that traverse eye from site of impact
- Retinal whitening is seen few hours after injury at periphery or over posterior pole
- Berlin's edema:
  — Retinal whitening at posterior pole
  — Cherry red spot may be seen
- Mechanisms for retinal whitening:
  — Photoreceptor damage
  — Extracellular edema
  — Glial swelling
- Condition usually clears in 3-4 weeks
- Prognosis —Variable
  May achieve BCVA 20/20 after resolution of macular edema
  May be left with visual disability with permanent macular scarring
- Treatment- Short course of oral steroids indicated for faster recovery.

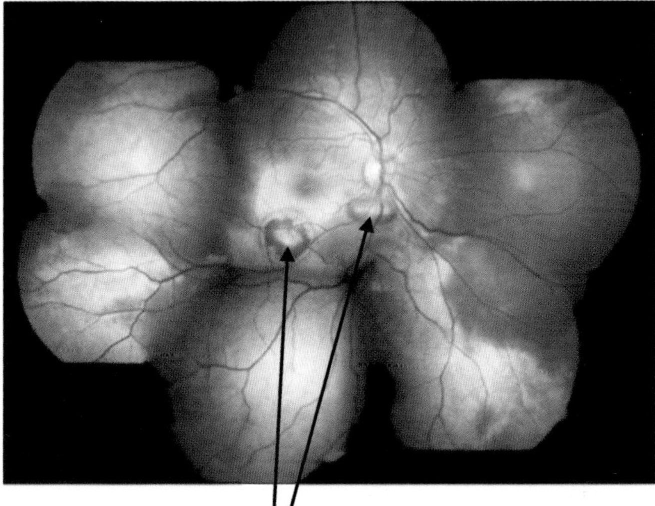

Fig. 3: Berlin's edema with mounds of subretinal hemorrhage

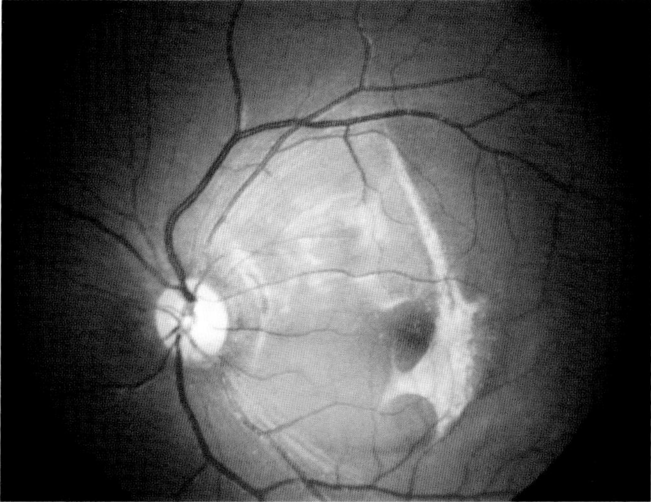

Fig. 4: Resolved Berlin's edema with subretinal scar

CHOROIDAL RUPTURE

- Mechanism:
  - Compression along A/P axis and stretching in horizontal axis
  - Sclera is strong enough and retina is distensible enough to resist rupture
  - Tears occur in Bruch's membrane, RPE and choriocapillaris which are less elastic
  - Trauma may also cause direct necrosis of choroids leading to choroidal rupture
  - Clinical picture
  - Crescent shaped
  - Concentric to optic disc
  - Usually single. May be multiple (25%)
  - Temporal to optic disc in 80% cases
  - There may be associated subretinal, intraretinal or choroidal hemorrhage
  - CNVM may develop at site of choroidal rupture
- Visual acuity:
  - Depends on site of involvement
  - Permanent visual impairment if fovea is involved
  - Treatment—No treatment unless CNVM develops

POST-TRAUMATIC MACULAR HOLE

- Mechanism:
  - Contusion necrosis
  - Vitreous traction
  - Mostly preceded by commotio retinae
- Treatment:
  - Observe for 2-3 months before offering surgery as hole may close spontaneously
  - Macular hole surgery (vitrectomy with ILM peeling and C3F8 gas inj).

OPTIC NERVE AVULSION

- Mechanism:
  - Extreme forward displacement/rotation of globe
  - Forceful backward dislocation of optic nerve from scleral canal
  - Backward pull on optic nerve by penetrating orbital injury
  - Sudden IOP increase causing rupture of lamina cribrosa

Clinical Features

- Total loss of vision
- RAPD

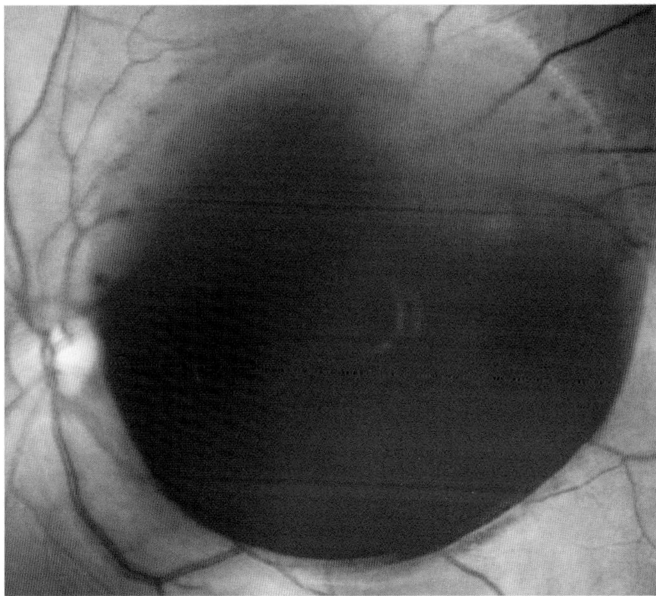

Fig. 5: Blunt injury—Massive preretinal hemorrhage

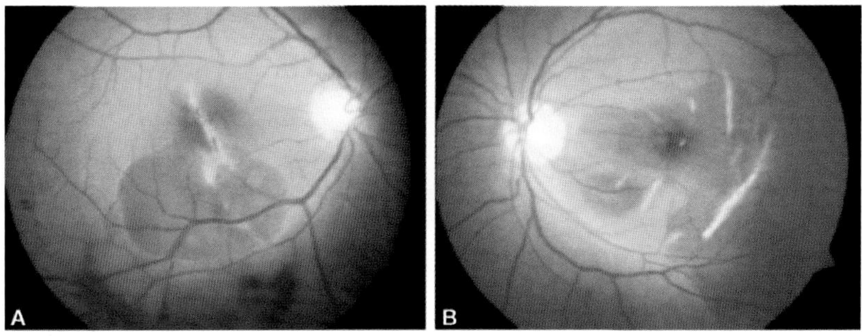

Figs 6A and B: Choroidal rupture with subretinal hemorrhage.
Note that they are typically concentric and on temporal side of optic disc

- Fundus:
  - — Vitreous hemorrhage
  - — Hemorrhage over optic disc
  - — Disc pallor–late presentation.

SCLERAL RUPTURE

- Site:
  - — Parallel to limbus
  - — Under recti insertions
- Signs:
  - — Bloody chemosis
  - — Deep AC
  - — Hyphema
  - — Vitreous hemorrhage.

Retinitis Sclopetaria

- Shock waves are generated by high speed object passing in the orbit
- When object passes close to sclera, these shock waves produce large areas of choroidal and retinal rupture and necrosis and this condition is called retinitis sclopetaria
- Clinical features- Extensive retinal and subretinal hemorrhages

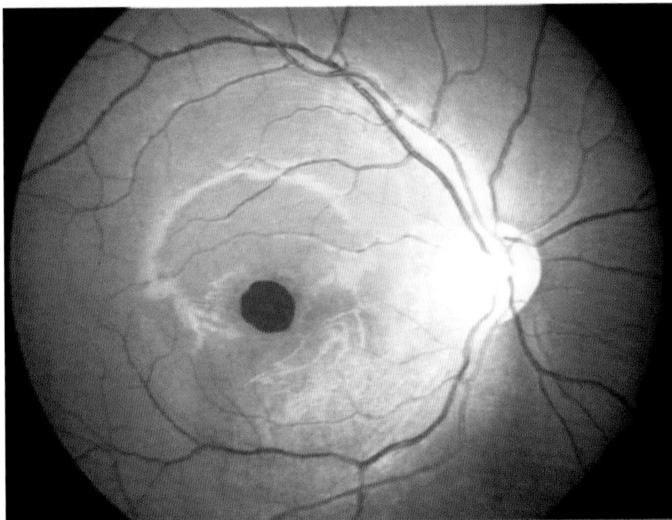

Fig. 7: Post-traumatic macular hole

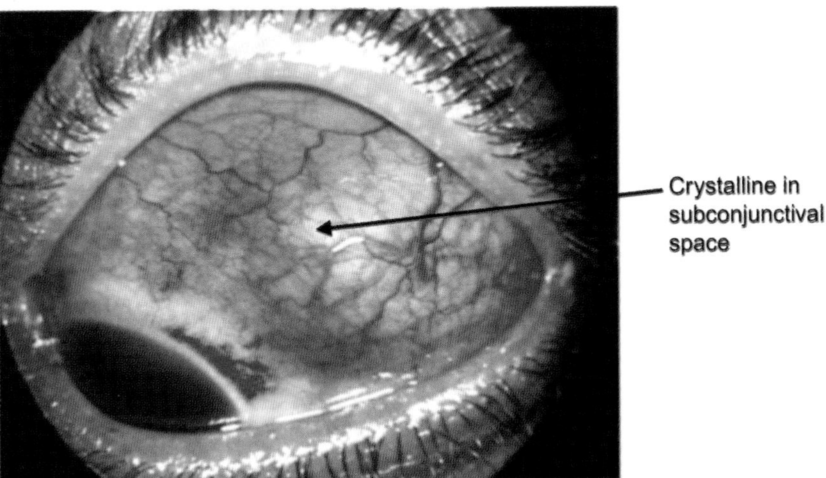

Fig. 8: Blunt trauma—phacocele with vitreous hemorrhage

PENETRATING TRAUMA

Penetrating Injury

Only entry wound.

Perforating Injury

Both entrance and exit wounds.

Manifestations

- Retained IOFB
- Vitreous hemorrhage
- Retinal detachment
- Post traumatic endophthalmitis
- Sympathetic ophthalmia

POST-TRAUMATIC ENDOPHTHALMITIS

- 2-7% of penetrating injury
- 7-31% of injury with IOFB
- Higher risk in rural setting
- The mean interval from injury to the onset of endophthalmitis
  - — *Bacillus cereus* and streptococci—1-2 days
  - — *S. epidermidis* and gram-negative organisms—3-4 days
  - — Fungi—1-2 months
- Risk factors
  - — Delayed presentation > 72 hours
  - — IOFB removal delayed > 1 week
  - — Iris prolapse
  - — Lens disruption
  - — Vitreous in wound
  - — Hyphema
  - — Soil contamination
  - — Contaminated IOFB
- EVS study not applicable to post traumatic endophthalmitis because More virulent organisms involved
  - — Multiorganismal
  - — Young age of patient
  - — Open wound
  - — Delay in diagnosis—Associated trauma may mask/confuse
- Evaluation

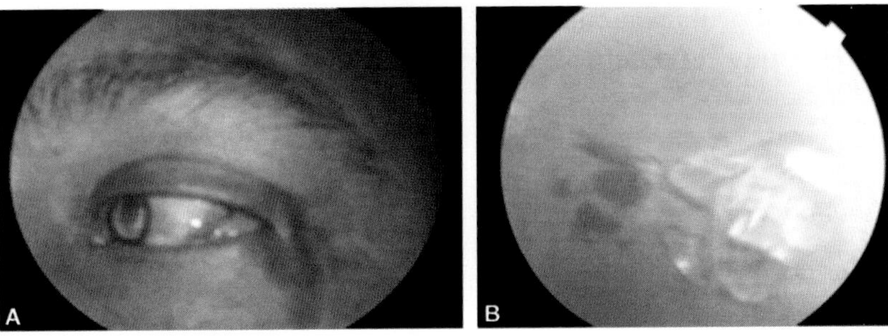

Figs 9A and B: Left eye photograph—External site of IOFBs entry temporally multiple glass foreign bodies in vitreous cavity with retinal hemorrhages

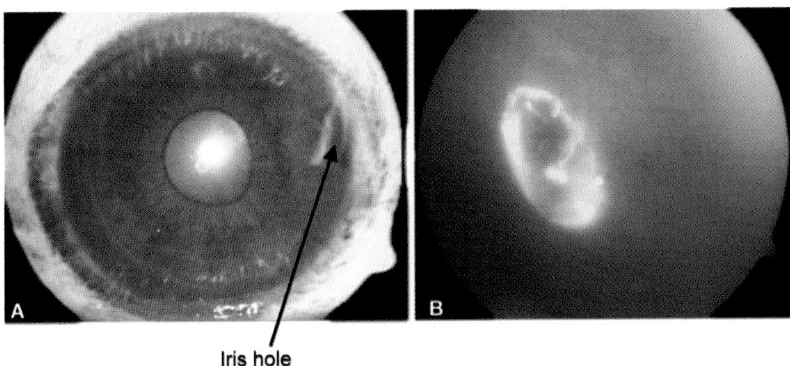

Figs 10A and B: Iris hole created by the foreign body lying over the retina

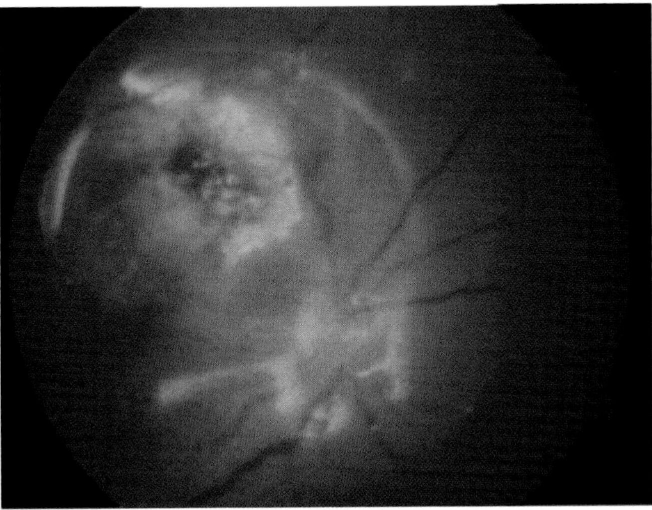

Fig. 11: Fundus photo right eye—Impacted metallic IOFB along superotemporal arcade

History of ocular trauma:
- — Hammering steel , working with baling wire, or working in an industrial setting
- — Penetrating injury with a plant substance or soil-contaminated foreign body
- — X-ray orbit—To R/O IOFB

- US B scan—if fundus not well visualized, to look for
  - — Retained intraocular foreign body
  - — Density of the vitritis
  - — Retina is attached or not
- CT/MRI
  - — In cases of suspicion of retained IOFB not picked on US B scan and X-ray
- Intravitreal antibiotics alone
  - — Have a limited efficacy in post-traumatic endophthalmitis and such cases need early vitrectomy followed by intravitreal injection of antibiotics.
- Vitrectomy
  More complete vitrectomy
  6 mm infusion cannula
  PVD induction
  IOFB removal
  Treatment of retinal breaks
  Tamponade—SO preferred
- Management
  - — Treat ruptured globe (if present).
  - — Tetanus immunization
  - — Intravenous systemic antibiotics including vancomycin or ciprofloxacin and an aminoglycoside or a third-generation cephalosporin. Consider clindamycin for *Bacillus* species.
- Topical antibiotics:
  - — Fortified vancomycin/moxifloxacin
  - — Fortified amikacin
- Topical cycloplegics
- Oral steroids
- Early pars plana vitrectomy with intravitreal antibiotics.

Prognosis

In post-traumatic endophthalmitis is strongly influenced by the nature of the injury and the extent of initial damage.

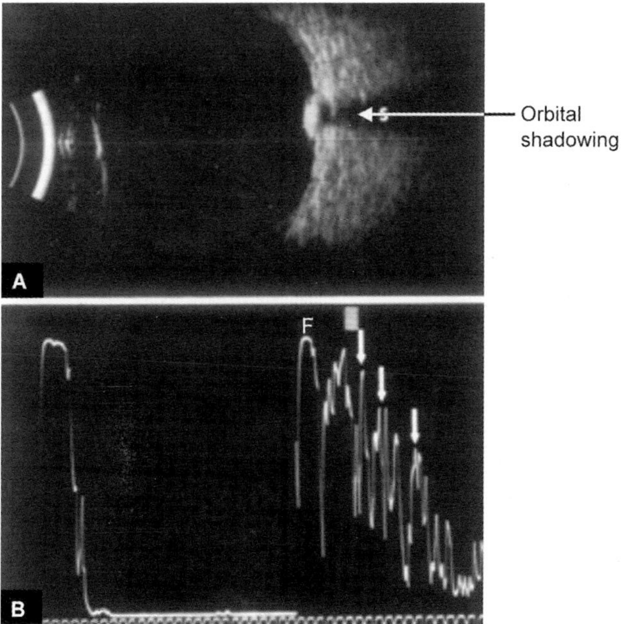

Figs 12A and B: US B scan—Metallic IOFB over retina. Note: High reflective surface with orbital shadowing

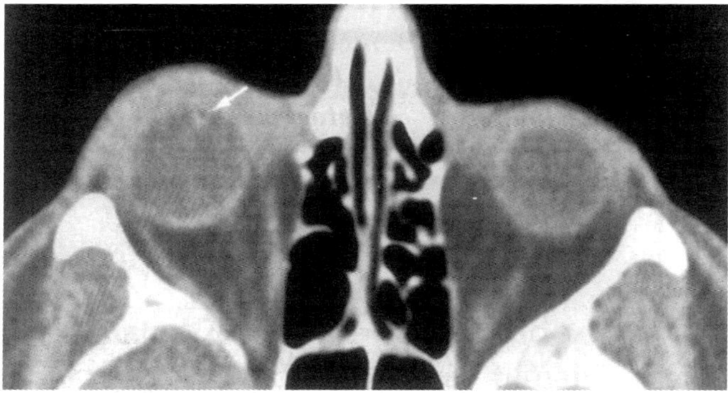

Fig. 13: CT scan showing a small IOFB lying in anterior vitreous cavity which could not be picked on US B scan

RETAINED IOFB

Primary Goal in Mx

To prevent/treat associated
- Endophthalmitis
- RD
- Late metallosis.

Evaluation

- Is there a foreign body?
- Is the foreign body intraocular or intraorbital?
- Are there multiple IOFBs?
- Exactly where inside the eye is the IOFB situated?
- Whether associated conditions are present (e.g. endophthalmitis, vitreous hemorrhage, retinal detachment)?

History

SLE –Severe inflammation in AC (Fibrin, hypopyon)

Indirect Ophthalmoscopy

- Retinal phlebitis
- Vitreous exudation.

USG—B-scan

- Best indirect method to find associated damage
- Do not attempt if open globe
- False positive—Gas bubble
  False negative—Small, wooden, vegetable matter.

Plain X-ray

- Can miss vegetative IOFB
- Not helpful in localization.

CT Scan—Gold Standard

- Indications
  - Doubtful IOFB not picked on U/S and X-ray
  - Exact localization of IOFB
  - Can miss plastic or even metallic IOFB if wide cuts (3 mm) are used or eye moves during procedure (spiral CT is better).

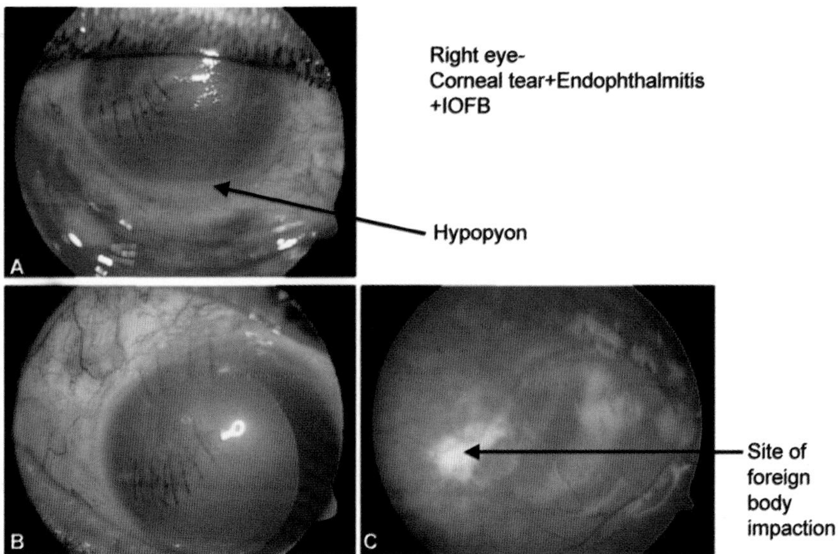

Figs 14A to C: Vit + B B + EL + IOFB removal + SOI done postoperative—2 months—Retina on, BCVA 6/36

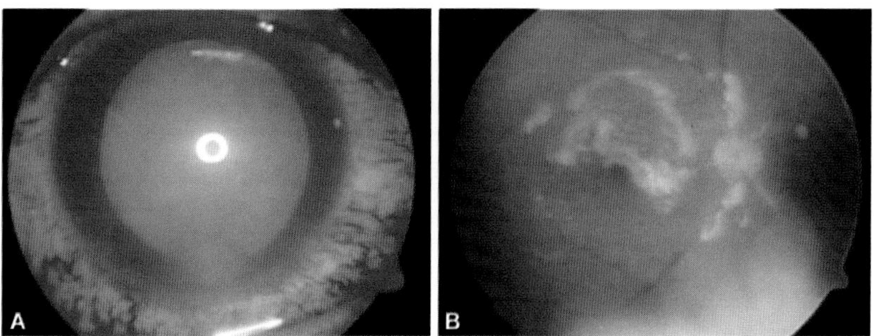

Figs 15A and B: Post-traumatic endophthalmitis. (A) Preoperative photograph showing AC exudation, self sealed small inferior corneal tear with early catarctous lens, (B) Patient underwent vitrectomy, buckle, IOFB removal, silicon oil injection and intravitreal inj. of antibiotics postoperative photograph showing sclerosed vessels emerging from optic disc with mild disc pallor

MRI—Rarely required

- C/I in metallic IOFB.

Management

Timing to perform surgery as soon as corneal clarity permits:
- Less chances of endophthalmitis
- Less incidence of PVR
- Less chances of multiple retinal lesions
- Careful watch for infection if surgery delayed for few days.

Steps of Surgery

- Clean and close still open original wound
- Prepare three pars plana incisions for vitrectomy
- Complete vitrectomy
- Free IOFB from remaining vitreous strands and/or capsule
- Extend the sclerotomy or make corneoscleral groove.
- Take contact with IOFB using IOM and forceps
- Remove foreign body using intraocular forceps (shake hand technique).

Risk of traumatic endophthalmitis with IOFB can be reduced if:
- Primary wound repair within 24 hours
- Topical and IV antibiotics to be started within 24 hours
- Open globe injury with high risk of developing endophthalmitis - Intravitreal antibiotics injection immediately following primary repair with planning for early vitrectomy with IOFB removal.

SYMPATHETIC OPHTHALMIA

A rare, bilateral granulomatous uveitis of acute onset, associated with either a perforating eye injury in the region of the ciliary body or a retained foreign body in the eye.

Etiology

The exact cause is unknown
Related to sensitivity (i.e., a reaction) to uveal pigment.

Symptoms

The injured eye becomes inflamed first, and the other eye follows (i.e., "sympathetically").
Photophobia, redness, and blurred vision
Some cases experience floaters and pain.

The history of trauma differentiates this condition from other types of granulomatous uveitis; other differentiating factors include its bilateral, diffuse, and acute nature.

Management

Consider enucleation of unsalvagable open globe within 14 days to prevent SO.

Local corticosteroids and atropine with systemic corticosteroids should be administered immediately if sympathetic inflammation has been diagnosed.

Untreated, sympathetic ophthalmia can progress to complete bilateral blindness over a period of months or years.

Conclusion

- The initial management of a traumatized patient comprises of the steps to minimize further trauma, minimize infectious risks and minimize psychological trauma.
- Perforating injuries of the globe with retained intraocular posterior segment foreign bodies most frequently result from occupational activities. Use of safety glasses while at workplace should be made mandatory to avoid such injuries.
- Open globe injury should have primary wound repair at the earliest so as to minimize chances of developing endophthalmitis.

CHAPTER
FOURTEEN

WHITE DOT SYNDROME

Shaifali Singla, Lalit Verma, Avnindra Gupta,
Dinesh Talwar, HK Tewari (India)

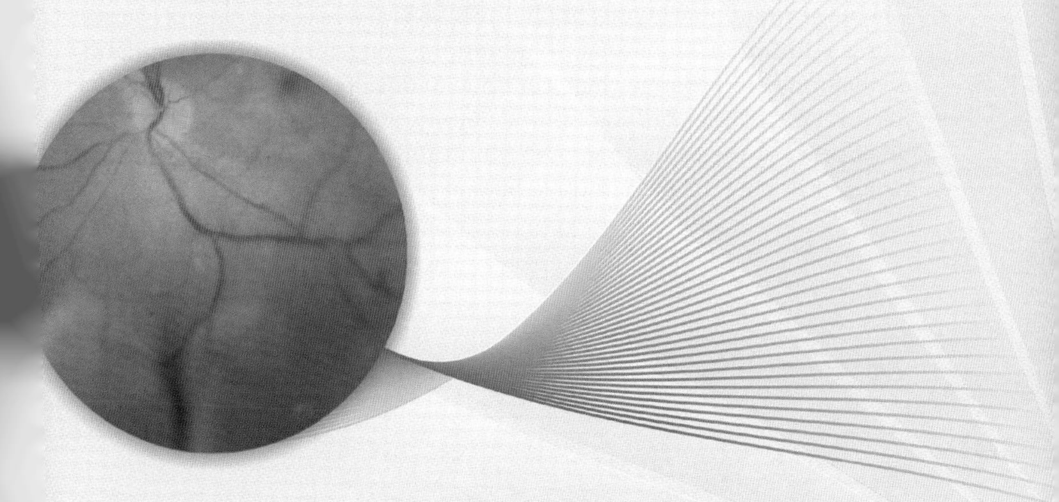

INTRODUCTION

The acquired inflammatory disorders affecting the retina, retinal pigment epithelium, and choroid of otherwise young healthy adults in the second to fifth decade have been grouped under white dot syndromes also known as inflammatory multifocal chorioretinopathies.

Symptoms

- Prodromal symptoms: Prior viral or flulike syndrome—occurs in approximately one-third of patients
- Early stage: Acute decrease in visual acuity, Blotchy scotomata, Photopsia, Metamorphopsia/micropsia, Photophobia
- Late stage: Mild visual impairment (20/25 to 20/40) is common, significant visual loss (20/200) is rare.

Signs

Patients should have a complete eye examination, including visual acuity, pupillary reactions, slit-lamp examination, and dilated indirect ophthalmoscopy.

- Early stage: Visual acuity may be normal; if the macula is involved, vision can decrease, anterior chamber reaction if present is mild, vitreous cells may be found in up to 50% of eyes that are affected.
- Retinal findings are the main feature of the disease: Multiple subretinal yellow-white lesions are seen in both eyes (Figs 1 and 2). In some cases, the lesions are unilateral with involvement of the second eye either within a short period of time or after an extended period. New lesions may occur in the affected eye as old lesions begin their resolution.
- Optic nerve involvement: Blurring of disk margins, hyperemia, edema, and superficial hemorrhages may be found.
- Late stage: Individual lesions resolve over several weeks as a natural course, along with other signs of inflammation. Long-term retinal pigment epithelium (RPE) changes may continue to develop long after recovery.
- Recurrences: These tend to occur bilaterally, although both eyes may not be affected at the same time. Long-term follow-up studies suggest that recurrences may develop in up to 50% of patients.

Case:

An 18-year-old girl presented with decreased vision in her both eyes for the last 4-5 days. Her vision was 6/60 in both eyes. On examination, anterior segment was normal and there were no retrolental cells. Fundus examination showed multiple yellowish placoid-like lesions in her both eyes at the posterior pole, more concentrated at the central macula with hyperemia of the disk.

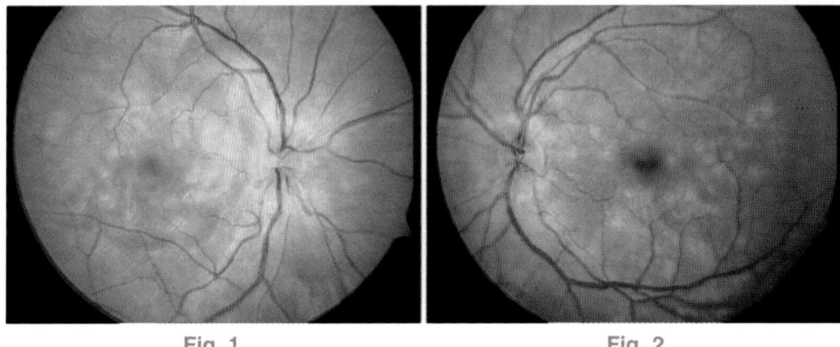

Fig. 1 Fig. 2

Figs 1 and 2: Both eyes showing multiple placoid lesions at the posterior pole

INVESTIGATIONS

- Fluorescein angiography (FFA) and Indocyanine green angiography (ICGA): Usually characteristic of the individual disease entities.
- Optical coherence tomography (OCT): In the acute phases, the OCT reveals a mild hyperreflective area above the RPE and, in the later phases, a nodular hyperreflective lesion on the plane of the RPE.
- Other tests:
  - Electroencephalography may show diffuse slowing of wave patterns.
  - Electroretinogram (ERG) findings may be minimally subnormal.
  - Electro-oculogram (EOG) findings may have substantial reduction of light-to-dark ratio studies, which show diffuse functional abnormality of the RPE.
  - Visual fields may show paracentral scotomata early; some visual defects may be permanent.
  - Dark adaptation may show delay in the acute phase, which can return to normal with time after recovery from the acute lesions.
  - The Stiles-Crawford effect shows early profound disorientation of the photoreceptors.

Medical Treatment

The treatment is somewhat controversial; however, the consensus is that no treatment seems to alter the course of the ocular lesions. The fundus lesions appear to run a relatively short self-limited course, which probably results from a one-time insult to the capillaries comprising the choroidal lobules. Corticosteroids for a short time can be given if fovea is compromised and vision is poor.

DIFFERENTIAL DIAGNOSIS

1. Acute posterior multifocal placoid pigment epitheliopathy (APMPPE)—usually bilateral, yellow white placoid discrete lesions in the fundus are characteristic, FFA shows early hypofluorescence followed by hyperfluorescence in late phase.
2. Multiple evanescent white dot syndromes (MEWDS)—usually unilateral, white dots concentrated in the macula and sparing fovea are characteristic. Disk edema is more frequent. FFA shows early and late hyperfluorescence of white dots (wreath like configuration), visual field reveals enlargement of blind spot.
3. Birdshot retinochoroidopathy—not an acute onset, older patients, more vitreous reaction and retinal vascular leakage. Multiple cream colored

She didn't have any history of fever or other illnesses before this episode. On doing fundus fluorescein angiography, there were multiple hypofluorescent spots in the early phase corresponding with the placoid lesions.

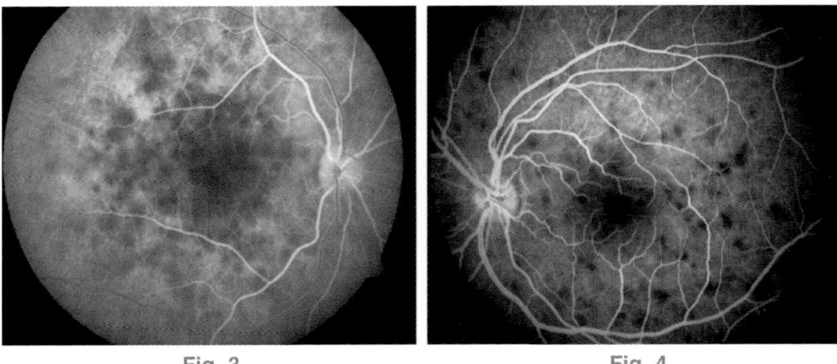

Fig. 3 Fig. 4

Figs 3 and 4: Fundus fluorescein angiography—Early phase showing hypofluorescent areas around foveal avascular zone corresponding to placoid lesions in the same patient as in Figures 1 and 2

These hypofluorescent spots became hyperfluorescent in the late phase. Leakage at the disk was also present.

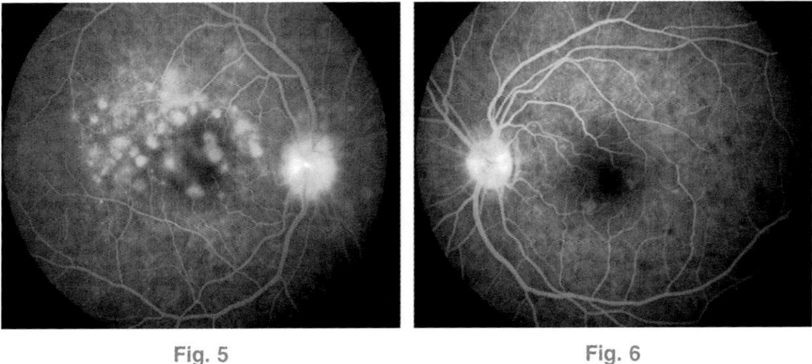

Fig. 5 Fig. 6

Figs 5 and 6: Late phase of the angiogram showing hyperfluorescent areas with leakage at the disk more so in the right eye as compared to the left eye

lesions less than one disk diameter scattered throughout the fundus with associated cystoid macular edema. HLA-A29 is positive in 90% of the patients.

4. Serpiginous choroiditis—chronic, episodic, progressive disease, bilateral. Serpentine lesions begin at the posterior pole and spread in a centrifugal fashion towards periphery. FFA shows early hypofluorescence and mid to late hyperfluorescence with variable staining in the center of the lesion. Foveal destruction eventually occurs, and central vision is lost in 20% or more of the eyes.
5. Multifocal choroiditis and panuveitis—usually bilateral at presentation, vitreous cells are present, extensive subretinal proliferation of retinal pigment epithelium with fibrosis or clumping is seen. Fibrosis in the form of napkin holder may surround the disk. FFA reveals early blockage by acute, active, yellow lesions in the choroids, with late staining of the lesions.
6. Progressive subretinal fibrosis and uveitis—extremely rare condition, chronic vitreous inflammation is present. White, fibrotic subretinal lesions, which enlarge and coalesce to involve most of the retina and choroid are characteristic.
7. Punctate inner choroidopathy—effects myopic women, small yellow-white lesions at the posterior pole with overlying serous retinal detachment. FFA shows early hyperfluorescence with staining in the late phase.
8. Acute retinal pigment epithelitis—discrete cluster of small dark spots surrounded by a halo of depigmentation at the level of retinal pigment epithelium in the macula. FFA shows hypofluorescent areas surrounded by hyperfluorescence. ERG and cortical evoked responses are normal.
9. Acute macular neuroretinopathy—majority of the patients have bilateral involvement, rarely reoccurs. Several small wedge shaped lesions surround the fovea and has inner retinal infarction in the central macula.
10. Sarcoidosis—occasionally present as deep small white lesions.
11. Diffuse unilateral subacute neuroretinitis—young adult, white dots on fundus examination, progressive loss of vision and visual field.

PROGNOSIS

Over all prognosis is good. Patient regains normal vision after the first episode but recurrent attacks and subsequent involvement of the fovea may lead to decreased visual acuity in some.

As she had sudden onset of vision loss and characteristic fluorescein angiography we made a diagnosis of white dot syndrome. As the lesions were just near to the fovea and there were severe vision loss we started her on short course of oral corticosteroids starting with 40 mg per day and then tapering off over 3 weeks. On follow-up over 4-6 weeks her vision improved to 6/6 in both eyes and fundus lesions regressed with no residual effect.

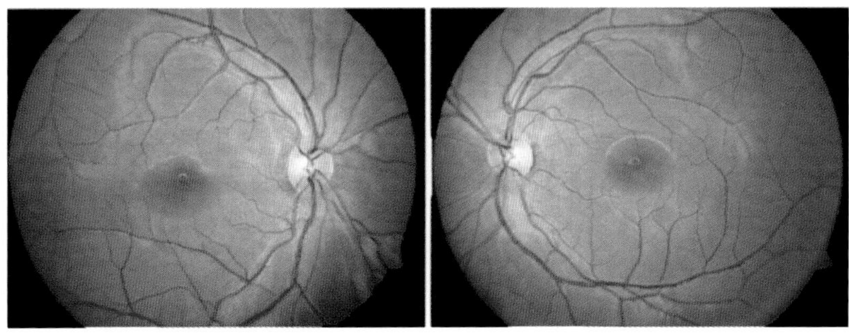

Fig. 7 Fig. 8

Figs 7 and 8: Same patient at 6 weeks follow-up showed regression of the lesions and fundus becomes normal

CHAPTER FIFTEEN

MISCELLANEOUS

- **MYELINATED NERVE FIBERS**
  Emanuel Rosen (UK)
- **OPTIC DISK DRUSEN**
  Emanuel Rosen (UK)
- **OPTIC NEURITIS**
  Emanuel Rosen (UK)

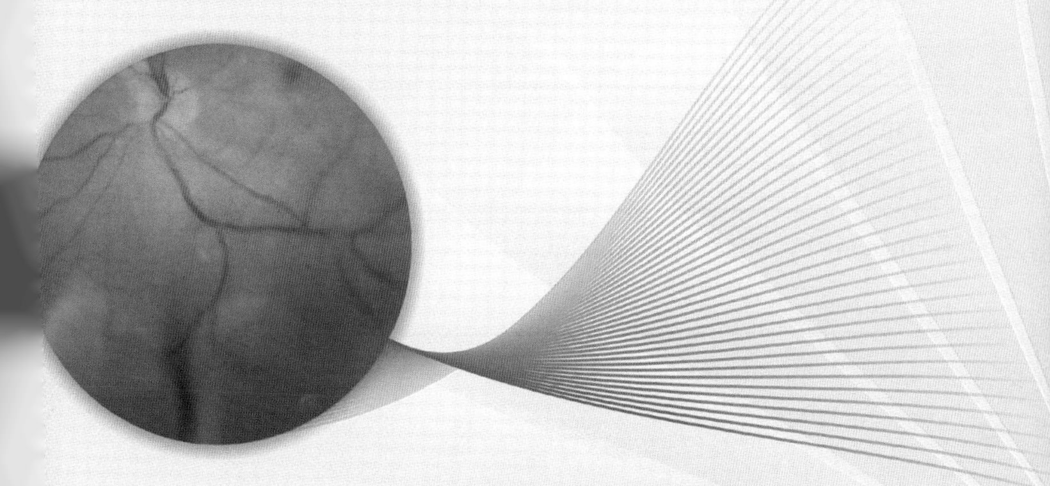

Myelinated Nerve Fibers

Emanuel Rosen (UK)

INTRODUCTION

Anatomical variant which can be confused with retinal exudation and papilledema by the uninitiated.

CLINICAL SIGNS AND SYMPTOMS

- Appear at birth or in early infancy
- Do not change subsequently
- No effect on visual acuity unless rare macular fibers involved
- White patches with feathered edges
- Obscure underlying blood vessels
- 33% occur in region of optic nerve head

COMPLICATIONS

- Rare macular fibers affect visual acuity.

PATHOGENESIS

- Lipid drops coalesce around axons to form myelinated medullary nerve sheath
- Myelination of optic nerve fibers commence at chiasm about 7 months gestation
- Myelination progresses towards eye but stops at lamina cribrosa and completes at 1 month after birth.

ASSOCIATIONS

- None

INVESTIGATIONS

- Imaging by retinal photography.

DIAGNOSIS

- Clinical appearance.

DIFFERENTIAL DIAGNOSIS

Papilledema in mild peripapillary myelinated fibers
Commotio retinae in peripheral myelinated fibers

EPIDEMIOLOGY

- Affects 0.5% population
- Males > females
- Inheritance as autosomal recessive or dominant trait

TREATMENT AND PROGNOSIS

- None

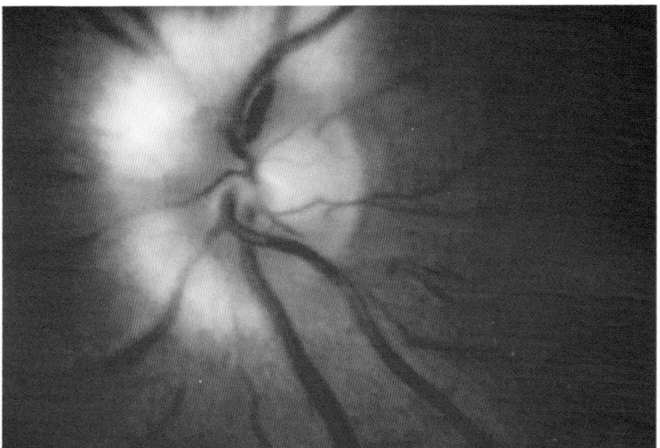

Fig. 1: Myelinated nerve fibers at optic nerve head

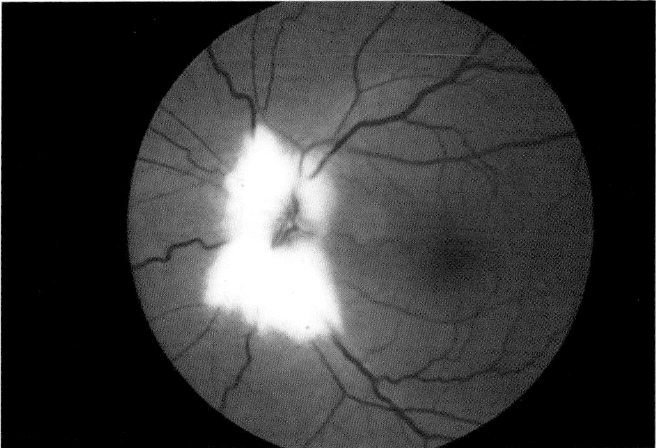

Fig. 2: Myelinated nerve fibers surround optic nerve head demonstrating radiating nerve fibers with myelin sheath

Optic Disk Drusen

Emanuel Rosen (UK)

INTRODUCTION

Benign space occupying lesions in the optic nerve head which may mimic other causes of disk swelling (see DD) can cause progressive visual field loss.

CLINICAL SIGNS AND SYMPTOMS

- Usually seen on routine evaluation
- Can be associated with sudden loss of vision and visual field defects
- Invisible or buried drusen associated with elevation of the disk
- Irregular ocular disk margin
- No central cup
- Occasional lumpy appearance of disk

COMPLICATIONS

- May be associated with or complicated by choroidal neovascularization

PATHOGENESIS

- Drusen composed of mucoprotein matrix consisting of acid mucopolysaccharides and RNA

Differential Diagnosis

- Chronic papilledema can be misdiagnosed
- Causes of disk elevation
- Intracranial origin
- Static appearance over many years

INVESTIGATIONS

- Visual field testing
- Imaging

Diagnosis

- Clinical diagnosis on ophthalmoscopy
- Imaging
  - Fundus fluorescein angiography shows autofluorescence of drusen

- Ultrasound examination drusen appears as highly reflective lesions in the optic nerve on orbital ultrasound
- CT scan drusen appears as small white spots in the distal optic nerve with the same density as bone

Differential Diagnosis

- Bilateral disk drusen could give bitemporal field defect and simulate chiasmal compressive lesion

TREATMENT AND PROGNOSIS

- No therapy available
- Monitoring of the condition to afford patients a prognosis and illustrations
- Defects may appear on visual field testing which may be slowly progressive

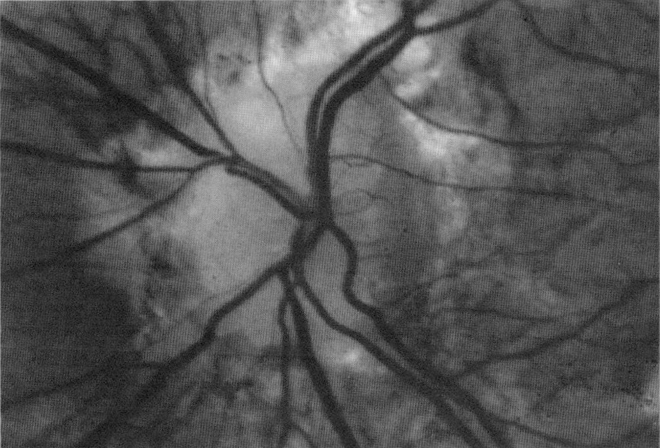

Fig. 1: Optic disk drusen with peripapillary RPE atrophy

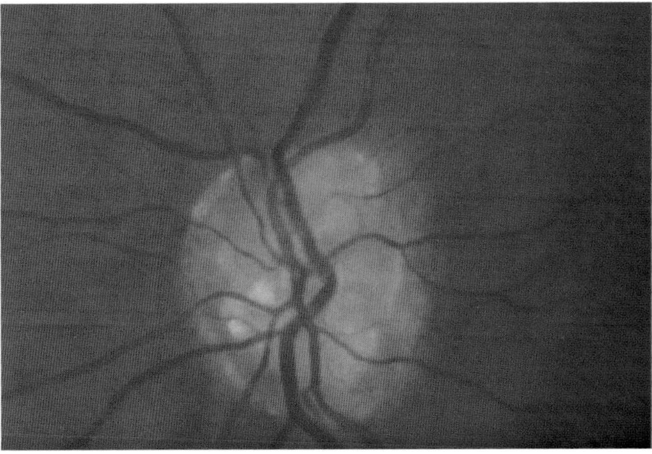

Fig. 2: Optic disk drusen these lesions will autofluorescence

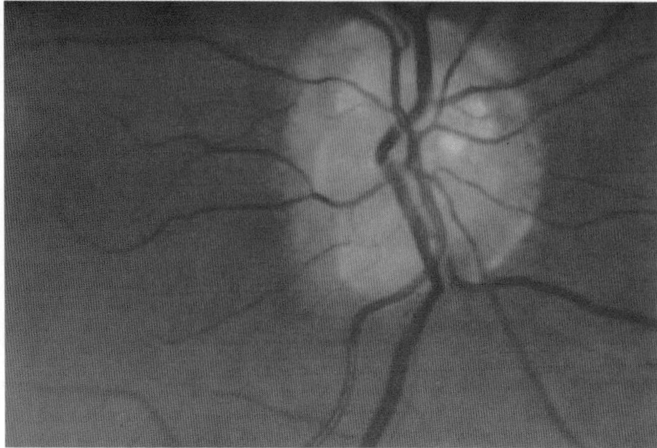

Fig. 3: Optic disk drusen may lead to nerve bundle field defects

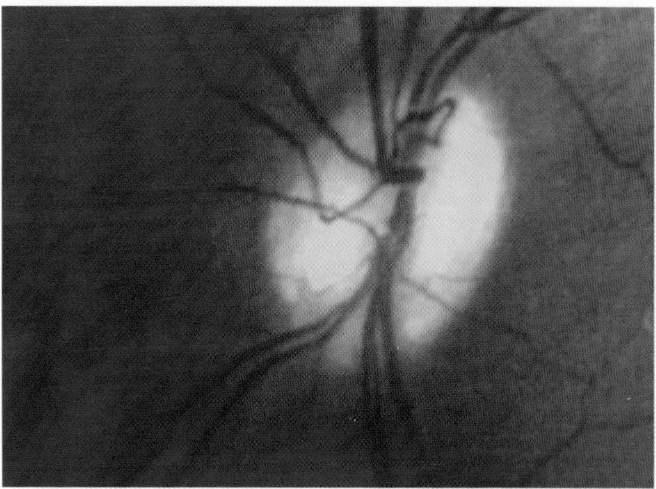

Fig. 4A: Optic disk drusen may lead to nerve bundle field defects

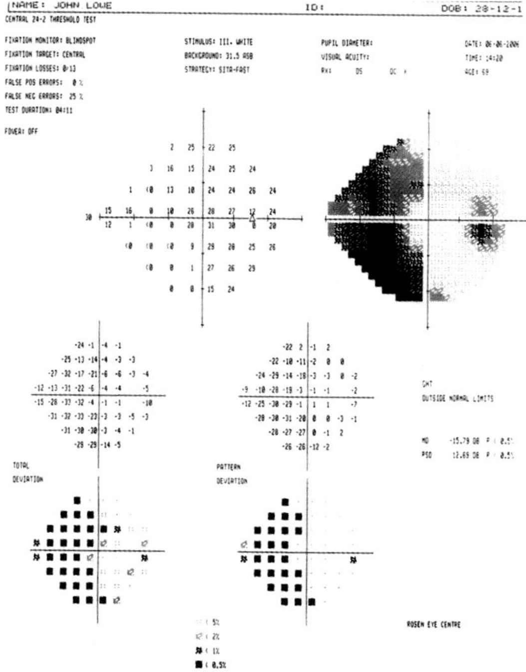

Fig. 4B: Optic disk drusen visual fields showing hemianopic unilateral nerve bundle field defect

Optic Neuritis

Emanuel Rosen (UK)

INTRODUCTION

Optic neuritis occurs in typical and atypical forms. The former is a consequence of demyelinating disease and may show a prompt response to high dose steroid therapy but with little or no effect on eventual visual outcome. Atypical forms are due to a variety of inflammatory diseases and may show a lasting and beneficial effect of high dose short term steroid therapy.

CLINICAL FEATURES

- Clinical appearance typically starts with pain on eye movement 3-5 days followed by vision loss
- Vision loss can progress over 5-10 days
- Within 1-2 months vision improves
- Color vision is affected out of proportion to acuity
- Typical defect is a central scotoma although other defects are seen with altitudinal loss occurring in 10% of cases
- Unilateral onset in vast majority of cases second eye can be involved at a later date
- Both eyes are very rarely affected simultaneously
- A relative afferent pupillary defect is seen in involved eye unless there has been a previous episode of optic neuritis in the fellow eye
- Disk edema occurs one-third of the time, normal disk two-thirds of the time (retrobulbar optic neuritis)
- Posterior vitreous cells or peripheral periphlebitis occasional observation

May occur as 3 variants

- As an isolated demyelinating process and frequently the first episode of multiple sclerosis
- A subsequent attack in a patient with multiple sclerosis
- Part of a systemic, inflammatory or infectious process

HISTORY

- Previous demyelinating episodes such as double vision, hemiparesis, sensory deficit, bowel or bladder difficulties or vertigo

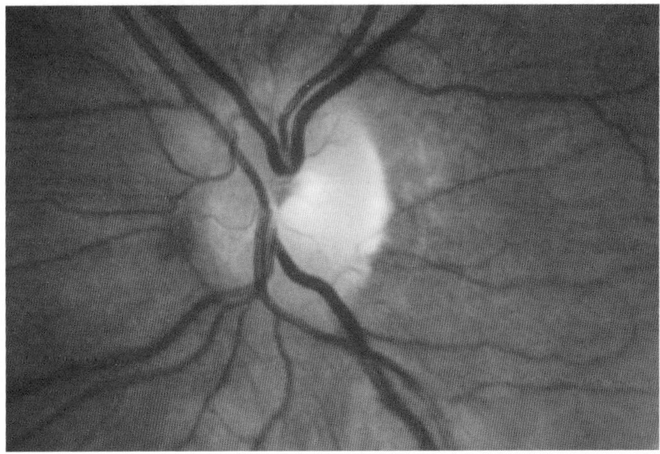

Fig. 1A: Retrobulbar neuritis showing slight blur upper nasal disk margin – see FFA

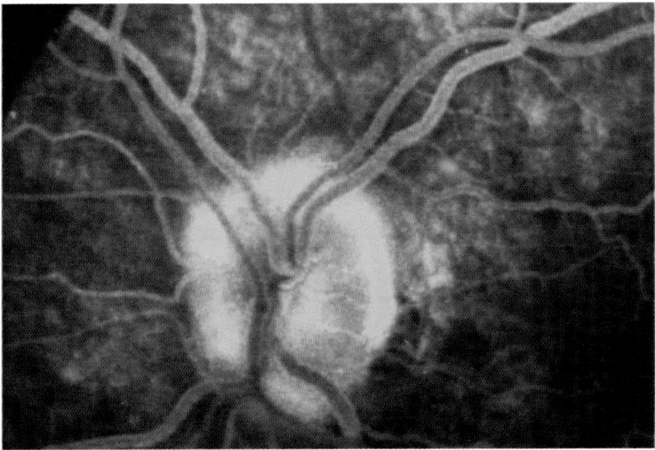

Fig. 1B: FFA retrobulbar neuritis diffuse leakage of dye around disk margin confirming retrobulbar inflammation

PROGNOSIS

- 90% of patients recover 6/12 or better vision by one year
- 36% of patients develop multiple sclerosis within 5 years

PATHOGENESIS

- An autoimmune disorder
- Gender distribution, most patients are female
- Age at onset, average age 30

Diagnosis

- Involuntary, testing not necessary in patients who fit the classical clinical description of optic neuritis

Differential Diagnosis

Other causes of optic disk swelling including pseudo-papilledema, inflammatory optic neuropathies. Also can include malingering.

IMAGING

- Not necessary in patients with classic optic neuritis but fundus fluorescein angiography may show leak of dye around otherwise normal margins of optic nerve head in retrobulbar neuritis.

PATHOLOGY

- Initially there is a lymphocytic perivascular infiltrate with destruction of the myelin and preservation of axons
- More severe involvement ? loss will occur
- At a later stage ? clean up and virus occurs

Differential Diagnosis

- In older patients the initial presentation of ischemic optic neuropathy can be similar to optic neuritis
- Typically less improvement over time in patient with ischemic optic neuropathy
- Rapid improvement at one month obtained on review so should lead to additional evaluation (atypical optic neuritis)

MANAGEMENT

- Medical therapy: Corticosteroids provide no benefit to long-term visual outcome
- Intravenous: Methyl prednisolone may lead to an improvement earlier than natural history but rarely sustained

Index

W